LATEST CONTRIBUTIONS TO
CROSS-CULTURAL PSYCHOLOGY

LATEST CONTRIBUTIONS TO CROSS-CULTURAL PSYCHOLOGY

Selected Papers from the Thirteenth International Congress of the International Association for Cross-Cultural Psychology

Edited by

J.-C. Lasry
J. Adair
K. Dion

Published for the International Association for Cross-Cultural Psychology

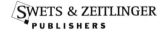

SWETS & ZEITLINGER
PUBLISHERS

LISSE   ABINGDON   EXTON (PA)   TOKYO

Library of Congress Cataloging-in-Publication Data

International Association for Cross-Cultural Psychology.
  International Congress (13th : 1996 : Montréal, Québec)
    Latest Contributions to cross-cultural psychology : selected
  papers from the Thirteenth International Congress of the
  International Association for Cross-Cultural Psychology / edited by
  Jean-Claude Lasry, Kenneth L. Dion
        p.   cm.
    Includes bibliographical references and index.
    ISBN 9026515472
    1. Ethnopsychology--Congresses.   I. Lasry, Jean-Claude.
  II. Dion, Kenneth L.   III. Title.
  GN502.I56   1996a
  155.8--dc21

Printed in The Netherlands by Krips, Meppel

ISBN 90 265 1547 2

Latest Contributions to Cross-Cultural Psychology

Jean-Claude M. Lasry, John G. Adair & Kenneth L. Dion (Eds.)

The XIIIth Congress of International Association for Cross-Cultural Psychology (IACCP) was held at the University of Montreal, from August 12 to 16, 1996, in Montréal, Quebec, Canada. There were more than 330 participants, from 40 different countries, who gathered in Montréal to present 340 papers or posters. For the second time in twenty years, the IACCP congress was held in North America, the first venue having been Queen's University, Kingston, Ontario, also in Canada. Hommage must be paid to the IACCP founders who made sure the venues of the international congresses would really be cross-cultural.

The present volume consists of contributions to the IACCP congress, twenty-four articles selected through the peer review process, authored by scholars representing the thematic and geographical diversity of cross-cultural psychology, from Australia to Zimbabwe. The papers are grouped under six sections, reflecting issues of current concern in cross-cultural psychology: 1) values and national identity, 2) acculturative stress and its resolution following immigration or migration, 3) personality and social behavior across cultures, 4) work/organizational psychology issues, 5) developmental/educational psychology topics, and 6) conceptual and methodological papers devoted to a metal-theoretical look at the evolution of the cross-cultural approach and to the ethics of cross-cultural research.

Prof. Janak Pandey's *presidential address* summarizes findings from a series of experimental and survey studies on the perception of, and coping with, environmental stressors, particularly crowding. The section of *Values and Identity* includes two articles. Ali and Northover studied the culture conflict experienced by young Asians living in the UK, depicted as being torn between the traditional culture of their ethnic minority and the culture of the British post-modern society. Feather and Adair compared samples of Australian and Canadian university students on their attitudes towards national identity, national favoritism (the Culture Cringe), global self-esteem, values and the tendency to cut down 'tall poppies' or people who occupy positions of high status.

The *Immigration and Acculturation* section comprises six contributions. Brami and Lasry surveyed samples of college students in Montreal, and showed that second-generation immigrant students more frequently adopted integration as a style of acculturation than students born outside Canada. Their data validated the orthogonality of the acculturation model. Based on a cultural anthropological approach, Eldering presents her research on female-headed Hindustani families in Surinam and the Netherlands, and identifies issues that need more attention in future research within the context of Berry's acculturation framework. In a 1995 study of Black South Africans, Hocoy showed apartheid resulted in psychological damage but also in responses of resilience, coping and strength. Black women were at a higher risk for marginalisation than Black men. Neto's sample of Portuguese second-generation adolescents living in Paris were not lonelier than their counterparts living in Portugal. Depression and social difficulty were the adjustment problems of Filipina domestic workers studied by Ward, Chang and Lopez-Nerney, who found that depression was associated with poor work conditions and weak identification as a Filipina. The last paper in this section deals with the concepts of enculturation and acculturation that Weinreich relates to ethnic identity and patterns of identification.

Another six papers constitute the *Personality and Social Behavior across Cultures* section. Benet-Martinez explored the indigenous Spanish personality constructs with a combined emic-etic perspective and found a seven-factor solution that closely resembled the North American Big Seven factor model. The cultural influence on attitudes and beliefs about suicide was investigated in Sweden, Japan and Slovakia by Eisler, Yoshida and Bianchi, with a scale assessing beliefs in intrapsychic, interpersonal and societal causes, as well as personal attitudes and normative beliefs. Gallois and her colleagues compared intergenerational communication patterns, and particularly filial piety, in young adults from eight nations, four Western (U.S., Australia, Canada and New Zealand) and four Asian/Southeast Asian (South Korea, Hong Kong, Philippines and Japan). Kiasuism describes a cultural preoccupation in Singapore, with never allowing oneself to lose out on any opportunity to get more, to be better than others. Ho, Monroe and Carr developed the first reliable scale to measure this concept and administered it to Singaporean and Australian students. According to Verna, relationship orientation, familialism and belief in hierarchy are dominant themes of Indian collectivism, which she found related positively to psychological well-being, but only in a socially supportive environment. The final paper in this section has implications for counseling. Horstmanshof and Reddy surveyed English speaking, non-English speaking and Asian sojourners in Australia. They found that satisfaction with the current situation was the most important factor influencing homesickness, but that personality type and cultural background also influenced means of coping with it.

The next section includes three articles with *Organizational/Work Psychology*. Lebanese and Anglo-australian participants were compared by El-Hayek and Keats on characteristics and motivation toward leadership. Hofstede's construct of individualism and collectivism, and Mitsumi's PM theory of leadership were used to discuss their findings. Kanungo, Aycan, and Sinha tested the Model of Culture Fit among workers in the United States, Canada and India. The three studies they reported confirmed the prediction that the socio-cultural environment and enterprise characteristics have a significant influence on managers' assumptions about human resource management. Sun and Bond developed an instrument to assess downward and upward influence tactics used in Chinese organizations. The Influence Tactics Profile, which includes items from the American and Chinese cultures, yielded two factors with high congruence across both influence directions.

Educational and Developmental Psychology is the theme of two contributions. Thomas argues for a culture sensitive pedagogy to complement the basic learning requirements common to all schooling. While acknowledging the emergence of a global culture, Thomas underlines the challenge of balancing the emic and etic dimensions in the new forms of teaching, and in accommodating global ideas and contextual needs. Vedder compared school children with different socialization traditions in the Netherlands, Curaçao and Sweden in terms of their social competence. The scale measured similar aspects of social behavior in all three countries where definitions of socially competent behavior varied slightly.

The last section of this volume includes three articles to *Conceptual/ Methodological Issues*. Exploring the relationship between cross-cultural psychology and anthropology, Gabrenya argues that, in cross-cultural psychology, the levels of analysis problem reflects the difficulty of conceptualizing the place of the individual in culture and society. He proposes six means to help improve the quality of research. In his brief report, Triandis provides a personal account of the events surrounding cross-cultural psychology's early interest in research ethics. Davidson's article also deals with cross-cultural research ethics, particularly with the report prepared by Tapp, Kelman, Triandis, Wrightsman and Coelho in 1974. The ethical guidelines from the Tapp et al. report are shown not to provide researchers with ways of resolving dilemmas arising from carrying out research in one's own culture, nor with conflicting Western and non-Western systems of ethics.

Before concluding, I would like to reiterate my gratitude to M. Henri Colas and Mme Carol Langevin, of Congrès Coplonar Inc., the Congress Secretariat, who helped to plan, organize and carry out the details of the XIIth congress. I would also like to thank Helen Kandarakis, the Scientific Program coordinator, as well as the Proceeding editorial assistants: Taryn Tang, Sophia Macrodimitris and Chantal Arpin.

The following colleagues deserve our sincere appreciation for helping us edit this volume: Bruce Avolio, John W. Berry, Deborah L. Best, Michael Bond, Richard Brislin, Irek Celejewski, Austin T. Church, Richard Clément, Barry Corenblum, Graham Davidson, Lutz Eckensberger, Norman S. Endler, William K. Gabrenya, Cindy Gallois, Charles Elwig, Harry Hui, Rabindra N. Kanungo, Rolf Kroger, Clarry Lay, Kwok Leung, Walter Lonner, R. R. MacRae, Don McCreary, Elizabeth Nair, Anita Wan-ping Pak, Ype H. Poortinga, José Miguel Salazar, Ute Schoenpflug, Norbert K. Tanzer, Donald M. Taylor, Harry Triandis, Kim Uichol, Maureen Vandermas-Peeler, Colleen Ward and Marta Young.

Finally, the help of Rinus Verkooijen (Tilburg University) in the final stage of the editing is gratefully acknowledged.

Jean-Claude Lasry
Chair, IACCP96

Table of Contents

Socio-Cultural Dimensions of Experience and Consequences of Crowding

Janak Pandey

ABSTRACT

This chapter summarizes findings from a series of experimental and survey studies on the perception and coping with environmental stressors, particularly crowding. Crowding is critical within India and other countries of South Asia, where the cultural context is collectivistic and people are more affiliative and interdependent. The results suggested that prolonged prior experience of living in a crowded home together with a sense of control, empower people to experience less negative consequences to enable them to cope with these stressors. The results indicated an apparent contradiction: Females were more upset by crowding, yet wanted to have more people and more children in their homes. It was concluded that understanding of cultural forces is necessary to explain coping with environmental stressors.

This chapter brings together and summarizes the salient findings of a series of previously published experimental and survey research related to the perception of, and coping with, environmental stressors such as crowding, air pollution, noise, and garbage in a variety of rural and urban settings in South Asia, particularly in India. The research program has been an ongoing collaborative effort of my students, and colleagues from Bangladesh, Pakistan, Nepal, and the United States. Most of the respondents in our studies have been common people, from typical middle class to extremely poor slum dwellers, belonging to both rural and urban neighbourhoods.

We chose to study environmental stressors and their varied consequences in South Asia for many reasons. First, the overwhelming majority of people in this region live in densely populated cities and villages and face severe economic and environmental stressors. More than one-sixth of the world's population lives in South Asia, where the average level of density is more than four times higher than in North America. Therefore, it is easier to examine, in this context, the effects of both extreme levels of high density and experiences of prolonged density on individuals. The pressures of increasing population, urbanization, and industrialization, are becoming unmanageable in Asia and this is likely to continue for several decades. For example, the controversial plague panic in October, 1994, caused a national alarm in India (India Today, October 31, 1994). A second reason for studying environmental stressors in South Asia is the range of sources of, and the variations in, socio-cultural uniqueness that exist in South Asia. Because of the large differences between economic classes, there is probably more variability in density levels and types of housing in India and in its neighbouring countries than in most other countries, and certainly more than in those investigated in North America. Due to the tradition of extended families living within one household, crowding may occur not only outside but also inside some homes.

The countries in South Asia are predominantly rural. Furthermore, in the primarily collectivistic cultural context of this region, personal inter-dependence is greater than it is in the individualistic West. This inter-dependence means that people are likely more affiliative, more interested in group harmony, more concerned with belongingness, and more willing to tolerate greater numbers of people (Kim, Triandis, Kagitcibasi, Choi & Yoon, 1994; Ruback & Pandey, 1996).

Residential Crowding Experience and Reactivity to Laboratory Crowding

In research literature, an important distinction is made between physical density and the psychological experience of crowding. However, most studies have been concerned with objective crowding, thereby de-emphasizing the psychological experience of crowding (Freedman, 1975; Hillery & Fugita, 1975; Paulus, Annis, Seta, Schkade, & Matthews, 1976). In the mid-eighties, we specifically designed a study to investigate the cross-situational effects of prior long-term crowding experience in the home on task performance in a crowded and in an uncrowded laboratory setting (Nagar, Pandey, & Paulus, 1988). Findings of some previous studies had indicated that crowding in a residential environment could be associated with negative reactions to others in different social settings (Baum & Valins, 1977; Paulus, 1980). In contrast, several other studies had demonstrated that previous crowding experience could increase tolerance toward others in other crowded settings (Paulus, 1988; Wholwill & Kohn, 1973). These latter findings suggested that having lived in crowded residential environ-ments for a prolonged period of time might help individuals learn to adjust to or to cope with a crowded situation. The main thrust of our study was to investigate the influence of the degree of crowding experienced in the home environment on respondents' reactions to crowded and uncrowded settings in the laboratory.

This study had important cultural and cross-cultural implications. If the generally high level of crowding experienced in India made Indians less responsive to crowding, then no effects of laboratory manipulations of crowding should be observed. The relatively large size of Indian families seemed well suited for testing the impact of residential crowding. Of course, cultural socialization, norms, and behavioural patterns might serve to mitigate the impact of home crowding (Altman & Chemers, 1980). We thought that if impacts of home crowding experience were obtained, this would suggest that such cultural features were not sufficient to eliminate crowding effects.

Male and female subjects, who had previously been classified as having had a prior continuous experience of high or low population density as measured by the Residential Crowding Scale, participated in a factorial experiment with high or low laboratory density (by changing the number of subjects in the lab room), under conditions of high, low or no noise. During the experiment, the subjects completed three cognitive tasks of differential difficulty (simple anagrams, complex anagrams, reading comprehension). Their reported feelings and perceptions of the experiment were also recorded. It was found that the presence of environmental stressors had a deleterious impact on story comprehension and complex anagram tasks but had no effect on the simple anagram task. In addition, respondents exposed to these stressors exhibited negative affect. The effect of noise and crowding appeared to be additive.

The results further indicated that respondents with high levels of prior experiences of crowding were less negatively affected by high lab density on the cognitive tasks (comprehension of story) presented early in the experimental session than were respondents who had low levels of prior experience of crowding. They also exhibited more positive affect. Thus, the influence of past experience of crowding on reactivity to different density conditions might depend not only on the level of density but also on the length of prior crowding exposure. Basically, individuals who differed in their experience of crowding also differed in the adaptation or tolerance level that they brought to other crowded situations. The findings also implied that continuous exposure to even low density in the home and neighbourhood may deplete this tolerance level. Although prior experience of crowding influenced reactivity to lab variations of density, it did not influence reactions to lab variations in noise. These findings supported our contention that long-term crowding experiences should prepare one for dealing with a variety of similar high-density experiences but not necessarily for other environmental stressors.

Perceived Control and Gender Differences in Response to Crowding

Consistently across various studies in rural and urban settings, the role of perceived control and of the magnitude of gender differences in response to crowding have been identified. In North America, such studies show fairly consistently that a sense of control over the environment is important in counteracting the negative effects of crowding (e.g. Rodin, Solomon, & Metcalf, 1978). There is strong evidence that perceived control acts as a main effect, such that individuals with more perceived control experience less mental distress and fewer physical symptoms than do persons with less perceived control. For example, based on a survey of 1,582 individuals in Chicago, Gove and Hughes (1983) found that the notion of perceived control explained more of the variance on most dependent variables than did their objective measure of density. There is quite a bit of debate on the generalizability of this Western-based conceptualization of control. People of different cultures have different views about the way people deal with the world in general and with adverse situations in particular. For example, traditional Hindu thought contains the belief that situational factors are more important than dispositional factors in determining behaviour (Miller, 1984) and that individuals should accept things as they are. Traditional beliefs in fatalism may make people accept events as they come, and inhibit individuals' desire to control the environment. Moreover, traditional beliefs place more emphasis on controlling one's emotions than on controlling the environment. We included perceived control in our research to test whether perceived control and household density were related to physical and mental health.

Individuals who have little control over environmental stressors and who have few resources to cope with them may be especially susceptible to their aversive consequences. The poor, women, elderly, and children are included in this vulnerable category. Because of their generally lower status and lessor power, particularly in traditional societies, women would also be expected to react more negatively than men to environmental stressors. Cultures differ with respect to expectations about gender roles. Because of the nature of the traditional Indian household (Sinha, 1988), it was expected that husbands would have more perceived control than would wives, a discrepancy that might explain other differences between spouses within a household. Gender differences in psychological traits are generally greater when there are greater differences in the roles of men and women, and role differences appear to be greater among the Muslims than among non-Muslims (Williams, Best, Haque, Pandey, & Verma, 1982). In typical households, particularly in villages, women are responsible for cooking, housekeeping, and taking care of children, as well as helping the men in other work. Women spend more time with others in the household, and therefore, should be more aware of the costs of high density levels, although they may also enjoy high levels of affiliation.

The Omnibus Project

As an initial investigation of crowding in rural settings, we analyzed a pre-existing data set (available at the Advanced Centre of Psychology, Allahabad University). These data, known as the Omnibus Project, consisted of interviews with residents of six villages near Allahabad. These interviews were conducted in 1986 by trained interviewers familiar with the local dialect. A total of 481 interviews were conducted with 279 males and 202 females. In each household, a male researcher interviewed the male head of the household and a female researcher interviewed the female head of the household. In most cases these individuals were married couples.

In each of six villages approximately 80 persons were interviewed (range: 77-83). The villages consisted of three developed and three less developed villages. The six villages were in three pairs based on their proximity to each other, so as to control for soil quality and other factors related to geography. The Omnibus survey interview instrument contained one item measuring perceived lack of control: "To what extent do you experience a lack of control?" Responses were made on a four point scale ranging from very little (1) to a great extent (4) and were reverse scored for analysis. Lack of control was significantly related to happiness, $r(475) = .13$, $p < .01$, economic well-being compared to others in the village, $r(472) = -.18$, $p < .01$, health now as compared as to what it was five years ago, $r(472) = .13$ $p < .01$, and a composite physical health score, $r(457) = .17$, $p < .01$. In other words, respondents with more perceived control tended to be happier, better off economically, in better health compared to five years ago, and healthier at the present time. A constructed measure of density (number of people in the household divided by the number of rooms in the house) was negatively correlated with relative economic well-being, $r(474) = -.21$, $p < .01$, and with a composite psychological health measure, $r(479) = -.11$, $p < .05$. There was no relationship between density and perceived lack of control, $r(471) = .04$, n.s.

These data suggested that perceived control might have some effects, but the effects would be small. In part, this may have been a function of the fact that only one question was used to measure perceived control. The data also suggested that density had some effects, but that these were not strong. However, together with prior studies, the data motivated us to pursue further investigations of crowding.

Interviews with Urban Residents

The Allahabad neighbourhood survey included a larger scale in which detailed information about living conditions and personal feelings were obtained to test how the relative difference between household members, in their perceived control over the environment, might affect their physical and mental health (Ruback & Pandey, 1991). Perceived control was operationalized in terms of control over aspects of the home and family, and that also provided an indirect measure of relative power in the family. Given the nature of traditional Indian households, we expected that women, especially those in the lower socio-economic status families, would have relatively lower levels of perceived control than men, and that the greater the difference, the worse the women would feel.

A number of factors led us to predict that women would respond more negatively to long term crowding than would men. First, women spend more time in crowded stressful situations in the home than do men. Second, if we assume that perceived control inhibits the stress associated with crowding, then women might suffer more from long term crowding because they have less control over their environment than do men. A third possibility is that women have less social support from household members than do men and therefore, suffer more than men do because they have fewer buffers to the stress.

We interviewed 167 couples, 334 individuals living in the city of Allahabad. The respondents' ages ranged from 18 to 86 years. They lived in households containing from 2 to 23 people. The number of children in the household ranged from 0 to 9. Most of the respondents were Hindu and lived in nuclear families; the remainder lived in multigenerational families. Although 43% of the respondents had at least some college education, 17% were illiterate. Household density (persons per room) ranged from .20 to 9.00, with median household density (2.00) more than three times the density level found in comparable studies in North America (e.g., Mdn = .65 was reported by Gove & Hughes, 1983). Within each of the households in the study, a male researcher interviewed the husband and a female researcher interviewed the wife.

In this study we included a large number of variables, both to control for possible spurious correlations and to investigate the relationship among high utility dependent measures. The variables in the study were in six categories. First, we included many background variables such as religion, caste, occupation, education, income, type of family (nuclear, joint, extended joint), and the type of environment in which respondents were raised. These variables were included primarily to serve as statistical controls for the relationship between density and the major dependent measures.

The second category of variables concerned measures of crowding and correlates of crowding. For each house, we obtained measures of the type of house, the number of rooms, the amount of area the structure covered, the amount of area in the compound, the distance between the house and the road, and the distance between the respondent and the nearest family. We also had observers rate the amount of garbage beside the home, the amount of noise in the area, and the adequacy of the drainage system. In addition, we examined the impact of scarce resources such as the extent to which facilities were shared (e.g., water tap, toilet).

The third group of variables dealt with interpersonal relationships between spouses, among family members, with children, and with neighbours. The idea behind these measures was that interpersonal behaviour from positive (social support) to negative (aggression) might be affected by crowding.

Fourth, we collected several measures of physical health, including symptomatology and visits to the doctor. We also collected measures of psychological well-being and depression. Finally, we had respondents complete a life-events scale so that we could put the stress from crowding in perspective with other possible sources of stress.

The fifth group of variables assessed subjects' control over their environment and themselves. We included these variables because research from the Western world suggests that perceived control is a mediator of the relationship between high density conditions and the feeling of being crowded (see, e.g., Rodin, 1976; Rodin et al., 1978; Ruback & Carr, 1984; Stockdale, 1978). Our choice of these multiple measures in each of the six categories was governed by our desire to show that crowding fits into a larger context of societal problems.

Overall, husbands had marginally more perceived control over the environment than did the wives. For both husbands and wives, this perceived control was positively related to feelings about the children, the house, the neighbourhood, and mental distress. Consistent with our hypothesis, the greater the difference in perceived control between husband and wife, the more physical symptoms the wife reported, the more mental distress she experienced, the more negative she felt about her children, her house, and her neighbourhood, the more quarrels she reported having with adults in her house, and the more she punished her children. For husbands, the difference between their perceived control and that of their wives was significantly related to only one variable, the extent to which the husbands rated their neighbourhood more positively. As predicated, husbands had more relative power in lower socio-economic households. That is, a greater difference in perceived control was associated with less property, lesser education of the husband, lesser education of the wife, and more children.

Correlations indicate that household density was related to perceived control over the environment for females but not for males, and more strongly related to dependent measures for female than for male respondents. For both males and females, higher density was related to lower ratings of their house, less interaction with their spouses, more punishment of the children, and more quarrels with neighbors. In addition, for females, higher density was related to lower ratings of children and greater ratings of quarrels with adults in the household and with neighbors.

Study of Males and Females in Rural Household
India, like most developing countries, is predominantly rural with more than 80% of the population living in rural settings. Research findings based on

city dwellers is less representative of the population, and therefore, we decided to go to the villages again for our next research (Ruback & Pandey, 1996). The major objective was to investigate whether rural women, compared to rural men, reacted more negatively to long term crowding.

The questionnaire used for the city respondents was suitably revised. Male and female researchers separately interviewed the male and female heads of household in each of 159 homes in three villages (different from those of the Omnibus Survey) of Allahabad district. The respondents ranged in age from 18 to 93 years. Almost all of them (94%) were Hindu with the remainder being Muslim, and most of these were of backward castes (64%), or of scheduled castes (17%). Although most of the women (80%) were illiterate, only 26% of the men were unable to read.

Most of the respondents had lived in the village for many years. Virtually all men had lived in the village their entire life whereas most of the women had lived in the village only since they had been married. Even though the women had spent less time in the village compared to the men, they probably had similar experiences in their parent's home as marriages took place between individuals of the same social and economic status. Most of the people lived in joint families (52%), or extended joint families (5%), rather than in nuclear families (43%). Males spent longer hours per day ($M = 9.75$) outside the house than did females ($M = 4.09$).

The number of people in the households ranged from 2 to 19 ($M = 7.04$). The number of adults in the house ranged from 2 to 11 ($M = 3.84$), while the number of children in the house ranged from 1 to 18 ($M = 4.62$). Household density ranged from .25 to 8.00 ($M = 1.89$). Density was significantly related to both number of people, and number of rooms. Similar to the findings of the earlier study, household density was significantly correlated with only some of the variables, and of these more for females than for males. Higher density was related to (a) a lower rating of places of activity, the supply of resources, and the amount of space in the house, as well as the house as a whole; and (b) higher ratings of perceived crowding and of the number of people in the house.

On most of the dependent variables, within households, men's and women's scores were significantly correlated. Within the households, the fact that men as compared to women, had a greater belief that they controlled their lives, and had less of a belief that God controlled their lives is consistent with the fact that in most households men do have more power regarding economic and other important decisions. Moreover, that women believed their lives were controlled by God is consistent with the norms of the culture in that women are responsible for all religious rituals in the house.

In general, men rated their house more positively. They rated the places where they ate, rested, and slept more favourably and they judged the supply of resources in the house (food, water, beds, etc.) to be more adequate. That men rated their living conditions more favourably than women did is consistent with the fact that men get the best resources in the household. In terms of interaction with others in their homes, men as compared to women, reported that both men and women were supportive and they did more positive things with their family and their neighbors. Probably, women experience continuing stress because they must adjust to their husbands' families, whereas husbands, because they do not have to make such adjustments, are likely to have harmonious relationships within the family. Men and women did not differ in their ratings of the positive aspects of their children, but women saw significantly more negative aspects in their children than men did, no doubt because women had much more contact with their children than did the men.

Several of the questionnaire and observational measures were related to physiological measures. Women with higher blood pressure readings reported more mental distress and more physical symptoms, gave lower ratings to the supply of resources in their home, and liked their house less. In spite of the fact that women reacted negatively to their home, their answers to questions about the level of crowding and the number of people in the household indicated that women did not consider these to be problems. Women thought more people could live in the house, both in terms of maximum number and comfort. Women's blood pressure readings were significantly related to only one variable, the maximum number of people they thought could live in the house, $r(25) = -.57$, $p < .01$, and were marginally related to the number of people who could live in the house. Women had lower pulse readings, perhaps indicating that some type of adaptation to others had taken place. Regarding the number of children, men were more likely to say that there were too many children.

In brief, in spite of the fact that women were more likely than men to be upset by the effects of crowding, they were more likely (a) to believe that their homes could comfortably house a greater number of people and (b) to want more children. However, all the analyses were bivariate. In order to ensure that the effects were not spurious, multivariate analyses were conducted. Across the ANCOVAS, the gender difference remained significant on virtually all of the variables, even when the other factors were statistically controlled. The significant gender effect was the only one that showed such consistency across variables.

Thus, consistently, our findings supported the apparent contradiction that females were more upset by crowding, and yet they also actually wanted to have more people and more children in the house. There could be several reasons for this contraction. First, it may be that women enjoy high levels of social interactions more than men do, regardless of any other factor. Second, it may be that women are not aware of the problems associated with high social density, and they desire more people in their household because they do not know the negative effects. Third, it may be that women recognized that high social density was a problem, and that there were other countervailing considerations that required them to want more people in their household. In other words, regardless of the psychological costs, the cultural demands on women, particularly in rural India, might drive them to be primarily concerned with social relationships. Women are upset and dissatisfied with their inferior position, over which they have no control. Because it is the husband's home, they see the presence of others as due to him. Women under stress in the family seek consoling interactions with other persons.

It is reasonable to believe that the cultural pressures causing women to desire more people in the household would be due to many reasons. For example, the pressure on women to have children immediately after marriage, and the preference for sons due to economic and religious considerations, may motivate them for a larger family. Interestingly, this preference for males still exists even though there will soon be a shortage of women; the current gender ratio of females to males is 929 to 1,000 (Chaudhary, 1992).

The fact that women had less perceived control than men may be indicative of the fact that their self-concept is closely tied to others. Other research suggests that when their self-efficacy is high, women in India want smaller families, even when other factors are held constant (Mukherjee, 1979). By implication, women who lack this sense of control and self-efficacy are bound to suffer. It is obvious that greater attention must be paid to the powerful cultural factors to educate people regarding environmental and economic stressors. At the recent Conference for the South Asia Region, WHO decided that there should be a change of emphasis from technology to behaviour, and as I have stated above, without understanding cultural forces, understanding of behaviour would be an elusive task.

References

Altman, I., & Chemers, M. M. (1980). *Culture and environment.* Monterey, CA: Brooks/Cole.

Baum, A., & Valins, S. (1977). *Architecture and social behaviour: Psychological studies of social density.* Hillsdale, NJ: Erlbaum.

Chaudhary, M. D. (1992). Population growth trends in India: 1991 census. *Population and Environment: A Journal of Interdisciplinary Studies, 14,* 3148.

Freedman, J. L. (1975). *Crowding and behaviour.* San Francisco: Freeman.

Gove W. R., & Hughes, M. (1983). *Overcrowding in the household: An analysis of determinants and effects.* New York: Academic Press.

Hillery, J. M., & Fugita, S. S. (1975). Group size effects in employment testing. *Educational and Psychological Measurement, 35,* 745-750.

Kim, U., Triandis, H. C., Kagitcibasi, C., Choi, S.-C., & Yoon, G. (1994). *Individualism and Collectivism: Theory, method, and applications.* Thousand Oaks: Sage Publications.

Miller, J. G. (1984). Culture and the development of everyday social explanation. *Journal of Personality and Social Psychology, 46,* 961-978.

Mukherjee, B. N. (1979). *Prediction of family planning and family size from modernity value orientation of Indian women.* Papers of the East-West Population Institute (No. 61). Honolulu, Hawaii: East West Centre.

Nagar, D., Pandey, J., & Paulus, P. B. (1988). The effects of residential crowding experience on reactivity to laboratory crowding and noise. *Journal of Applied Social Psychology, 18,* 1423-1442.

Paulus, P. B., Annis, A. B., Seta, J. J., Schkade, J. K., & Matthews, R. W. (1976). Density does affect task performance. *Journal of Personality and Social Psychology, 34,* 248-253.

Paulus, P. B. (1980). Crowding. In P. B. Paulus (Ed.), *Psychology of group influence* (pp. 245-289). Hillsdale, NJ: Erlbaum.

Paulus, P. B. (1988). *Prison crowding: A psychological perspective.* New York: Springer-Verlag.

Rodin, J. (1976). Density, perceived choice and response to controllable and uncontrollable outcomes. *Journal of Experimental Social Psychology, 12,* 564-578.

Rodin, J., Solomon, S., & Metcalf, J. (1978). Role of control in mediating perceptions of density. *Journal of Personality and Social Psychology, 36,* 989-999.

Ruback, R. B., & Carr, T. S. (1984). Crowding in a women's prison: Attitudinal and behavioural effects. *Journal of Applied Social Psychology, 14,* 57-68.

Ruback, R. B., & Pandey, J. (1991). Crowding, perceived control, and relative power: An analysis of household in India. *Journal of Applied Social Psychology, 21,* 315-344.

Ruback, R. B., & Pandey, J. (1996). Gender differences in perception of household crowding: Stress, affiliation, and role obligation in rural India. *Journal of Applied Social Psychology, 36,* 417-436.

Sinha, D. (1988). Changing family scenario in India and its implication for mental health. In P. R. Dasen, J. W. Berry, & N. Sartorius (Eds.), *Health and cross-cultural psychology. Towards application.* Newbury Park, CA: Sage.

Stockdale, J. E. (1978). Crowding: Determinants and effects. In L. Berkowitz (Ed.), *Advances in experimental social psychology (Vol. II).* New York: Academic Press.

Wholwill, J., & Kohn, I. (1973). The environment as experienced by the migrant: An adaption level view. *Representative Research in Social Psychology, 4,* 135-164.

Williams, J. E., Best, D. L., Haque, A., Pandey J., & Verma, R. K. (1982). Sex-trait stereotypes in India and Pakistan. *Journal of Psychology, 111,* 197-181.

Values and Identity

Distinct Identities: South Asian Youth in Britain

Nasreen Ali
University of Manchester
United Kingdom

&

Mehroo Northover
University of Ulster
United Kingdom

ABSTRACT

"Culture conflict" is a popular term used to describe second generation young British Asians depicted as facing the dilemma of bipolar values. Supposedly, they must choose either the constraining norms of Asian religions and life-styles of their migrant parents, and thus maintain ethnic identity, or adopt the relative freedom offered by Western values, mediated by teachers and peers at school, colleagues in the workplace, and the images and ideas diffused by television, radio and press. However, empirical evidence provides a more complex picture not so much of stark choice, but of conflicting identification patterns with parents, own community, and role models from the community at large. These are resolved by adopting separate pathways and evolving individual value systems. While all consider language to be an important feature of ethnicity, it is not found to be a determinant of ethnic identity.

Reflecting the previous colonial status of a number of European nations, Britain in particular has received a large number of immigrants over the past thirty years, many of them from the sub-continent of South Asia. Whereas the people from South Asia are diverse in culture, history and religion, and despite multicultural policies in the United Kingdom, this group has been ascribed a collective identity. In the press and among the general public there is some confusion over appropriate categorization of ethnic minorities in Britain (see Madood, 1995, and Gilroy, 1994). With the breakdown of the category 'black' to describe all 'non-white' people, there is an ongoing debate as to whether this will lead to two designations - African-Caribbean and Asian. In the light of increasing Muslim 'visibility' (Ali, 1997) a third category of Muslim may be necessary.

In the detail of this paper we shall be distinguishing between sub-groups among South Asians but when covering aspects of the culture which are shared by all sub-groups, we will be using the category of South Asian with the acknowledgment that this is also an inadequate term. For the purpose of this paper is not to focus on the sub-cultural identities within this group, but rather on the development of an identity among the young people which shares elements of British culture and the culture of their parents' generation. Both types of values are discussed later in this paper.

Geographically, the original migrants and their offspring are spread over the entire United Kingdom, in sparse communities in some areas as in Northern Ireland or in dense pockets in the inner cities such as in Sparkbrook in Birmingham, in Leicester and in Bradford. Technological advances in communication have added a fresh dimension to these relationships between the ethnic minorities from the Indian subcontinent and Western values, represented in British institutions and systems of law, social and health services and education. Cross-cultural psychologists recognize that processes of identity change can best be understood in relation to social context and this is particularly significant for South Asians in Britain. Here the context is not only the community in Britain but also the close ties and communication with the home countries of their parents. Communication by telephone, electronic mail and transport has never been swifter between South Asians in Britain and their kin in India, Pakistan and Bangladesh. A constant supply of videos, films and music from these sources to Britain has also increased the impact of the 'home' culture on the communities in Britain although the influence is not uniform across individuals or sections of South Asians.

Migration of different sub-cultural groups to Britain has to some extent helped to bring about changes at different levels in the various groups of young South Asians in their relations with each other and with British society in general. For example, at the level of music and dance, South Asians and African Caribbeans have contributed to each other's musical tradition and to the general youth culture in Britain which embraces African-Caribbean *reggae* as well as Punjabi *bhangra* in a fusion of musical styles.

Conceptual Foundations to the Study

The media and general public in the UK simplify this structural complexity in terms of a single Asian ethnicity and through the metaphor of conflict. South Asian youth is depicted as being torn between the traditional culture of the ethnic minority and the culture of a post-modern society entering an era of global communication and competition. This is claimed to be reflected in the younger generation who experience and desire the attractions of Western freedoms while held firmly in the grip of traditional and constraining values. They are often represented in the media as caught in the dilemma of bipolar choices between the values of their parents' generation from the Indian subcontinent and those of the mainstream of British society —the former seen as orthodox and the latter as progressive— the conflict between two cultures.

Another notion closely associated with South Asians and other ethnic minority groups is that of low self-esteem and low self-evaluation. Some social psychological theories tend to encourage the notion of low self-esteem under certain circumstances and especially when a group sees itself ascribed to an unjustly inferior social position. Tajfel's theory of social identity and intergroup relations (1981) suggests that under certain conditions (many of which would apply to Asian British families) categorization by groups (us and them) leads the subordinate group to turn inward on itself seeking favourable comparison for itself by promoting and lauding aspects of its own culture such as its own language or valued customs. This promotion of a valued and distinctive characteristic would help in distinguishing the group and its members from the mainstream and other minority groups. Implicit in this theory is the notion of divergence which carried to its logical conclusion must lead to conflict (see also Giles and Johnson, 1981 for the role of language in inter-group competition and the gaining of favourable self-esteem).

The inference of low self-evaluation of minority ethnic groups made by the superordinate group has been disproved in a number of studies using the theoretical framework of Identity Structure Analysis (see Northover, 1988; Kelly, 1989 among others). Here the distinction between the 'etic/emic' perspectives is useful. Weinreich (1996a) has made the distinction between 'ego-recognized' and 'alter-ascribed' identity. Ascriptions of identity characteristics to subordinate groups arise from taking an 'etic' view of a group, that is, adopting analytic concepts of ethnicity which transcend the specificity of cultures. Adopting an 'emic' view is to be concerned with culturally specific attitudes and values. Ego-recognized identity is the group's concept of itself and its self-evaluation. Social identity theorists take the etic view, ascribing a group's self-evaluation by reason of the socio-economic status of its members while the group members evaluate them-selves and others from their own stand-point, maintaining an ego-recognized identity.

Berry's (1988) model of acculturation describes 'acculturation' as culture change that results from continuous, first-hand contact between two distinct cultural groups. He points out that while originally proposed as a group-level phenomenon, acculturation is now recognized as also being an individual phenomenon. At this second level, acculturation refers to change in an individual (both overt and covert traits) whose cultural group is collectively experiencing acculturation. He continues to point out that while mutual changes are implied in this definition, in fact most changes occur in the non-dominant group as a result of influences from the dominant group. Thus it is assumed that it is the non-dominant groups that psychologically adapt to the context.

Berry's theory of acculturation in a cross-cultural perspective (1986) sets out a matrix of acculturation based on two central issues, contact-participation and cultural maintenance. When posed simultaneously, he maintains that four varieties of acculturation may be posited, these being integration or assimilation and separation or marginalisation. Moreover, any behavior is a candidate for shift during acculturation according to Berry (p. 40) and "as contact continues identity changes may be monitored by a variety of techniques which can provide evidence of simple shifts and for identity conflict and confusion (related to acculturative stress)".

Although Berry sees acculturation as a process, inherent within his definition is that it is a one-way process by which the minority becomes like the superordinate majority by foregoing elements of its own identity (Ali, Ellis, & Weinreich, 1996b). Further, his perspective of value change in ethnic minorities lacks the conceptual quality which would give a flavor of the developmental processes of change in identity structure, self-concepts and aspirations of a culturally specific nature. In South Asian communities contact and support from within, differences within and between each community, socio-economic religious and political differences give rise to differing contestations of identity. Such constructions of the social world are not for monitoring but for understanding within the framework of a theory which allows for the incorporation of the community's own perceptions of itself.

However, identity cannot remain fixed in the face of contextual change. Ghuman (1993) shows Hindus, Muslims and Sikhs in Britain have adapted in varying degrees to the values of the younger generation, which in turn are influenced by Western values of the society at large. Study of the many subcultural and religious divisions within the South Asian group would reveal developmental processes of individuals and their responses to the changing social demands of the 60's through to the 90's. Such responses to the social and historical contexts are apparent in most migrant communities.

Eldering's study (1995) of Hindustani Surinamese in the Netherlands also shows that

"the interaction between the public and private domains may have different outcomes. Important factors in this process are the economic and power structures of society, the attitude of the culture groups in contact, their numerical strength, their daily life setting, and the social cohesion of ethnic communities".

Under the conditions prevailing in the Surinamese plantations, the Hindustanis found that the caste system lost its economic function hence its influence. Further changes in values were effected through the loss of community cohesiveness through a second migration to the Netherlands, illustrating the influence of social and economic environments on communities.

Ghuman (1991) in his study of South Asians has collected valuable comparative data in 1974 and 1987 on such traditional opinions as "parents and children should live on their own", "a woman's place in the home", "learn to speak our own language", "our women should wear English clothes" and found that the 1987 sample had moved toward greater agreement with the Western view of such values. Such evidence of change, however, does not highlight whether redefinitions of identity have taken place by foregoing aspects of own ethnic group identity or changes in psychological processes involved in the redefinitions of identity.

Bernabe, Clement and Lamontagne (1979) have suggested a hierarchical model of theory building and empirical study which proposes that at any given time, the metatheoretical level feeds into theoretical achievement which in turn leads to empirical achievement. Empirical achievement feeds directly into theoretical achievement hence indirectly feeding into the general metatheoretical framework. While Bernabe et al.'s epistemological model presents a sound perspective on the role of empirical evidence in meta-theory, such a perspective tends towards an abstract approach to research and lacks the concepts for capturing empirical evidence.

In order to understand the processes of redefinition of identity which have taken place within South Asian communities it seems necessary to understand the psychological processes at work and to locate the individual's identifications with significant others in own and the other ethnic groups. Such an exploration would produce a contexualised profile of a group of people adapting to their social environment.

Identity Structure Analysis: The Theoretical Framework of the Research Studies

No single methodology or theory can encompass such processes of psychological, sociological and economic change. It has to be supplemented from other research sources, interviews, television and video documentaries and informed coverage in the quality press. However, the psychological processes experienced by individuals need the intervention of psychological theorists to explain such change. Further, empirical evidence should lead to fresh theoretical insights rather than constraining empirical data within the bounds of rigid and formulaic explanations of human behavior.

While Identity Structure Analysis (Weinreich, 1980, 1983b, 1989) cannot provide an all-encompassing general theory, it provides a theoretical framework which incorporates concepts which have been empirically tested. Propositions are derived from field studies which can also be tested and modified or incorporated into the general theoretical framework. This framework lends itself to the formation of hypotheses, and testing these using the existing identity concepts. Moreover, the concepts of ISA have been operationalised using algebraic formulae and dedicated computer programs enable the collection and analysis of data.

Within ISA, the concept of *situated identity* is highly suitable in exploring the identity of young South Asians who live in a multicultural environment. Conceptually, ISA sees identity as situated, that is that, alternative self-images may be engaged in by an individual when cueing into different social contexts (*me as I am when I am with my own/other group*). Such alternative identity states may be regarded as aspects of one's overall identity, in which how one behaves, presents oneself and experiences one's situated self differs according to the social context (Weinreich, Kelly, & Maja, 1986). Identity in this view constantly presents different facets of self as one is associated with new encounters and terminations.

Individuals living in multicultural societies will experience new encounters and decide to terminate or redefine personal meanings in other interactions. Drawing on a number of strands from antecedent theories including Erikson's work on identity (1963), Weinreich has elaborated the single concept of identification by replacing it with two modes of identification, *role model* and *empathetic identification*. The first type concerns itself with the aspirational needs of people, the desire to *idealistically identify* with these positive role models and desire to emulate the qualities perceived in these others. Empathetic identification on the other hand, is the perception of sharing qualities perceived in others which may be good or bad characteristics. Individuals may also form *contra-identifications* with others perceived as negative role models and seek to dissociate from perceived qualities.

A further notion of *conflicts-in-identification* is introduced. While culture conflict in popular thinking often refers to conflict when torn between two cultures, using the ISA notion of *identification conflicts* with significant others allows us to move away from this popularist and negative perception of culture-conflict. Identification conflicts occur when empathetic identification is multiplied by a desire to dissociate (contra-identification) from negative qualities perceived in another person or group.

The term conflict-in-identification is here replacing the rather loose and ambiguous term 'identity conflict' and replaces it with the notion of identification conflicts with significant others within one's own or other groups. In ISA terms, an increase in empathetic identification with own or other group may occur when individuals behave in ways which are quite different from when they are with some other group, while nevertheless feeling attached to their own group (Weinreich, 1986). This increase or decrease in empathetic identification is thus dependent on social context or *situated identity*. For example, this may apply when individuals are speaking and interacting in their own language or in English with members of their own group or other groups (Northover, 1988). It is clear then that, whereas 'identity' conflict' could be used to refer only to some general notion of conflict associated with a person's self image, a person's conflicts in identification can be located precisely in relation to particular individuals and groups. Therefore use of the term conflicts-in-identification enables a shift to be made from the generality of unspecified identity conflict, to specific identification conflicts with others.

Individuals formulate their own opinions on a range of topics, such as dress, music, boy and girl friends, and in the case of South Asian youth, may forge conceptions of themselves which are neither approved by their parents, nor by their native white peers. If this is the case, they have to withstand considerable psychological conflict (Weinreich, 1997). ISA regards individuals' conflicts-in-identification with others as being an important psychological impetus for personal change. In contradistinction to the popular notion of identity conflict between Asian youth and their parents which has been so often portrayed negatively. ISA sees a degree of conflicted identifications with others as a resource rather than a liability.

Some research on the identity of South Asians and other minorities links the popular notion of identity conflict with low self-evaluation. The term *self-evaluation* also needs clarification. Ascriptions of identity characteristics to subordinate groups arise from taking an 'etic' view of a group (see Weinreich, Bond, & Luk, 1996) that is, adopting analytic concepts of ethnicity which transcend the specificity of cultures. Adopting an 'emic' view is to be concerned with culturally specific attitudes and values. Ego-recognized identity is the group's concept of itself and its self-evaluation. Social identity theorists take the etic view, ascribing a group's self-evaluation by reason of the socio-economic status of its members while the group members evaluate themselves and others from their own stand-point, maintaining an ego-recognized identity.

When a spread of partial identifications with other role models and groups are experienced, this results in a degree of *identity diffusion*. ISA conceptualises identity diffusion as the degree of difficulty in resynthesising childhood and later identifications, that is a difficulty in incorporating new identifications and resolving conflicts-in-identification which are dispersed over a number of significant others (Weinreich, Bond, & Luk, 1996). In some circumstances, high identity diffusion may be accompanied by very low self-evaluation and the individuals concerned may be in states of identity crisis. However in other circumstances, individuals may exhibit identity diffusion as a result of having identification conflicts and yet have moderately favourable self-evaluation. Identity diffusion, as a lack of a completely coherent sense of cultural grounding, may be detrimental to one's sense of well being but may alternatively be the impetus for redefinition of self and thereby maintenance in updated form of one's ethnic identity (Weinreich, Bond, & Luk, 1996). Identification conflicts or the absence of identification conflicts with significant others is the focus of the three research studies presented below.

In Weinreich's (1989, p. 70) empirical research, exploring identity structures of individuals and groups has its beginnings in theoretical assumptions and concepts which he has operationalised using algebraic translations and encapsulated within the IDEX computer programs. Theoretical process postulates (ISA) provide the framework for understanding individual and group identity processes.

"This view of theory-building allows for serious consideration to be given to those aspects of human behavior which are to a degree autonomous and innovative. It points to the importance of placing rational thought and action in relation to irrational processes. It places theorizing within the social context of people's transactions with others and with societal institutions" (Weinreich, 1989, p. 71).

ISA is an economical means of exploring individual and group identities whereby people evaluate themselves and others when judged by a set of values forming part of their belief system. An ISA instrument is generated from initial interviews with small, representative groups and is tailor-made to encompass the values expressed by the group which are presented to the respondent as bipolar constructs. The instrument consists of a set of bipolar constructs and a set of entities. Since primary identifications with family or ethnic group remain dominant through life (Northover, 1988), significant others such as parents and friends are nominated among the entities. Others, such as elders of the community, religious leaders, teachers, media figures, colleagues at school and at work may also be introduced to reflect the social constellation of individuals who might influence or be influenced through socialisation and interaction. An instrument optimally consists of about 20 entities and 18 or 20 constructs.

The respondent determines his or her own favored pole of each construct by the rating given to the entity *ideal self* (*me as I would like to be*), thus expressing a personal ideological stance. Billig (1991) says that any attitude is "more than an expression in favor of a position; it is also implicitly or explicitly an argument against the counter-position" (p. 113). The selected pole of any construct thus also expresses a value opposed to the counter-value.

When a respondent consistently rates an approved entity on the same favored pole of a construct, he or she expresses the evaluative aspect of cognitive judgment. Negatively appraised entities are assigned to the opposite pole. This represents cognitive-affective consistency expressed as high *structural pressure* (+70 and over). Values come under pressure when there is a recognition that people significant to oneself now differ in relation to certain personal aspirations and there is a cognitive-affective inconsistency in appraising these entities and results in low structural pressure. Low structural pressure (SP) indicates that the value is conflicted owing to the cognitive-affective inconsistencies between a person's principles and his/her appraisal of individuals in the social world.

Core Features of Asian Youth Identity

South Asian communities are developing varied patterns of identity within each generation and from one generation to the next. While the original migrants have had to adapt at least physically to their new environment, for the youth who have been born and brought up in Britain, their own ethnic group is not the only source of socialisation. In such instances partial identifications with the other ethnic group may occur.

If indeed the South Asian youth in the research highlighted below are going through a process of 'culture conflict', it is assumed that they will have higher identification with majority culture entities and high identification conflicts with representations of their own ethnic group. The assumption would also be that they would have low self evaluation.

Research illustrates the complexity of structures within the samples. By using the value system of the responding groups rather than an imposition of values judged to be positive or negative by the researchers, some understanding of the identity structures of the sample can be obtained. Read together with the numerous other studies using a variety of methodologies and featuring psychometric scales, observation and interviews conducted on this group in British society, a more varied and multidimensional picture of identity may be obtained.

Using the above concepts, Kelly's study (1989) of Muslim Pakistanis and Greek Cypriots in Britain argues that the general expectation regarding both communities is the disjunction popularly called 'culture conflict' between the values of the older and younger generations of any group recently migrating to another culture. However, in the early stages of his research, Kelly became aware that a distinction had to be drawn between those in the Muslim samples who displayed greater or lesser empathetic identification with the indigenous culture, which he then refers to as the 'progressive' and 'orthodox' groups respectively. This in itself is a useful distinction so that estimates of the parameters of identity can be differentiated within groups as well as between groups of respondents, thus refining the notion of a monolithic and stereotypical mass into one of individuals and differentiated identities following differing pathways toward a redefinition of identity.

The need for such redefinition is a salient feature of groups faced with certain ethnic values which fly in the face of the mainstream belief system.

Such a value may be that "boys and girls should be able to mix freely" - a value subscribed to by progressives in Kelly's sample. He also found no support for the proposition of self-devaluation which appears to be implicit in Tajfel's theory. However, Kelly found (p. 85), while all groups including the indigenous sample display high levels of positive self-evaluation (as defined by the ISA framework), the male indigenous group had the highest levels of self-evaluation ($M = 0.889$) while the progressive female Muslims had the lowest ($M = 0.723$). The *identity diffusion* or overall spread and intensity of conflicts-in-identification with others is also greatest for the progressive Muslims.

Kelly explains this higher level of conflict-in-identification of the progressive group as being with own ethnic group representatives involved in the Mosque, the Muslim Center and other networks. Situated with their own group members, the levels of diffusion increase further. The lower level of self-evaluation of this group in no way can be argued as a generalized process of self-devaluation (p. 89). It can however, be viewed

"as part of an ongoing process of redefinition in which the formation of new identifications (for example with representatives of the indigenous culture) play an increasingly important but turbulent part".

In understanding the psychological process of conflict-in-identification, a generalized notion of culture conflict can be disambiguated. While a perception of shared qualities with both one's own ethnic group and mainstream groups prevails, the simultaneous wish by respondents to dissociate from some of these qualities results in conflict-in-identification. In the case of progressives in this sample, the conflicted identification is greater with their own community than with the mainstream.

These conflicts-in-identification need to be resolved and Weinreich suggests that the pathways to re-definition of self may take different courses. He postulates that one means toward resolution of conflicts-in-identification may be re-evaluations of self in relation to the others but within the limitations of one's currently existing value system. This would mean that those people described as orthodox in the study would retain their ethnic values but might reduce their contra-identification with their own ethnic group. A further option would be to reduce any sense of sharing qualities with their mainstream counterparts. Choice of the latter option would mean lessening of the need to integrate into the mainstream and might eventually cause marginalisation from indigenous British people.

An alternative as postulated by Weinreich (1989) is the broadening of one's value system which would "establish a new context for one's self-definition" leading to fundamental changes in one's value system. This latter course would seem to be that adopted by the progressives leading to greater identification with members of the indigenous British group.

What has emerged from Kelly's study are empirical propositions with regard to a community in transition from its home culture to some form of accommodation with the values of the mainstream. The first proposition derived by Kelly concerns the salience of ethnicity in identity change through identification conflicts with their own ethnic group. He also points to part identification with the majority group's values from which arise a "new ethnic coherence" developed through self-esteem judged according to newly shared and self-chosen values.

This last proposition lends fresh insight into the notion of culture conflict. Far from being a group of confused and rootless people, the orthodox group of respondents is secure in its own cultural values, while the progressives, who may be those generally referred to as "confused and caught between two cultures", appear to emerge with a new strength and independence of outlook and values.

Some further insights into development and change among the South Asian community in Britain are found in a more recent study by Ali (1997). The focus of her research was the Kashmiri community in Luton. This community is particularly interesting with regards to their ego-recognized identification as 'Kashmiri' which has been subsumed by others under the alter-ascribed identifier 'Pakistani'. This further illustrates the complexity of categorization by those commentating on the communities from an etic perspective.

Results of the research show that the younger Kashmiris have higher empathetic identification with majority entities than the older respondents. However, for old and young Kashmiris, identification conflicts are highest with own ethnic group. Moreover, Kashmiri youth have higher identification conflicts with own group entities than the older respondents, which supports the idea that youth from ethnicised minorities have highest identification conflicts with their own group. These differences are accounted for as reflecting the younger Muslims' dual socialisation with their own ethnic group and later identifications with white majority society. This means that their primary allegiances are first grounded in their own ethnic groups, but their subsequent socialisation presents alternative views, which when adopted in part, conflict with their earlier identifications with their own group. An alternative explanation may be suggested and argued that identification conflicts are their plight in a discriminatory society. However, if this explanation were to be supported, then young Kashmiris would internalize the derogatory view of their own ethnic group held by the majority society leading to devalued self images (Ali, Ellis, & Weinreich, 1996).

Self-evaluation fell within the high range for older men ($M = 0.83$), older women ($M = 0.81$), young male ($M = 0.73$) and young female ($M = 0.40$) Kashmiris. These figures combined with moderate levels of identity diffusion for older men ($M = 0.26$), older women ($M = 0.31$), young male

(M = 0.29) and young female (M = 0.40) indicate that identification conflicts are acting as a resource for redefinition of identity towards updated identification.

Ali's research once again shows a pattern and variety and change within an ethnicised community. The younger generation's greater engagement with mainstream values is apparent in both Kelly's and Ali's research demonstrating fresh responses from the community to the social context. This may be a result of the change of attitude to the country of origin as well as the country of migration. Ghuman (1993; 7) has reported that the early migrants thought of Britain as a temporary phase in their lives, convinced they would return home eventually. Despite staying on permanently, their values and identification with their own country are indications of their attachment to the home country. On the other hand, the younger generation are conscious of being part of British society and being engaged in redefining their identity by reappraising their values drawn from both cultures thus resolving conflicts-in identification with their primary/ethnic group.

Language is seen as an important element of individual and group identity and frequently mentioned by all ethnic groups as a mark of ethnicity. Theories of language accommodation (see Giles et al in a number of studies) are one evidence of the use of language to express attraction or divergence between a speaker and interlocutor. If as argued by Weinreich empathetic identification with individuals and groups is responsive to context, there should be a raised level of conflict-in-identification among ethnicised minority members when situated in social contexts, that is, with their own or other group. Moreover, language being a shorthand or social semiotic and an expresser of identity, would by its use raise empathetic identification with one's own group as a mental representation of primary identifications with own group members. This inner representation of early identifications, it has been argued by Northover (1988), is accompanied by a shift in those values encoded in the language of home. Similarly, English in the case of South Asians, would encode the values of the wider society and identifications with individual members of the British group.

This innate notion of the importance of language was put to the test by Northover (1988) with Gujarati/English bilinguals of Asian British ethnicity and adolescent status living in the inner city areas of Birmingham and Leicester. Using different methodologies, Ervin-Tripp (1964) reported a condition of dual identities in the case of bilingual bicultural subjects in their two languages. Whereas Ervin-Tripp found significant changes of persona in the context of their two languages, she was unable to explain whether this was a special case of bilingualism among biculturals or simply the effect of language. Evidently, she lacked a theoretical approach to her experimentation whereas the concepts posited by Weinreich, can afford explanations of shift in identifications and values in terms of situated identity.

The sample of respondents in Northover's study (using the framework of ISA) consisted of young men and women from Hindus (M19, F17) and Muslims (M4, F12) in Birmingham and Leicester. They were presented with an identity instrument in English which was also translated into Gujarati and presented to the respondents at suitable intervals, care being taken in the design to minimize as far as possible, the effect of time and order of language on the respondents. As with Kelly's sample, the respondents were divided into two groups on the basis of the construct "feels English" (called Anglo-oriented or progressive)/"doesn't feel at all English" (described as Indo-oriented or orthodox). This construct was designed as a crucial indication of the respondents' identification with English people they encountered.

While all the respondents agreed that language was important to them, the effect of the context of Gujarati or English was not uniform across the sample of Hindu and Muslim boys and girls, nor was it consistent with the notion that use of one's familial language will increase favourable identification with one's own ethnic group. The explanation for this result can be found in Northover's theoretical proposition that language is an encoder of identifications with influential others and in the case of bicultural bilinguals such as the South Asian youth in the sample, significant modifications in empathetic identifications with own group would occur in their two languages of Gujarati and English.

The results showed that some values were modified in the context of Gujarati (GL) compared with the English language (EL) context. For example, Anglo-oriented (progressive) girls had significantly different values on the construct "Housework for both men and women" contrasted with "Housework for females only". The progressive group favored housework for both men and women in both languages, but in Gujarati, the structural pressure on the construct was low (10.07 on a scale of -100 to +100 structural pressure). In the English language on the other hand, the value appeared to be much more consistently and stably held at a structural pressure of 52.27. In this instance, these progressive girls are uncertain and inconsistent in the use of the evaluative dimension of housework to be shared by both sexes in GL, but quite positive in EL. It appears that in the context of GL, the girls revert to an ethnically-oriented view of sex roles.

Table 1 illustrates conflict-in-identification of Anglo-oriented (progressive) girls with English people in the context of Gujarati (GL) and English (EL). The context of GL causes these girls greater conflict-in-identification for although they generally favor British values and have high levels of empathetic identification with English people, the language of primary

Table 1. Conflict-in-Identification of Anglo-Oriented (Progressive Girls) (N = 20)

Target Entity	Gujarati language	English language	F	df	p
Own ethnic group	0.49	0.45	8.04	1, 19	<0.01
English people	0.44	0.36			

Note. Effect of language context (Gujarati and English) on the perception of the South Asian females.

Table 2. Conflict-in-Identifiation of Muslim Girls (N = 20)

Target Entity	Gujarati language	English language	F	df	p
Own ethnic group	0.40	0.24	6.57	1, 19	<0.025
English people	0.40	0.42			

Note. Effect of language context (Gurajati and English) on Muslim girls among South Asians.

socialisation Gujarati, and Gujarati is the carrier of primarily important empathetic identifications with family and community. Increased empathetic identification through GL leads to greater conflict-in-identification.

Indo-oriented or orthodox girls would be expected to show an increase in empathetic identification with their own group thus raising the level of conflict-in-identification. They also show a significant increase of conflict-in-identification in the Gujarati language in relation to Gujaratis (Table 2). For these girls, with an orientation towards their own group, speaking in the ethnic language of their favored group increases empathetic identification significantly. However, in rating English people, conflict-in-identification hardly differs between the two languages and is of a high level in both GL and EL. One must conclude that, while the girls favor the ethnic group feeling they are not at all English, nevertheless they feel strongly enough on certain mainstream values, acquired through socialisation at school with English teachers and peers, to have approved of certain values encoded in English.

Moderation of values seems to take place in the context of language in the case of Asian British girls and boys, but changes are not always consistent with their orientations to British values among progressive (Anglo-oriented) girls or Indian values among the orthodox (Indo-oriented) ones. Both groups of progressives and orthodox appear to have strong empathetic identifications with their own group while accepting certain values from the mainstream.

Discussion

The three studies above highlight the problem of homogenization and the use of blanket categories such as 'South Asian', to describe complex psychological processes which seek to minimize psychological stress in the case of a physically (through skin color) and culturally distinct group. Language appears to add a further element of differentiation, and as a carrier of social identity and an encoder of cultural norms and values, it has an additional impact on situated identity. Ervin-Tripp's original surmise was that bicultural bilinguals were a special case of bilinguals, but the explanation for the phenomenon must come from theoretical antecedents which are provided in the studies discussed here.

It is clear that there is no essential notion of identity amongst the youth in the above studies. It follows therefore that South Asian Youth in Britain will not be homogeneous in their identifications with their own ethnic group or with white majority culture due to significant differences between individuals. Nor are they homogeneous in terms of their identifications with their own and other ethnic groups. Various experiences of socialisation, religious affiliation and relationships with significant others in one's life are all important factors in the process of identity formation and reformation, and therefore any broad categories should be used with caution.

What is common to the South Asian youth in the cited studies is the value they place on their own ethnic groups' norms and beliefs. It is clear that they are reappraising their own group values and beliefs with those of the majority society. Their identity has taken on broad aspects of the majority culture, but they are doing so without forgoing aspects of their own ethnic group identity.

Conclusion

Research is in contradistinction to the commonly held perceptions of culture conflict within South Asian communities in Britain. Increased conflicts-in-identification occurring through redefinitions and more updated versions of ethnicity may set younger individuals away from the older generation, but this does not suggest the alternative of a complete identification with the superordinate white majority. Differences in identification conflicts between the generations is not about culture conflict but rather a process of identity development.

Notions of homogeneity of a single South Asian British community do not stand up to investigation in the psychological and sociolinguistic studies discussed in this paper. The heterogeneous nature of this group is evident and each perspective by researchers has emphasized diversity, change and adaptation. It is clear that what is required are more refined concepts of identity to deal with the complexity of identity formation. The conceptual framework of ISA has been presented as one possible conceptual approach that may be useful for the study of identity within the multicultural context.

References

Ali, N. (1997). *Community and individual identity of the Kashmiri community in the United Kingdom.* Unpublished research in preparation for a PhD thesis. University of Luton.

Ali, N., Ellis, P., & Weinreich, P. (1996a, April). *Kashmiri British identity: Generational identifications.* Paper presented at the British Psychological Society's Conference at Brighton.

Ali, N., Ellis, P., & Weinreich, P. (1996b). *Enculturation and the maintenance of ethnic distinctiveness.* Paper presented at the British Psychological Society's Conference at Brighton, April, 1996.

Bernabe, J., Clement, R., & Lamontagne, C. (1979). Social rite practice and perceptual information processing. In W. Callebaut, M. Demey, R. Pinxten, & F. Vandamme (Eds.), *Theory of knowledge and science policy.* Ghent: Communication and Cognition.

Berry, J. (1986). Multiculturalism and psychology in plural societies. In L. H. Ekstrand (Ed.), *Ethnic minorities and immigrants. A cross-cultural perspective.* Lisse: Swets & Zeitlinger.

Berry J. W. (1988). Acculturation and psychological adaptation: a conceptual overview. In J. W. Berry & R. Annis (Eds.), *Ethnic psychology: Research and practice with immigrants, refugees, natived peoples, ethnic groups and sojourners.* Amsterdam: Swets & Zeitlinger.

Billig, M. (1995). *Ideology and opinions.* London: Sage.

Eldering, L. (1995). Child-rearing in bi-cultural settings: A culture-ecological approach. *Psychology and Developing Societies, 7,* 133-153.

Erikson, E. (1963). *Childhood and society.* New York: W.W. Norton.

Ervin-Tripp, S. (1964). Language and TAT content in bilinguals. In *Language acquisition and communicative choice.* Stanford: Stanford University.

Ghuman, P. A. S. (1991). Best and worst of two worlds? A study of Asian adolescents. *Educational Research, 33,* 121-132.

Ghuman, P. A. Singh (1993). *Coping with two cultures.* Clevedon: Multilingual Matters.

Giles, H., & Johnson, P. (1981). The role of language in intergroup relations. In J. Turner & H. Giles (Eds.), *Intergroup behaviour.* Oxford: Basil Blackwell.

Gilroy (1994). *Black atlantic.* London: Verso.

Kelly, A. J. D. (1989). Ethnic identification, association and redefinition: Muslim Pakistanis and Greek Cypriots in Britain. In K. Liebkind (Ed.), *New identities in Europe.* London: Gower.

Madood, T. (March, 1995). *The end of a hegemony: From political blackness to ethnic pluralism.* Paper presented for the CRE Seminar Constructing and Deconstructing 'Black Identity'.

Northover, M. (1988). *A theoretical and empirical investigation of ethnic identify and bilingualism: Gujarati/English British youth.* Unpublished D Phil dissertation. Belfast: University of Ulster.

Tajfel, H. (Ed.) (1981). *Human groups and social categories.* Cambridge: Cambridge University Press.

Weinreich, P. (1980). *Manual for identity exploration using personal constructs.* Bristol: ESRC.

Weinreich, P. (1983a). Emerging from threatened identities: ethnicity and gender in redefinitions of threatened identity. In G. Breakwell (Ed.), *Threatened identities.* Chichester: Wiley.

Weinreich, P. (1983b). Psychodynamics of personal and social identity: theoretical concepts and their measurement in adolescents from Belfast sectarian and Bristol minority groups. In A. Jacobsen-Widding (Ed.), *Identity, personal and socio-cultural.* Stockholm: Almquist and Wicksell International.

Weinreich, P., Kelly, A. J. D., & Maja, C. (1986). *Situated identities: Conflicts in identification and own group preference in racial and ethnic identifications: rural and urban Black youth, South Africa.* Paper presented at the 8th Congress of the International Association for Cross-Cultural Psychology, Istanbul.

Weinreich, P. (1989). Variations in ethnic identity: Identity Structure Analysis. In K. Liebkind (Ed.), *New identities in Europe.* London: Gower.

Weinreich, P., Luk C. L., & Bond, M. (1996). Ethnic stereotyping and Identification in a Multicultural Context: 'Acculturation', self-esteem and identity diffusion in Hong Kong Chinese University students. *Psychology and Developing Societies, 8,* 107-169.

National Identity, National Favoritism, Global Self-Esteem, Tall Poppy Attitudes, and Value Priorities in Australian and Canadian Samples

Norman T. Feather   &   John G. Adair
The Flinders University of South Australia   University of Manitoba
Australia   Canada

ABSTRACT

This study compared samples of Australian and Canadian university students with respect to attitudes toward tall poppies or high achievers, national favoritism as indicated by a tendency to favor the products and achievements of their own country, global self-esteem at the personal level, and value priorities. Measures of national identity and national identification were also obtained for the Australian sample. Results showed that both samples were similar in regard to national favoritism, tall poppy attitudes, and global self-esteem. In both samples, favoring the fall of tall poppies was negatively related to both self-esteem and national favoritism, and national favoritism was positively related to self-esteem. National favoritism and national identification were positively related in the Australian sample. Categorizing self as Australian rather than having some other national identity was associated with higher national favoritism and higher national identification, consistent with social identity theory. National favoritism scores were higher for Canadian Anglophones than for Canadian non-Anglophones. Australian students rated some universalistic, prosocial values such as equality, a world of peace, and a world of beauty as more important for self and conformity values as less important when compared with the Canadian students. Gender differences in value ratings were consistent with previous findings.

Over the past few years the first author has been collecting data concerned with national identification, in-group favoritism, attitudes toward high achievement, and values in a program of research involving a small set of different countries. This research was conducted with the assistance of colleagues in these countries and, in each case, the data have been obtained from student samples. The countries involved in the research are Australia, Canada, China, India, Indonesia, Malaysia, New Zealand, and the U.S.A. These countries were selected so as to provide for a wide range of comparisons across very different cultures.

The present paper reports some findings from Australia and Canada based upon data obtained from Flinders University in 1994 and by John

Adair from the University of Manitoba in 1992. The results from other countries will be reported as the data analysis proceeds.

The choice of variables that were included in these studies was dictated in part by the interests of the first author at the time but they are variables that are also of general interest to cross-cultural researchers. We will discuss each set of variables in turn and indicate the hypotheses that we were interested in testing.

National Identification and In-Group Favoritism

There is a small but developing research interest among social psychologists in the study of such topics as national identity, patriotism, and national favoritism (e.g., Billig, 1995; Bourhis, 1996; Cinnirella, 1997; Feather, 1993, 1994c, 1995a, 1996b; Mlicki & Ellemers, 1996; Schatz & Staub, 1997; Staub, 1997). The first author became interested in this topic as a result of examining a belief that often surfaces in the mass media in Australia. This is the belief that Australians suffer from a "cultural cringe," and tend to regard Australian products and achievements as of lesser value when compared with those produced by other developed countries. The first author developed a scale to measure cultural cringe (Feather, 1993) and included it in the study with Australian and Canadian students reported in the present paper.

The obverse of cultural cringe is the belief that the products and achievements of one's own country are superior to those of other developed countries. In recent publications the first author has focussed on this belief, assessing it by using the Cultural Cringe Scale but scoring the items in the scale in the reverse direction so as to provide a measure of national favoritism (Feather, 1994c, 1995a, 1996b). A consistent result obtained from these studies is that national favoritism is stronger among Australians who identify themselves as Australians rather than as belonging to some other national group. In addition, the Australian results show that national favoritism is positively related to strength of national identification as measured by items concerned with caring about being an Australian and pride in Australia. These two items were included in the present study but only in the Australian questionnaire.

Similar findings were expected for the Australian sample tested in the present study. These findings, that relate in-group favoritism at the national level to national identity and to strength of national identification, are consistent with the implications of social identity theory and its subsequent developments (e.g., Hogg & Abrams, 1988; Oakes, Haslam, & Turner, 1994; Turner, Hogg, Oakes, Reicher, & Wetherell, 1987).

Tall Poppy Attitudes

The first author's interest in attitudes toward high achievers developed from examining another commonly held and widely promulgated belief in Australia, namely that Australians like to cut down "tall poppies" or people who occupy positions of high status. He has conducted an extensive program of research into attitudes toward high achievers using a variety of research procedures (Feather, 1994a, 1996c). As part of this research program he devised a scale to measure tall poppy attitudes that provides two scores. One score, called "favor fall," indicates the degree to which a person favors the fall of tall poppies, cutting them down to size. The other score, called "favor reward," indicates the degree to which a person believes that tall poppies should be rewarded, with their achievements recognized in a positive way.

The Tall Poppy Scale also formed part of the Australian/Canadian study. It was included in order to determine whether the Australian students were distinctive in their tall poppy beliefs when compared with the Canadian students. There is already some evidence to indicate that Japanese students are more inclined to cut down high achievers when compared with Australian students (Feather & McKee, 1993), perhaps reflecting a more collectivist orientation in the Japanese culture (Triandis, 1995). Indeed, differences in tall poppy attitudes across nations may be useful information that is relevant to the individualism-collectivism distinction, with collectivist cultures more willing to bring tall poppies down to the group level.

Global Self-Esteem

Results from studies of tall poppies (Feather, 1994a, 1996c) showed that people who reported low self-esteem were more likely to favor the fall of tall poppies when compared with those who reported high self-esteem. In contrast, those who reported high self-esteem were more likely to favor rewarding tall poppies when compared with those who reported low self-esteem, although this relation tended to be weaker than the former one and occurred less consistently. We included the modified version of the Rosenberg Self-Esteem Scale (Rosenberg, 1965) as modified by Bachman, O'Malley, & Johnston (1978) in order to investigate whether these relations between global self-esteem and tall poppy attitudes would also occur for the Australian and Canadian students who participated in the present study.

Some findings from previous studies also suggest that there may be a weak negative relation between endorsement of a cultural cringe and self-esteem or, on the obverse side of the coin, a weak positive relation between national favoritism and self-esteem (Feather, 1996b). That is, people who report low personal self-esteem may be more likely to denigrate their nation's products and achievements (or display less national favoritism) when compared with those who report high personal self-esteem. We were also able to test this hypothesis in the present study.

The relations specified in the hypotheses involving tall poppy attitudes, national favoritism, and global self-esteem may partly reflect the effects of attitudes toward self that are the product of a person's own status and life experience (Feather, 1994a, 1996c). Those who have been successful in terms of their own goals and who have developed beliefs that they are competent and useful individuals would be expected to have higher self-esteem when compared with those who have been less successful. Their own higher standing on the ladder of success and competence may then lead them to want to see tall poppies rewarded and not cut down to size, and may also lead them to hold more favorable beliefs about the products and achievements of their nation. Those who have been unsuccessful in their life pursuits and who have developed negative views about their own competence and usefulness would be expected to have lower self-esteem. They may envy tall poppies, wanting to see them displaced from their high positions rather than rewarded because of their high status. They may also tend to hold more negative views about their nation's products and achievements, generalizing from their own status and experience.

Values

Research on values by social psychologists is of long standing but, until recently, it has been rather sporadic. In his Presidential address to the Society for the Psychological Study of Social Issues, Rokeach (1968) argued that the study of values had been neglected in favor of research on attitudes. Subsequently, he published his book *The Nature of Human Values* (Rokeach, 1973) in which he reported an extensive program of research that used his Value Survey. The first author began research into human values in Australia in the late 1960s and published the initial results in *Values in Education and Society* (Feather, 1975), a couple of years after Rokeach's book appeared. He has maintained an active interest in the study of values over subsequent years with a particular emphasis on relations between values, valences and actions, on cross-cultural similarities and differences in value priorities, and on relations between values and justice variables (e.g., Feather, 1986, 1990, 1992, 1994b, 1995b, 1996a). Hence, it is not surprising that a major focus of this study was to investigate value priorities for the Australian and Canadian samples.

Given the fact that we used student samples from two Western societies and that students in a particular age range (late teens/early 20s) probably share similar concerns regardless of culture, we expected to find some similarities in value priorities across the two samples. We were more interested, however, in differences in value priorities that might relate to differences in culture. To some extent this part of the research was exploratory, although some hypotheses can be formulated based on what we know about each culture. For example, the first author has proposed that there is a degree of conflict in the Australian culture between individualist, achievement values and collectivist, prosocial values, and also a tendency for Australians to favor equality and to react against high status and authority, especially if the high status is seen to be undeserved (Feather, 1994a, 1996c). An Australian concern with "mateship," friendship, and equal status relationships with others has also been noted (Feather, 1975, pp. 212-214). Triandis (1995) described the Australian culture as horizontal and individualistic in contrast to the American culture which he saw as vertical and individualistic. In his terms, "the vertical dimension accepts inequality, and rank has its privileges...the horizontal dimension emphasizes that people should be similar on most attributes, especially status" (p. 44).

Hofstede (1980) found that Australia and Canada were similar in relation to his cultural level dimensions of power distance, uncertainty avoidance, individualism, and masculinity, and that both were relatively high on the individualism dimension. Lipset (1990) described Canada as "a more class-aware, elitist, law-abiding, statist, collectivity-oriented, and particularistic (group-oriented) society than the United States" (p. 8). He also cited a summary by Berton (1982) that stated that Canadians "are law-abiding, deferential toward authority, cautious, prudent, elitist, moralistic, tolerant (of ethnic) differences, cool, unemotional, and solemn" (Lipset, 1990, p. 44). Lipset (1963a, 1963b) also related value patterns in Australia, the United States, Britain, and Canada to the sequence of historical events involved in the development of each democracy, but Baer, Curtis, Grabb, and Johnston (1996) reported evidence from a study of child-rearing values that was critical of his conclusions. They also cautioned against making too much of the national differences they obtained, noting that there was a lot of similarity in results across nations in regard to the qualities that people value in their children. Baer, Grabb, and Johnston (1990) also published a critical analysis and reassessment of Lipset's thesis concerning Canadians and Americans.

On the basis of these discussions, we expected to find that the Australian and Canadian students that we tested would be similar in regard to individualist, achievement values, but that the Australian students would assign higher importance to equality, and lower importance to conformity values that relate to deferential rules of conduct, when compared with the Canadian students. Berton's (1982) summary also suggests that the Canadian students may assign higher priority to values that imply a degree of control and constriction when compared with the Australian students.

Gender Differences

We included gender of participant as a variable in the study in order to determine whether any national differences that might be found were common to both male and female participants. We expected to replicate gender differences found with the Rokeach values that have been described by Feather (1987).

Method

Participants

The Australian sample in the present study consisted of 186 students (63 male, 121 female, 2 who did not specify gender) who were enrolled in the introductory course in psychology at the Flinders University in Adelaide, South Australia in 1994. The mean age of the sample was 22.56 years (*SD* = 6.58).

The Canadian sample comprised 310 students (129 male, 181 female) who were enrolled in the introductory course in psychology at the University of Manitoba, in Winnipeg, Manitoba, in 1992. The mean age of the sample was 19.78 years (*SD* = 5.16).

Procedure

These participants completed the 20-item Tall Poppy Scale, the 16-item Cultural Cringe Scale, a modified version of the Rokeach Value Survey (Rokeach, 1973) in which participants rated the importance for self of each of the 18 terminal and 18 instrumental values on a 7-point scale, and the 10-item modified version of the Rosenberg Self-Esteem Scale (Bachman et al., 1978; Rosenberg, 1965) as used in previous studies to measure global self-esteem (e.g., Feather, 1993). The order of presentation was Tall Poppy Scale, Cultural Cringe Scale, Rosenberg Self-Esteem Scale, and Rokeach Value Survey.

Participants completed the questionnaires anonymously and they were subsequently debriefed about the aims of the study.

Scales

The Tall Poppy Scale comprised 20 items such as the following: "It's good to see very successful people fail occasionally," "Very successful people sometimes need to be brought down a peg or two, even if they have done nothing wrong," "One ought to respect the person at the top." The scale provided two scores, favor fall and favor reward, each of which was based on 10 items. Participants answered each item by using a 6-point response scale labeled as follows: +1, I agree a little; +2, I agree on the whole; +3, I agree very much; -1, I disagree a little; -2, I disagree on the whole;

-3, I disagree very much. Subsequently, a constant of +4 was added to item responses so as to achieve a positive scale. Total scores for favor fall and favor reward could therefore range from 10 to 70. As indicated previously, both of these scores have been used in previous research on tall poppies (Feather, 1994a, 1996a). The internal consistency reliabilities (Cronbach *alphas*) for the two scales were as follows: favor fall (Australian, $\alpha = .80$; Canadian, $\alpha = .72$), favor reward (Australians, $\alpha = .74$, Canadians, $\alpha = .73$).

The Cultural Cringe Scale comprised 16 items such as the following (modifications for the Canadian sample are presented in parentheses): "The standard of manufacturing products in Australia (Canada) compares very well with the standard of similar products from overseas (in other countries)," "You can't really say that Australian (Canadian) achievements are good until they've been judged by overseas experts (experts outside of Canada)," "Australians (Canadians) tend to over-rate their own importance in the world." Eight of the items were positively worded and eight were negatively worded. The full 16-item scale as used in Australia is presented in Feather (1993). Participants responded to each item using the same 6-point response scale as they used for the Tall Poppy Scale. In the present study, items were not scored in the direction of cultural cringe but in the direction of national favoritism, with higher scores indicating that participants favored Australia's (Canada's) products and achievements (see also Feather, 1994c, 1995a, 1996b). Responses to each item were converted to a positive scale by adding a constant of +4. National favoritism scores could therefore range from 16 to 112. The internal reliabilities (Cronbach *alphas*) were as follows: Australians, $\alpha = .83$; Canadians, $\alpha = .82$). A mean score was computed for each participant by averaging across the 16 items, giving a possible score range from 1 to 7.

The modified version of the Rosenberg Self-Esteem Scale consisted of 10 items, each of which involved a statement (e.g., "I feel that I'm a person of worth, at least on an equal plane with others," "I am a useful person to have around"). Participants answered each item by checking one of five responses that related to how true they thought the item was for self, ranging from *never true*, through *sometimes true*, to *almost always true*. Responses were scored from 1 to 5 in the direction of positive self-esteem, and total self-esteem scores could range from 10 to 50. The internal reliabilities (Cronbach *alphas*) were as follows: Australian students, $\alpha = .87$, Canadian students, $\alpha = .87$.

The Rokeach Value Survey (Rokeach, 1973) was presented in rating format rather than in the usual ranking format. The rating scale for each of the terminal and instrumental values in the Rokeach Value Survey was divided into seven equal parts and it was labeled *Not important to me at all as a value* (scored 1), and *Extremely important to me as a value* (scored 7) at the end points, and *Moderately important* (scored 3) and *Very important* (scored 5) at the third and fifth divisions of the scale.

As in previous studies (e.g., Feather, 1993, 1995a, 1996b), a categorical measure of national identity was obtained by asking the Australian students to check from a number of national groups (Australian, British, Vietnamese, etc.) which one they considered themselves to be. These students also completed two items to assess the strength of their identification with the Australian nation. The two items were as follows: "In general, how much would you say being an Australian means to you? How much do you care about being an Australian?," and "How proud are you to be a member of the Australian nation?" Participants answered each item by using a 5-point Likert scale (see Feather, 1996b, p. 55, for details). Because scores on these two items were highly correlated ($r = .80$, $p < .001$), they were combined for each participant to provide a composite measure of identification with Australia that could range from 2 to 10.

Equivalent measures of national identity and national identification were not included in the Canadian questionnaire, which was administered two years prior to the Australian one. However, the Canadian students were asked whether English was their first language (Yes/No), so as to classify them into Anglophones versus non-Anglophones. Canadian research typically sorts participants according to Anglophone/Francophone but, within the Manitoba sample, there were so few of any non-English language group, that all participants who indicated that their native language was not English were grouped together as non-Anglophones.

Participants in both samples provided information about whether they were born in Australia (Canada) or elsewhere, and also about the country where their fathers were born (Canadian sample), or the country where each parent was born (Australian sample).

Results

Means and SDs

Table 1 presents the means and *SD*s for favor fall, favor reward, self-esteem, and national favoritism for the Australian and Canadian samples, and the mean and *SD* for national identification for the Australian sample. The first four variables in Table 1 were analyzed by using 2 x 2 multivariate analysis of variance (MANOVA) with nation (Australia, Canada) as the first factor and gender (male, female) as the second factor. Because there was a three year difference in age between the two samples, age was included as a covariate in the analysis.

The analysis showed that the multivariate or omnibus *F*s were statistically significant for the main effect of gender, $F(4, 460) = 11.93$, $p < .001$, and

Table 1. *Mean Scores, SDs, and Intercorrelations for Variables for Australian and Canadian Students*

Variable	Australian students		Correlations				
	Mean	SD	Favor fall	Favor reward	Self-esteem	National favoritism	National identification
Favor fall	34.74	10.30	--	-.41***	-.31***	-.32***	-.02
Favor reward	49.01	8.49	-.36***	--	.13	.08	.28***
Self-esteem	41.10	5.80	-.16**	.09	--	.28***	.14
National favoritism	5.29	0.84	-.21*	.12*	.20***	--	.36***
National identification	7.45	2.01	--	--	--	--	--
Canadian students	Mean		36.27	49.10	40.52	5.20	--
	SD		8.45	7.95	5.58	0.79	--

Note. n.s. for the correlations ranged from 172 to 180 for the Australian sample and from 305 to 308 for the Canadian sample. Correlations for the Australian sample are above the diagonal; for the Canadian sample, they are below the diagonal. Tests of significance are two-tailed; *p* < .05, **p* < .01, ***p* < .001.

for the interaction of nation and gender, $F(4, 460) = 2.40$, $p < .05$. The omnibus F for the main effect of nation was not statistically significant.

The means in Table 1 show that participants in both countries were more inclined to favor rewarding tall poppies than to favor their fall from positions of high status, and also that they displayed a positive attitude toward their country's products and achievements, i.e., there was no evidence of a cultural cringe. Mean scores for national favoritism were above the midpoint (4) of the scale.

The statistically significant gender differences obtained from the MANOVA were as follows: (a) Female participants were less in favor of the fall of tall poppies when compared with male participants, $M = 34.63$ and 37.46 respectively, $F(1, 463) = 14.69$, $p < .001$, and more in favor of rewarding tall poppies, $M = 50.03$ and 47.72 respectively, $F(1, 463) = 6.69$, $p < .01$; (b) National favoritism scores were higher for female participants when compared with male participants, $M = 5.30$ and 5.11 respectively, $F(1, 463) = 8.01$, $p < .01$, and global self-esteem scores were lower, $M = 39.92$ and 42.05 respectively, $F(1, 463) = 13.33$, $p < .001$.

The nation by gender interaction was statistically significant only for favor fall, $F(1, 463) = 5.72$, $p < .05$. The gender effect described previously was larger for the Australian participants.

Correlations
Table 1 also shows that statistically significant correlations were obtained in both samples between favor fall and favor reward and between favor fall and self-esteem. These findings replicate previous results (Feather, 1994a, 1996b). In addition, statistically significant negative correlations were obtained for both samples between favoring the fall of tall poppies and national favoritism, and statistically significant positive correlations between national favoritism and self-esteem. A statistically significant positive correlation was obtained for the Australian sample between national favoritism and national identification, replicating previous results (Feather, 1994c, 1996b). National identification was also positively and significantly related to favoring the reward of tall poppies in the Australian sample.

The correlations just noted remained statistically significant after controlling for age and gender by using partial correlation. However, the positive correlation between favoring the reward of tall poppies and self-esteem then became statistically significant in both samples: for the Australian sample, $r(161) = .17$, $p < .05$; for the Canadian sample, $r(299) = .13$, $p < .05$.

National Favoritism, National Identification, and National Identity
National favoritism was related to national identity, as was the case in previous studies (Feather, 1993, 1994c, 1995a, 1996b). Those students in the Australian sample who identified themselves as Australian had significantly higher national favoritism scores when compared with those students who reported some other national identity, Ms = 5.35 and 4.99 respectively, $t(174)$ = 2.10, p < .05. The former students with reported Australian identity also had higher national identification scores when compared with the latter students; Ms = 7.72 and 6.00 respectively, $t(182)$ = 4.45, p < .001.

The results also showed that those students in the Canadian sample who reported English as their first language (Anglophones) had significantly higher national favoritism scores when compared with those students who reported some other first language (non-Anglophones), Ms = 5.31 and 4.56 respectively, $t(272)$ = 5.73, p < .001.

These findings were further supported by the results of analyses for each sample that separated students in relation to whether they were born in Australia (or Canada) or born in some other country. Students who reported Australia (or Canada) as their birthplace had significantly higher national favoritism scores when compared with students who reported some other country as their birthplace. The means for national favoritism were 5.35 and 4.90 respectively for Australians reporting born in Australia compared with born elsewhere, $t(173)$ = 2.42, p < .05. The means were 5.34 and 4.66 for Canadians reporting born in Canada versus born elsewhere, $t(239)$ = 5.65, p < .001.

National favoritism scores were also higher for those Australian students whose parents were either both born in Australia (M = 5.40) or who had one Australian-born parent and one parent born in another country (M = 5.58), when compared with those Australian students whose parents were both born in another country (M = 4.92); $F(2, 172)$ = 7.87, p < .001. National identification scores were also higher for those Australian students with Australian-born parents (M = 7.69) or with parents of Australian/other origin (M = 8.00), when compared with those Australian students whose parents came from another country (M = 6.75); $F(2, 179)$ = 5.16, p < .01. Canadian students with fathers born in Canada had higher national favoritism scores when compared with those Canadian students whose fathers were born in another country. The respective means were 5.34 and 4.90, $t(304)$ = 4.67, p < .001. Information was not available concerning the birthplace of the mothers for the Canadian sample. Nor were national identification scores available.

Table 2. *Mean Ratings and Univariate Fs for Terminal Values for Australian and Canadian Male and Female Students*

Terminal value	Australian students		Canadian students		Univariate F	
	Male	Female	Male	Female	Nation	Gender
A comfortable life	5.00	4.79	5.06	5.16	.60	.20
An exciting life	5.73	5.63	5.55	4.92	16.54***	8.38**
A sense of accomplishment	5.55	5.90	5.30	5.69	4.87*	7.92**
A world at peace	5.25	6.09	4.88	5.85	2.94	39.40***
A world of beauty	4.87	5.60	4.46	4.61	20.56***	9.10**
Equality	5.73	6.18	5.24	5.95	7.72**	18.99***
Family security	5.85	6.23	5.89	6.24	.01	10.79***
Freedom	6.25	6.38	6.05	6.18	3.83	1.51
Happiness	6.22	6.56	6.15	6.42	3.76	10.57***
Inner harmony	6.03	6.34	5.12	5.47	48.37***	7.17**
Mature love	6.15	6.04	5.85	5.82	4.65*	.27
National security	4.20	4.65	4.69	5.04	5.00*	6.04*
Pleasure	5.35	5.28	5.32	5.41	.26	.00
Salvation	3.48	3.48	4.06	4.41	9.26**	.70
Self-respect	5.50	6.21	5.65	5.95	.11	18.86***
Social recognition	4.05	4.12	4.57	4.46	5.14*	.02
True friendship	6.27	6.56	6.19	6.29	4.68*	4.55*
Wisdom	5.72	5.99	5.49	5.43	6.27*	.78

Note. For Australian students, $N = 60$ females, $N = 117$ for males; for Canadian students, $N = 129$ for males, $N = 181$ for females.

*p < .05; **p < .01; ***p < .001.

Table 3. Mean Ratings and Univariate Fs for Instrumental Values for Australian and Canadian Male and Female Students

Instrumental value	Australian students		Canadian students		Nation	Univariate F
	Male	Female	Male	Female		Gender
Ambitious	4.73	5.08	5.27	5.33	6.02*	2.42
Broadminded	5.79	6.10	5.34	5.37	25.86*	1.81
Capable	5.31	5.63	5.41	5.34	.70	1.33
Cheerful	5.23	5.67	5.33	5.34	1.43	2.78
Clean	3.66	3.98	4.63	4.88	35.47***	3.49
Courageous	5.48	5.53	5.44	5.43	.31	.02
Forgiving	5.18	5.57	5.12	5.22	2.47	3.56
Helpful	4.89	5.59	4.76	5.20	4.58*	18.81***
Honest	5.69	6.29	5.53	6.07	2.37	21.62***
Imaginative	5.31	5.01	4.66	4.33	17.76***	4.44*
Independent	5.63	5.90	5.28	5.55	6.29*	4.22*
Intellectual	5.29	5.50	5.25	5.51	.02	3.59
Logical	5.18	4.88	4.98	4.91	.15	1.75
Loving	5.61	6.08	5.78	6.06	.00	9.37**
Obedient	3.73	3.23	4.07	4.14	11.50***	2.15
Polite	4.48	4.74	5.15	5.17	12.03***	.97
Responsible	5.10	5.61	5.73	5.98	15.03***	10.60***
Self-controlled	4.68	4.69	5.43	5.16	14.44***	.90

Note. For Australian students, $N = 62$ females, $N = 119$ for males; for Canadian students, $N = 128$ for males, $N = 181$ for males.
$*p < .05$; $**p < .01$; $***p < .001$.

Mean Value Ratings

Tables 2 and 3 report the mean importance ratings for each of the 18 terminal and 18 instrumental values for the Australian and Canadian samples. The ratings for each set of values were analyzed using 2 x 2 multivariate analysis of variance (MANOVA) with nation (Australia, Canada) as the first factor in the analysis and gender (male, female) as the second factor. Age was again included as a covariate in the analysis.

The multivariate or omnibus Fs were statistically significant for the main effects of nation and gender but the omnibus F for the nation by gender interaction effect was not statistically significant. The respective omnibus Fs for the nation effect were as follows: terminal values $F(18, 465) = 5.58$, $p < .001$; for the instrumental values, $F(18, 468) = 6.42, p < .001$. The respective omnibus Fs for the gender effect were as follows: terminal values, $F(18, 465) = 5.26$, $p < .001$; instrumental values, $F(18, 468) = 4.83, p < .001$.

These results in Table 2 show that students in both samples rated true friendship, happiness, freedom, and family security as high in importance on the average, and pleasure, social recognition and salvation as low in importance. The results in Table 3 show that students in both samples rated being honest and loving as high in importance on the average, and being clean and obedient as low in importance.

The results also show that the following values were rated as significantly higher in importance by the Australian students when compared with the Canadian students: an exciting life, a sense of accomplishment, a world at peace, a world of beauty, equality, inner harmony, mature love, true friendship, wisdom, being broadminded, being imaginative, and being independent.

In contrast, the following values were rated as significantly higher in importance by the Canadian students when compared with the Australian students: national security, salvation, social recognition, being ambitious, being clean, being obedient, being polite, being responsible, and being self-controlled.

These value differences occurred for both male and female participants. They suggest a greater emphasis by the Australian students on values that Schwartz (1992) would classify as belonging to the stimulation and universalism value types and more emphasis by the Canadian students on values that he would classify as belonging to the security and conformity value types.

The analysis of gender differences showed that the male participants rated the following values as significantly higher in importance when compared with the female participants: an exciting life and being imaginative. The female participants rated the following values as more important: a sense of accomplishment, a world at peace, a world of beauty, equality, family security, happiness, inner harmony, national security, self-respect, true friendship, being helpful, being honest, being independent, being loving, and being responsible. Evident in these differences is a stronger emphasis by male participants on values that Schwartz (1992) would classify as stimulation values and more emphasis by female participants on values that he would classify as belonging to the benevolence, universalism, and security value types.

Discussion

These results provide new information about Australian/Canadian similarities and differences in regard to social attitudes and values. Students from both countries were similar in their attitudes toward tall poppies or high achievers and in their levels of national favoritism. Thus, there was no evidence from this comparative study to support the commonly held view that Australians are distinctive in wanting to see tall poppies cut down to size or to support the belief that Australians suffer from a cultural cringe.

Note, however, that students in both samples were more in favor of rewarding tall poppies than in seeing them fall, a difference that is consistent with an individualistic, achievement emphasis in both the Australian and Canadian cultures. We would expect this difference to be attenuated in more collectivist cultures where standing out from the group meets with disapproval and where there may be more pressure to bring tall poppies down to the same level as others.

Future analyses will involve comparisons with other nations that have been included in this cross-cultural program, and it may be the case that countries that are clearly different from Australia and Canada with respect to cultural dimensions and construal of self will be associated with differences on some of the variables, as occurred, for example, when Australian and Japanese students were compared in regard to tall poppy attitudes (Feather & McKee, 1993).

The results also showed that the two samples were similar in personal self-esteem and in some of their value priorities. However, there were some differences in value priorities that were consistent with hypotheses and that might reflect cultural effects. The tendency for the Australian students to assign less importance to conformity values and more importance to equality when compared with the Canadian students is consistent with social and historical analyses of the Australian culture that describe Australians as egalitarian in outlook and as having a tendency to react against restrictive forms of authority and rules of conduct that are seen to be associated with superior social class, high status, and pretentiousness (e.g., Feather, 1975, pp. 201-231). When compared with the Australian students, the Canadians gave stronger endorsement to values concerned with control, conformity, salvation, ambition, and recognition, and they rated universalistic, prosocial values concerned with peace and beauty, and values that related to the inner life of harmony, imagination, and wisdom as less important. It is possible that some of the value priorities held by the Canadian students may reflect the influence of their powerful U.S. neighbor. However, it is likely that the value patterns for each sample are the product of many influences, some of which may be shared by the Australian and Canadian cultures and some that are distinctive to each culture. Specifying common and distinctive influences across cultures that determine similarities and differences in basic values will involve multidisciplinary research inputs.

The results from both samples showed that favoring the fall of tall poppies was negatively related to global self-esteem, replicating previous findings that have been discussed elsewhere (Feather, 1994a, 1996c). Favoring the reward of tall poppies was positively related to self-esteem in both samples, but the correlation was statistically significant only after controlling for the effects of age and gender. As indicated previously, a significant positive relation between these variables has been found in some studies (e.g., Feather, 1991; Feather, Volkmer, & McKee, 1991), but not consistently. However, in both samples, national favoritism was positively related to self-esteem and negatively related to favoring the fall of tall poppies. The positive relation between national favoritism and personal self-esteem replicates a previous finding (Feather, 1996b). Considered together, these results show that both students with more negative views of self and students with more negative beliefs about the products and achievements of their country were more inclined to favor the fall of tall poppies or high achievers when compared with students with higher levels of self-esteem and students with higher levels of national favoritism. They also show that the absence of a cultural cringe (or higher national favoritism) was associated with stronger self-esteem.

The results were consistent with social identity theory (Hogg & Abrams, 1988; Oakes et al., 1994; Turner et al., 1987) in showing that the in-group bias that was reflected in higher national favoritism was a function of self-categorization that related directly to reported group membership (Australian sample). Categorizing oneself as Australian was accompanied by a degree of in-group favoritism. Thus, those Australian students who reported Australian identity were also more in favor of Australia's products and achievements when compared with students who identified with some other national group. The former students also reported stronger identification with Australia, and national favoritism was positively related to the strength of this identification. These results replicate previous findings (Feather, 1994c, 1995a, 1996b).

The higher national favoritism reported by students who categorized themselves as Australian carried through when students were categorized in relation to their country of birth (Australia or elsewhere) and in relation to the country of origin of their parents, replicating previous results (Feather, 1994c, 1995a). Moreover, stronger identification with Australia was more evident among Australian students who had Australian-born parents or at least one Australian-born parent when compared with Australian students whose parents were both born outside of Australia.

These findings for the Australian students suggest that both group processes relating to social identity and acculturation processes involving different socialization experiences had effects on national favoritism and national identification.

Evidence that could be interpreted in terms of social identity processes was not available for the Canadian sample because, as indicated previously, these students did not complete measures of national identity and national identification. National favoritism scores were higher for those Canadian students who reported that English was their first language, who were born in Canada, and who had fathers who were born in Canada when compared with Canadian students who were non-Anglophones, who were not born in Canada, and who had fathers who were not born in Canada. These findings probably reflect acculturation differences. They may also reflect the effects of social identity but more research is needed on this topic.

We end with a caveat. The present results should be qualified in terms of the samples that we used. The samples were convenience samples from two universities in Australia and Canada and they are not necessarily representative of each country's men and women or even of their male and female university students. Both countries involve regional and cultural diversity. Wider samples have been taken in the Australian research on the variables included in our study (eg, Feather, 1994a, 1995a) but it is clear that further sampling of different segments within each country is required before results can be generalized. However, studies like the present one have value by establishing both the theory and the measures that may be appropriate for more extensive testing with probability samples in survey research.

References

Bachman, J. G., O'Malley, P. M., & Johnston, J. (1978). *Adolescence to adulthood: Change and stability in the lives of young men.* Ann Arbor, MI: Institute for Social Research.

Baer, D., Curtis, J., Grabb, E., & Johnston, W. J. (1996). What values do people prefer in children? A comparative analysis of survey evidence from fifteen countries. In C. Seligman, J. M. Olson, & M. P. Zanna

(Eds.), *The psychology of values: The Ontario symposium* (Vol. 8, pp. 299-328). Mahwah, NJ: Erlbaum.

Baer, D., Grabb, E., & Johnston, W. J. (1990). The values of Americans and Canadians: A critical analysis and reassessment. *Social Forces, 68,* 693-713.

Berton, P. (1982). *Why we act like Canadians.* Toronto: McClelland & Stewart.

Billig, M. (1995). *Banal nationalism.* London: Sage Publications.

Bourhis, R. Y. (1996). Canadian and Québécois national identity. *International Journal of Psychology, 31,* 475.

Cinnirella, M. (1997). Towards a European identity? Interactions between the national and European social identities manifested by university students in Britain and Italy. *British Journal of Social Psychology, 36,* 19-31.

Feather, N. T. (1975). *Values in education and society.* New York: Free Press.

Feather, N. T. (1986). Cross-cultural studies with the Rokeach Value Survey: The Flinders program of research on values. *Australian Journal of Psychology, 38,* 269-283.

Feather, N. T. (1987). Gender differences in values. In F. Halisch & J. Kuhl (Eds.), *Motivation, intention, and volition* (pp. 31-45). New York: Springer-Verlag.

Feather, N. T. (1990). Bridging the gap between values and actions: Recent applications of the expectacy-value model. In E. T. Higgins & R. M. Sorrentino (Eds.), *Handbook of motivation and cognition* (Vol. 2, pp. 151-192). New York: Guilford Press.

Feather, N. T. (1991). Attitudes towards the high achiever: Effects of perceiver's own level of competence. *Australian Journal of Psychology, 43,* 121-124.

Feather, N. T. (1992). Values, valences, expectations, and actions. *Journal of Social Issues, 48(2),* 109-124.

Feather, N. T. (1993). Devaluing achievement within a culture: Measuring the cultural cringe. *Australian Journal of Psychology, 45,* 182-188.

Feather, N. T. (1994a). Attitudes toward high achievers and reactions to their fall: Theory and research concerning tall poppies. In M. P. Zanna (Ed.), *Advances in experimental social psychology* (Vol. 26, pp. 1-73). San Diego, CA: Academic.

Feather, N. T. (1994b). Human values and their relation to justice. *Journal of Social Issues, 50(4),* 129-151.

Feather, N. T. (1994c). Values, national identification and favouritism towards the ingroup. *British Journal of Social Psychology, 33,* 467-476.

Feather, N. T. (1995a). National identification and ingroup bias in majority and minority groups: A field study. *Australian Journal of Psychology, 47,* 129-136.

Feather, N. T. (1995b). Values, valences, and choice: The influence of values on the perceived attractiveness and choice of alternatives. *Journal of Personality and Social Psychology, 68,* 1135-1151.

Feather, N. T. (1996a). Reactions to penalties for an offense in relation to authoritarianism, values, perceived responsibility, perceived seriousness, and deservingness. *Journal of Personality and Social Psychology, 71,* 571-587.

Feather, N. T. (1996b). Social comparisons across nations: Variables relating to the subjective evaluation of national achievement and to personal and collective self-esteem. *Australian Journal of Psychology, 48,* 53-63.

Feather, N. T. (1996c). Values, deservingness, and attitudes toward high achievers: Research on tall poppies. In C. Seligman, J. M. Olson, & M. P. Zanna (Eds.), *The psychology of values: The Ontario symposium* (Vol. 8, pp. 215-251). Mahwah, NJ: Erlbaum.

Feather, N. T., & McKee, I. R. (1993). Global self-esteem and attitudes toward the high achiever for Australian and Japanese students. *Social Psychology Quarterly, 56,* 65-76.

Feather, N. T., Volkmer, R. E., & McKee, I. R. (1991). Attitudes towards higher achievers in public life: Attributions, deservingness, and affect. *Australian Journal of Psychology, 43,* 83-91.

Hofstede, G. (1980). *Culture's consequences: International differences in work-related values.* Beverly Hills, CA: Sage.

Hogg, M. A., & Abrams, D. (1988). *Social identifications: A social psychology of intergroup relations and group processes.* London: Routledge.

Lipset, S. M. (1963a). *The first new nation: The United States in historical and comparative perspective.* New York: Basic Books.

Lipset, S. M. (1963b). The value patterns of democracy: A case study in comparative analysis. *American Sociological Review, 28,* 515-531.

Lipset, S. M. (1990). *Continental divide: The values and institutions of the United States and Canada.* New York: Routledge.

Mlicki, P. P., & Ellemers, N. (1996). Being different or being better? National stereotypes and identifications of Polish and Dutch students. *European Journal of Social Psychology, 26,* 97-114.

Oakes, P. J., Haslam, S. A., & Turner, J. C. (1994). *Stereotyping and social reality.* Oxford: Blackwell.

Rokeach, M. (1968). A theory of organization and change within value-attitude systems. *Journal of Social Issues, 24,* 13-33.

Rokearch, M. (1973). *The nature of human values.* New York: Free Press.

Rosenberg, M. (1965). *Society and the adolescent self-image.* Princeton, NJ: Princeton University Press.

Schwartz, S. H. (1992). Universals in the content and structure of values: Theoretical advances and empirical tests in 20 countries. In M. P. Zanna (Ed.), *Advances in experimental social psychology* (Vol. 25, pp. 1-65). Orlando, FL: Academic.

Schatz, R. T., & Staub, E. (1997). Manifestations of blind and constructive patriotism: Personality correlates and individual-group relations. In D. Bar-Tal & E. Staub (Eds.), *Patriotism in the lives of individuals and nations* (pp. 229-245). Chicago: Nelson-Hall.

Staub, E. (1997). Blind versus constructive patriotism: Moving from embeddedness in the group to critical loyalty and action. In D. Bar-Tal & E. Staub (Eds.), *Patriotism in the lives of individuals and nations* (pp. 213-228). Chicago: Nelson-Hall.

Triandis, H. C. (1995). *Individualism and collectivism.* Boulder, CO: Westview Press.

Turner, J. C., Hogg, M., Oakes, P., Reicher, S., & Wetherell, M. (1987). *Rediscovering the social group: A self-categorization theory.* Oxford: Basil Blackwell.

Author Note

The research described in this report was supported by a grant from the Australian Research Council. Correspondence concerning this article should be addressed to N. T. Feather, School of Psychology, The Flinders University of South Australia, GPO Box 2100, Adelaide 5001, Australia.

Immigration and Acculturation

Acculturation and Ethnic Identity among Sephardic College Students in Montreal

Paula S. Brami   &   Jean-Claude M. Lasry
Université de Montréal   Université de Montréal
Département de Psychologie   Département de Psychologie
and
Hôpital Général Juif S.M.B.D.
Département de Psychiatrie

ABSTRACT

The objectives of this paper are to assess the validity of the orthogonal model of acculturation, and to evaluate the influence of being first or second generation immigrants on styles of acculturation, as well as the impact of having attended an ethnic school on college students' ethnic identity. A sample of 76 immigrants students (43 females and 33 males) who had at least one parent born in Morocco was surveyed in four Montreal colleges.

The absence of correlation between the students' identifications with the culture of origin and with the two host cultures, validated the orthogonality of the acculturation model. Results show 93% of the respondants report a strong identification with Sephardic culture. However, more than half of the respondents favour the integration style of acculturation, meaning a strong identification with both Jewish and Canadian cultures. Second generation students are significantly more identified as Canadians or *Québécois* than first generation ones. Respondents who had attended Ashkenazic schools were less strongly identified with Jewish Sephardic culture than those who had attended either Sephardic schools or public schools. The influence of the family environment is discussed.

Acculturation and assimilation were terms used interchangeably in early immigrant studies. Assimilation was a unidirectional process, symbolized by the melting-pot metaphor: immigrants were to melt into the crucible of the nation, to emerge later as new citizens. Oetting and Beauvais (1991) have noted that "members from the dominant majority who were writing papers then saw their culture as superior and the minority culture as inferior". The earlier models thus "tended to be unabashedly prejudiced and value-laden" (p. 660). The concepts of assimilation and acculturation were later differentiated, and acculturation was defined as a reciprocal process: as the immigrants adapted to the host culture, they evolved, and so did the nation that welcomed them.

The assimilation paradigm underlies the linear and unidimensional models assessing the change immigrants were going through after their resettlement, and during their adaptation to their new environment (e.g., Eisenstadt, 1954; Gordon, 1964). The dominant majority's answer to the immigrants' goal of becoming rich and respected was to assimilate them into its culture. In this process, the immigrants have to relinquish their specific values and behaviors, as well as their cultural identity, in order to endorse the particular values and behaviors of the host majority, and to adopt the dominant cultural identity.

An Orthogonal Model of Acculturation
Several researchers struggled with the concept that identification with one's original culture was not contradictory to identification with the host country (McFee, 1968; Zak, 1973; Maykovitch, 1976). Berry (1980) was the first to propose a biaxial model of acculturation in which identification with the host culture coexists with identification with the culture of origin. Oetting and Beauvais (1991) went one step further in proposing the orthogonality of the axes, but they measured ethnic behaviors rather than cultural identification.

Berry (1980) identified four styles of acculturation (integration, marginality, assimilation and separation) based on the answers to two questions all immigrants should ask themselves: "*Is is considered of value to maintain relationships with the host society?*" and "*Is it considered of value to maintain one's cultural identity characteristics?*" As Lasry and Sayegh (1992) have pointed out, these two questions assess two different concepts: social relations and cultural identity. We modified Berry's questions in our development of a measure of ethnic identity which would apply equally to the home- and host-cultures. The two questions deal with the immigrants' feelings of identification with both cultures. We also dropped the wording "*Is it considered of value ...*" that elicits social desirability (de Sachy, 1997). The stem of the question is thus very simple: "*How much do you feel ...* (cultural group label)?", lending itself to answers for both axes. The ten-point answer scale ranges from 1 to 10, with "*not at all*" and "*completely*" at each end of the scale.

The orthogonal model developed also yields four modes of acculturation. *Integration* implies high identification with both cultures, while *marginalisation* reflects a low or non-existent identification with both cultures. *Assimilation* implies high identification with the host culture and a low one with the culture of origin. The converse mode is labelled *ethnocentrism*, a term which connotes positively a high identification with the immigrants' country of origin, while *separation* implies a value judgment emanating from the dominant majority's perspective.

Objectives

This study is part of a research project exploring interrelations between acculturation, ethnic identity and mental health among immigrant adolescents. The objectives of this paper are to assess the influence of being first or second generation immigrants on styles of acculturation, and to evaluate the impact of having attended an ethnic school on college students' ethnic identity. The main hypothesis postulates that students who have attended Jewish elementary or secondary schools will manifest a stronger Jewish identity than those who have attended public schools.

Ethno-cultural communities have long realised their survival depends on the transmission of their cultural heritage, as well as on their adaptation to the host society. Canada's and Québec's multiculturalism policies have facilitated the establishment and funding of ethnic schools in Montreal. Participants in the present study were college students who have attended an elementary or secondary ethnic school in Montreal. We focused on Jewish Sephardic students because more than half of them have received a formal Jewish education (Shahar, 1991). Sephardic Jews who have immigrated to Montreal come mostly from Morocco. In Hebrew, Sepharad means Spain, from which Jews were expelled in 1492, unless they converted to catholicism. Sephardic Jews represent about a third of the total Montreal Jewish community, which is mainly Ashkenazic, i.e. originating from Central Europe (Ashkenaz meaning Germany in Hebrew).

Method

Participants

Sephardic students attending four Montreal colleges (St-Laurent, Vanier, Dawson, Marianopolis and Jean-de-Brebeuf) were recruited through a Jewish student association. To be eligible, respondents had to have at least one parent born in Morocco. More than 60% of the 125 questionnaires handed out individually in school were returned in prestamped envelops.

The average age of the 76 students (43 female and 33 male) was 18 years; all were attending Cegep level I or II. About two-thirds of the respondents (64%) were second generation immigrants; of the first generation immigrants born outside Canada, most (18 out of 27) were born in Israel. Previous schooling was classified into four types: (a) Jewish Sephardic, (b) Jewish Ashkenazic, (c) Mixed Sephardic or Ashkenazic plus Public, and (d) Public.

Instruments

Acculturation Styles. Two questions were used to assess levels of identification with the culture of origin and with the host society: (1) *"How much do you feel Jewish Sephardic?"* and (2) *"How much do you feel Canadian?"* (Lasry & Sayegh, 1992) The crosstabulation of the two answers (on a ten-point scale) yielded four acculturation styles. An answer of 6 or more on both scales classifies the answer as integration, and of 5 or less, as marginalization. An answer of 6 or more on the Canadian identification scale and of 5 or less on the Jewish Sephardic scale, classified the answer as assimilation; the opposite scores classified the answer as ethnocentrism. Because the study was carried out in Montreal, a second host culture question assessed identification with the *Québécois* culture.

Ethnic Loyalty Scale. The scale used to assess ethnic loyalty was adapted from Zak (1973). Based on his factor analysis, 14 questions were selected from the 20-item scale designed to measure Jewish American identity. Seven of the items assessed Jewish Sephardic loyalty whereas the other seven assessed loyalty to the Canadian culture. The Cronbach alpha coefficients were high for both subscales (> .80), and were similar to those obtained by Zak in his 1973 study.

Situational Identity. Clément, Sylvestre and Noels (1991) designed a scale to measure the ethnic identity of Haitian immigrants in Montreal, in different daily situations. Twenty of these situations were selected to evaluate the students' identification with the Jewish Sephardic culture and with the *Québécois* culture. The answers were given on the same ten-point scale used for the acculturation questions. Examples of situations are: *"In my contacts with classmates, I feel ..."*, *"When I watch the TV news, I feel ..."*, *"When I am at home, I feel ..."*, *"In my way of living my emotions, I feel ..."*. Reliability coefficients in our study were as high (.97) as those obtained by Clément et al.

Other Measures. A ten-item scale to evaluate Jewish religious practices, was adapted from Dashefsky and Shapiro (1974); its internal reliability was .77. Other data collected in this study that will not be reported here comprise mental health (Ilfeld's Psychiatric Symptom Index, 1976), self-esteem (Rosenberg, 1979), social desirability (Graham, 1987), problems of adaptation (Sayegh & Lasry, 1993) and perceived discrimination (Mogghadam, Taylor, & Lalonde, 1988).

Results

The Pearson correlations between identifications to the culture of origin and host cultures were null or non-significant: feeling Jewish Sephardic

Table 1. Indices of Ethnic Identity of Montreal Jewish Sephardic College Students

	Score range	Cronbach α	M	SD
Ethnic Identification				
Jewish Sephardic	1-10	--	8.8	1.7
Canadian	1-10	--	6.2	2.9
Québécois	1-10	--	2.1	2.2
Ethnic Loyalty				
Jewish Sephardic	1-5	.82	4.3	.67
Canadian	1-5	.80	2.3	.83
Situated Identity				
Jewish Sephardic	1-10	.97	8.4	1.7
Québécois	1-10	.97	2.0	1.5

Note. Ethnic Identity scores are based on single items, hence Cronbach alphas coud not be calculated. The Ethnic Loyalty scales are based on 7 items, and the Situated Identity scales, on 20 items.

correlates .02 with feeling *Québécois*, and .11 with feeling Canadian. The two host country identifications were significantly correlated ($r = .41, p < .001$).

In Table 1 are presented three indices of ethnic identity: Ethnic Identification, Ethnic Loyalty and Situational Identity. The highest identification expressed by the students was to the Jewish Sephardic culture, on the three indices: on the identification score ($M = 8.8$), on the Loyalty scale ($M = 4.3$ on a five-point scale, or 8.6 on a ten-point scale) and on the Situational Identity scale ($M = 8.4$). Respondents identified moderately with the Canadian culture, as reflected in the identification score ($M = 6.2$) and the Ethnic Loyalty mean ($M = 4.6$). Identification with the *Québécois* culture is low, both on the identification score ($M = 2.1$) and on the Situational Identity mean ($M = 4.0$).

The same three identity indices are presented according to generation of immigration in Table 2. The Jewish Sephardic feeling of identity was not influenced by the students' birthplace (i.e., whether they were born in Canada or outside Canada) but was rather high on the three identity measures. Identification with the host cultures were affected by country of birth: students born in Canada felt more identified with Canadian or

Table 2. Ethnic Identity Means According to Generation of Immigration

Ethnic Indices (N =)	First generation (27)	Second generation (49)	t	p
Ethnic Identification				
Jewish Sephardic	8.6	8.9	0.91	n.s.
Canadian	5.3	6.8	2.17	.03
Québécois	1.6	2.4	1.90	.06
Ethnic Loyalty				
Jewish Sephardic	4.1	4.4	1.44	n.s
Canadian	2.0	2.5	2.34	.02
Situated Identity				
Jewish Sephardic	8.3	8.5	0.61	n.s.
Québécois	1.8	2.0	0.60	n.s.

Note. First generation students were born outside Canada, second generation students were Canadian-born.

Québécois culture than those born outside Canada ($M = 6.8$ vs 5.3, $p < .03$, or $M = 2.4$ vs 1.6, $p < .06$).

The vast majority of the students interviewed (93%) have adopted the two styles of acculturation indicating a strong identification with their culture of origin: ethnocentrism and integration. However, more than half of the respondents (55%) favour integration, which reflects a strong identification with both Jewish and Canadian cultures. Marginalisation and assimilation as modes of acculturation were rarely adopted (less than 7%) in our study.

The influence of ethnic schooling is presented in Table 3. In answering the question of ethnic identification, Sephardic children who had attended Ashkenazic schools (at the elementary or secondary level) mentioned they were less strongly identified with Jewish Sephardic culture than those who had attended Sephardic schools ($M = 8.0$ vs 9.4, $p < .002$), and than those who had gone through the public school system (vs 9.2 or 8.6, $p < .05$). The same pattern appeared more clearly with the Situational Identity scales: those Sephardic children who had attended Ashkenazic schools were less strongly identified with Jewish Sephardic culture than those who had attended either Sephardic schools or public schools ($p < .001$). The Canadian and *Québécois* identifica-

Table 3. Ethnic Identity Means According to Types of Schooling

Identity Indices (N)	Type of Schooling (N)				F	t A/B	t B/ACD
	A (28)	B (22)	C (13)	D (13)			
Ethnic Identification							
Jewish Sephardic	9.4	8.0	9.2	8.6	3.59*	3.16***	2.64***
Canadian	6.3	5.5	7.2	6.7	1.04		
Québécois	2.3	2.1	2.3	1.6	0.32		
Ethnic Loyalty							
Jewish Sephardic	4.5	4.1	4.3	4.1	1.54		
Canadian	2.3	2.4	2.3	2.3	0.05		
Situated Identity							
Jewish Sephardic	9.0	7.2	8.8	9.0	5.87***	3.75***	4.07***
Québécois	1.6	2.1	2.6	1.6	1.64		

Note. A = Jewish Sephardic; B = Jewish Ashkenazic; C = Mixed (Jewish + Public); D = Public
*p < .05; **p < .01; ***p < .001.

tions were not affected by the type of ethnic schooling on the three
identity measures.

Discussion

The orthogonal model of acculturation assumes the independance of its
two axes. The null or insignificant correlations reported in this study
between identification with the culture of origin and with the two host
cultures, validated the principle of orthogonality in the model. A similar
conclusion was reached with Lebanese immigrants in Montreal (Lasry &
Sayegh, 1992).

Young Sephardic students attending college in Montreal demonstrate a
very high level of identification with their original culture on the three
ethnic identity measures. Their Canadian identification is about average,
while their *Québécois* identification is quite low. In a survey of a multicultural district of Montreal, Kirmayer et al. (1996) found immigrants'
identification with *Québécois* culture was about half the level of their
Canadian one. Political parties in Québec have long known immigrants
prefer to identify with Canada rather than with Québec, a Canadian
province.

Our results show that identification with the Canadian host culture
increases from first to second generation while identification with the
Jewish Sephardic culture remains stable. This is reflected in a clear
increase in the adoption of integration as an acculturative style. The fact
that Canadian identification increases from first to second generation
underlines the importance of using a bidimensional model. In the unidimensional model, an increase in identification with the host country
would conversely mean a decrease in original culture identification. The
second axis in the bidimensional model allows for differentiating
integration from assimilation and marginalisation from ethnocentrism.
Our data show that second generation Sephardic (Moroccan) students feel
more part of Canadian life than their peers born outside of the country.

Students of Moroccan descent, whether born in Canada or elsewhere,
express a similarly strong degree of Jewish Sephardic identity. Phinney
(1990), and Rosenthal and Feldman (1992) also found that adolescents
strongly support the maintenance of their culture of origin (in spite of a
decrease in ethnic practices and behaviours with time). The absence of
differences between Canadian born and immigrant students, in terms of
Sephardic identity, is likely due to their very high level of ethnic
identification.

Contrary to our expectations, students who frequented the public
school system did not express a weaker degree of Jewish Sephardic

identity than students who attended Jewish schools. The very high level of ethnic identification expressed by both groups might well be an explanation. The importance of family environment in the transmission of values and identity should not be overlooked, though, particularly in the case of Jewish identity, as religious practices are an integral part of this identity. Recent community surveys in Montreal (Shahar, 1991) have shown Moroccan Jews observe more religious practices than their Canadian born Ashenazic counterparts.

An unexpected difference appeared between college students having attended Jewish Ashkenazic schools and the three other groups of students. The former present a significantly weaker Jewish Sephardic identity, whether measured by the single acculturation question or by the 20-item Situational Identity scale. With a strong Sephardic identity (between 7 and 8, on a 10-point scale) and the highest level of religious observance, these Moroccan students, who have spent their elementary or high school years in an Ashkenazic environment, express a strong adherence to the basic tenets of Jewish culture, while manifesting a less intense attachment to their cultural specificity. Shuval (1966) has shown that Moroccans in Israel expressed self-rejection of their ethnic group when they introjected the negative stereotype existing in their milieu.

In conclusion, this research clearly supports the orthogonality of the bidimensional model of acculturation. While very strongly attached to their culture of origin, second generation Moroccan students manifested a higher degree of identification with the host culture, and thus a greater desire to integrate into the Canadian society, than first generation Moroccan immigrants. The similar level of Jewish identification between students coming from public schools and Jewish ethnic schools seems due to their very intense Jewish identity and to their family environment.

References

Berry, J. W. (1980). Acculturation as varieties of adaptation. In A. M. Padilla (Ed.), *Acculturation. Theory, models and some new findings* (pp. 9-25). Boulder, CO: Westview Press.

Clément, R., Sylvestre, A., & Noels, K. A. (1991). Modes d'acculturation et identité située: Le cas des immigrants haïtiens de Montréal. *Canadian Ethnic Studies, 33,* 81-94.

Dashefsky, A., & Shapiro, H. (1974). *Ethnic identification among American Jews.* Lexington, MA: Lexington Books..

De Sachy, R. (1997. *L'acculturation des immigrants ouest-africains francophones à Montréal: Conséquences sur l'identité et la santé mentale.* Mémoire de maîtrise inédit, Département de psychologie, Université de Montréal, Montréal, Québec, Canada.

Eisenstadt, S. N. (1954). Reference group behavior and social integration: An exploratory study. *American Sociological Review, 19,* 175-185.

Gordon, M. M. (1964). *Assimilation in American life: The role of race, religion, and national origins.* New York: Oxford University Press.

Graham, J. R. (1987). *The MMPI - A practical guide* (2nd ed.). New York: Oxford University Press.

Ilfeld, F. W. Jr. (1976). Further validation of psychiatric symptom index in normal population. *Psychological Reports, 39,* 1215-1228.

Lasry, J.-C., & Sayegh, L. (1992). Developing an acculturation scale: A bidimensional model. In N. Grizenko, L. Sayegh, & P. Migneault (Eds.), *Transcultural issues in child psychiatry.* Montréal: Editions Douglas.

Maykovitch, M. K. (1976). To stay or not to stay: Dimensions of ethnic assimilation. *International Migration Review, 10,* 337-387.

McFee, M. (1968). The 150% man, a product of blackfeet acculturation. *American Anthropologist, 70,* 1096-1107.

Moghaddam, F. M., Taylor, D. M., & Lalonde, R. N. (1988). Individualistic and collective integration strategies among Iranians in Canada. *Canadian Journal of Behavioral Science, 19,* 121-136.

Oetting, E. R., & Beauvais, F. (1991). Orthogonal cultural identification theory: The cultural identification of minority adolescents. *The International Journal of Addictions, 25,* 655-685.

Phinney, J. S. (1990). Ethnic identity in adolescents and adults: A review of research. *Psychological Bulletin, 108,* 499-514.

Rosenberg, M. (1979). *Conceiving the self.* New York: Basic Books.

Rosenthal, D. A., & Feldman, S. S. (1992). The relationship between parenting behavior and ethnic identity in Chinese American and Chinese Australian adolescents. *International Journal of Psychology, 27,* 19-31.

Sayegh, L., & Lasry, J.-C. (1993). Acculturation, stress et santé mentale chez des immigrants libanais à Montréal. *Santé mentale au Québec, XVIII,* 23-52.

Shahar, C. (1991). *Montreal Jewish community: Attitudes, beliefs and behavior.* Montreal: Department of Community planning, Federation CJA.

Shuval, J. T. (1966). Self-rejection among North African immigrants to Israel. *The Israel Annals of Psychiatry and Related Disciplines, 4,* 101-110.

Zak, I. (1973). Dimensions of Jewish American identity. *Psychological Reports, 33,* 891-900.

Acculturation Under Stress: Female-Headed Hindustani Families in the Netherlands

Lotty Eldering
Leiden University, Netherlands

ABSTRACT

Acculturation has been an important research topic for cultural anthropologists, sociologists and cross-cultural psychologists. Whereas cultural anhropologists chiefly pay attention to acculturation at group level, cross-cultural psychologists are predomianty interested in acculturative atitudes at the individual level. Presenting outcomes of a research on female-headed Hindustani families in Surinam and the Netherlands, based on a cultural anthropological approach, some issues that need more attention within Berry's acculturation framework, are highlighted. These issues concern the interaction between groups and individuals in the acculturation process, the relationship between attitudes towards acculturation and actual behavior, and the time dimension of acculturation.

Acculturation has been an important research topic for cross-cultural psychologists, cultural anthropologists and sociologists for several decades. Although it is often stressed that these disciplines should collaborate more, this rarely occurs, and each discipline has developed acculturation models for its own research community. In this contribution I will present some outcomes of our research on female-headed Hindustani families in the Netherlands (Eldering & Borm, 1996a). With this research based on anthropological insights, I wish also to highlight some issues that need more attention in future research within Berry's acculturation framework (Berry, 1990, 1997). In the next section I comment on this framework. The research on Hindustani families in the Netherlands is introduced in section two. In subsequent sections their marriage and divorce patterns will be compared with those in the Hindustani community in Surinam of about a generation ago.

Neglected Issues in Acculturation Research

Acculturation is a process of cultural change that starts when two cultural groups enter into continuous and direct contact. This process has been studied by cultural anthropologists and sociologists for many years. They have developed acculturation models with phases and possible outcomes (cf. Eisenstadt, 1954; Gordon, 1964). Whereas cultural anthropologists chiefly pay attention to acculturation at group level, cross-cultural psychologists are predominantly interested in acculturation from the perspective of individuals. Berry (1990, 1997) is developing a model for the study of psychological acculturation. In a recent discussion with colleagues, he states that his "model" is not yet a model in theoretical sense, but a framework, a 'skeleton' onto which various "bits of flesh" have been fitted (Berry, unpublished). Using our research on female-headed Hindustani families, I wish to highlight some issues that need more attention in future research within this framework. These issues concern the interaction between groups and individuals in the acculturation process, the relationship between attitudes towards acculturation and actual behavior, and the time dimension of acculturation.

Berry (1997) distinguishes three types of group-level factors that influence psychological acculturation: factors related to the society of origin, to the society of settlement and to the acculturating group. So far he has paid more attention to the influence of macro-level factors in the society of settlement, than to the meso-level interaction between acculturating groups and individuals. He emphasizes, for instance, the correlation between a policy and ideology of multiculturalism and positive adapatation of individual immigrants, but does not study this policy's influence at meso-level (Berry, 1997; Georgas, Berry et al., 1996). The acculturating group is not a homogeneous entity, but it often consists of subgroups or social categories with divergent interests, for instance religious or ethnic subgroups or men and women. Immigrating individuals predominantly live in families, whose members may differ widely in acculturation attitudes and degree of participation in the host society. This often leads to major conflicts between parents and children or husband and wife (Eldering & Knorth, 1996).

A second issue that merits more detailed study is the relationship between attitudes and behavior. A positive attitude towards integration or assimilation does not necessarily lead to behavioral changes. Social control within the family or the ethnic community may hamper the translation of attitudes into actual behavior. Women from traditional ethnic groups, for instance, may be more inclined to integrate or assimilate than their husbands, but do not find opportunities to do so. The reverse occurs, when behavioral change precedes attitudinal change, for example when girls from orthodox Muslim groups have to attend school after puberty even when their parents prefer them to stay at home (Eldering, 1995).

Finally, questions about when acculturation starts and what changes can be attributed to acculturation need to be discussed. Acculturation studies how individuals who have developed in one cultural context attempt to live in a new cultural context, according to Berry (1997). Many immigrants, however, already experienced substantial changes in their home country under the influence of the society to which they migrated later, although there was no question of direct contact in that period. This happens, for instance, when not all family members emigrate at the same time or when groups immigrate into a society that has colonized their country of origin for a long period (Moroccans in France, Hindustani in the Netherlands, Pakistani and East Indians in Britain).

Female-Headed Hindustani Families in the Netherlands

The Hindustanis[1] living in the Netherlands have a long history of migration. Between 1873 and 1917 their forefathers emigrated as indentured laborers from India to Surinam, a Dutch colony with a plantation economy, and in the 1970s there was a wave of Hindustani emigration from Surinam to the Netherlands, mainly for political reasons. About one third of the total Surinamese Hindustani population is currently residing in the Netherlands. At the request of a Surinamese Association (SRS) in The Hague the Center for Intercultural Pedagogics of Leiden University conducted a small-scale qualitative study on the situation of female-headed Hindustani families in The Hague in 1994 and 1995[2]. The association was concerned about reports that single Hindustani mothers were facing many problems in their day-to-day life.

Sample and Research Methods[3]
Because of the difficulty of getting access to the Hindustani community and of the issues to be studied, potential mothers for the research were contacted personally by a Hindustani intermediary, mostly a social worker. After an introductory visit in which the researcher explained the research objectives, the mothers were interviewed extensively about their

---

1 The indentured laborers who were brought to the Caribbean in the nineteenth century from India were known as East Indians in the British colonies and as Hindustanis in the Dutch. In the censuses of the modern Caribbean states their descendants are still recorded as East Indians (Guyana, Trinidad) and Hindustanis (Surinam). Descendants of African slaves are known and recorded as Creoles in Surinam.

2 This research was funded by the SRS, and by the Science Shop and Center for Intercultural Pedagogics, both of Leiden University.

3 A similar study investigated female-headed Moroccan families in the Netherlands (Eldering & Borm, 1996b).

life history, particularly their youth, marriage and divorce, and their current social position and problems with the children. The interview was based on the cultural-ecological model, which assumes that the social and cultural context in which a person lives strongly influences his or her well-being and risks of developing psychosocial problems (Eldering, 1995).

Although it was impossible to draw a random sample of female-headed Hindustani families, we selected a sample that reflected the Hindustani population in the Netherlands in region of origin (Paramaribo vs. rural districts in Surinam), religion (Hindu, Muslim or Christian), educational level and length of stay in the Netherlands. A total of 17 Hindustani mothers were interviewed: 16 divorced women and one unmarried mother, aged between 29 and 51. Twelve mothers were Hindus, four Muslims and one was Roman Catholic. Six women had had only elementary education, the remainder had followed at least a few years of secondary education. On average they had two or three children. In this paper I concentrate on the life history of the single mothers.

Unique Life Histories, Similar Patterns

Although the life history of each of the mothers interviewed, is unique, analysis of these cases showed many similarities in the field of education, marriage and divorce. Firstly, the mothers' parental families in Surinam had a positive attitude towards the education of their children, whether boys or girls. A girl's education was not intended primarily for a career, but to enable her to earn a living in case her husband died or left her.

"When your husband leaves you and the children, your school certificate will serve you as your second husband", as the mother of one of the women interviewed used to say. Parents were also keen to marry off their daughters soon after puberty. They were constantly worrying about the chastity and virginity of the girls and the honor (*izzat*) of the family. Education and marriage were competing values when they were adolescents in Surinam. Despite the high value the families attached to education, it was often not possible to continue education after elementary school and obtain a secondary school certificate. Lack of secondary education in rural areas, the risks faced by girls walking long distances to school and the fact that older girls had to help in the household were the main obstacles to continuing education. The low quality of the education in Surinam may also be held responsible for the school failure of these girls. When a girl failed at school her parents arranged a marriage for her as soon as possible.

The second common feature is that the marriages of most of the women interviewed were arranged with a man from the same ethnic and religious backgrounds (Table 1). Whereas marriages between a Hindu

Table 1. Intergenerational Changes in Marriage and Divorce

	Netherlands 1995[1]	Surinam 1961[2]
Marriage		
Ethnic endogamy	87%	95%
Religious endogamy	81%	> 85%
Living with husband's family	56%	60%
Divorce		
Percentage of divorce	-[3]	32%
Female-headed families	30-41%[4]	4%
Reasons for divorce		
Physical violence	68%	
Addiction (alcohol, drugs, gambling)	55%	9%
Adultery/ "outside wives"	55%	22%
Conflicts with in-laws	12%	17%
Abandonment without reason given	-	36%

Note. [1] Eldering and Borm, 1996a; [2] Speckmann, 1965; [3] Sample consisted exclusively of divorced mothers; [4] Hooghiemstra and Niphuis-Nell, 1995; Mungra, 1990.

and a Muslim were not accepted by the Hindustani community in Surinam, those between Hindus from the Sanatan Dharm and Arya Samaj had become acceptable, on the condition that the woman followed her husband's religion after marriage. Further, the joint family structure and parental control over the life of the couple was still strong at the time of their marriage. More than half of the women interviewed had lived for a time in their husbands' paternal household (Table 1); this was especially likely if the marriage had been contracted in Surinam. Although several women complained about being treated harshly by their in-laws, the husband's family appears to have had a certain control over his behavior —and especially his drinking behavior— as long as the couple were part of the joint family.

The man's addiction (mostly to alcohol and to a lesser degree to drugs and gambling), physical violence and his having "outside wives" appeared to be the major reasons for divorce (Table 1). Muslim women did not report alcohol problems in their husbands. About half of the women had also had conflicts with their in-laws. However, although these problems often began soon after the marriage was contracted, the women decided to file for divorce after an average of eight years of marriage. The reason they endured their lot for so many years has to do with their views about marriage and the role of a good wife. Both Hindu and Muslim women had been raised to see self-sacrifice, modesty and fidelity to their husbands as the highest virtues of a married woman. They had learned to accept a subordinate position vis-à-vis their husbands and their in-laws. The Hindu women often referred to the goddess Sita as their role-model (cf. Kakar, 1994). They felt irrevocably bound to their husbands after the Hindu marriage ceremony of *Saptapadi* ("the seven steps around the fire") and they saw it as their duty to endure hardship and abuse. Another reason why the women endured their husbands' addiction and physical abuse for so many years was shame: the shame of making the family's problems publicly known and of requesting help from relatives or social workers. Moreover, they often did not expect help from their parents. When the women complained about the behavior of their husbands, they were sent back by their parents or not believed. And because the Hindustani community in the Netherlands is characterized by closeness and its members have a strong reluctance to make problems public within or outside the community, the women may also have postponed their decision to end the marriage because they knew that they would be held in low esteem by the community after their divorce.

The acculturation process of the Hindustani women was strongly influenced by their marital problems. About two thirds of the women interviewed worked outside the home. Their work was not only necessary in order to pay the accumulating debts, it also functioned as a respite from their husbands' alcoholism and physical abuse.

Single Parent Families: Exceptions or Commonplace?
So far I have presented some outcomes of our small-scale study of female-headed Hindustani families. Since the Hindustani mothers in our research could not be selected randomly, it is relevant to know whether single mothers and their previous marriage problems are exceptional within the Dutch Hindustani community. Several researches show that about one third of the Hindustani families in the Netherlands are currently headed by a woman. The estimated percentages vary from 30 (Mungra, 1990) to 41% (Hooghiemstra & Niphuis-Nell, 1995). These percentages are much higher than we expected given the marriage ideology prevailing among Hindustanis. There seems to be a big discrepancy between this ideology and daily practice. Hindustani parents in the Netherlands still prefer their children to marry a person from the same ethnic and religious backgrounds, in a Hindu or Muslim ceremony

(Mungra, 1990). Alcohol addiction is a widespread problem within the Hindustani community in the Netherlands too, particularly among Hindus (SRS, 1989).

We may thus assume that many Hindustani women in the Netherlands encounter similar problems in their day-to-day life as the women we interviewed. Alcohol addiction, physical abuse and divorce appear to be pervasive problems within the Hindustani community in the Netherlands. Are these problems and the high percentages of divorce and female-headed families the results of acculturation in the Netherlands or did they already exist in Surinam? To shed more light on these issues I will compare the current situation of Hindustanis in the Netherlands with that of Hindustanis in Surinam about a generation ago.

Marriage and Divorce in Surinam about a Generation Ago

The Evolution of the Hindustani Community

Surinam was a Dutch colony for over three centuries — from the Treaty of Breda with the English in 1667 until independence in 1975. Until the beginning of the twentieth century Surinam was a plantation economy. In 1863, the year of the emancipation of the slaves, Surinam had about 53,000 inhabitants, more than 80% of whom were (emancipated) slaves originating from West Africa. To replace the slaves, nearly 35,000 Hindustani from Eastern Uttar Pradesh and Western Bihar in India were brought to Surinam from 1873 to 1917 to work as indentured laborers on the plantations. The number of women was less than half of the number of men (Eldering, 1995). The evolution of the Hindustani community in Surinam was marked by several stages. After a period of social disorganization and anomie upon the arrival of the first immigrants, the Hindustani tried to reconstruct their social and cultural life. The Brahmans played an important role in the reconstruction of religious life. The authorities encouraged the immigrants to settle permanently by offering them a gratuity of Dfl. 100 if they renounced their return passage and allowing them to rent land. In 1939 nearly all Hindustanis owned farmland. When they became farmers the Hindustanis gradually reconstructed the joint-family structure. Increasing urbanization and social differentiation marked the period after World War II. Education became an important vehicle of upward mobility, particularly for boys. This period showed an increasing social disintegration of the Hindustani community. The social control of the community and its leaders decreased, individual competition increased and marriage instability grew (Speckmann, 1965). A (forced) acculturation in marital affairs took place after the new Marriage Law for Hindus and Muslims came into force in

1940. It raised the minimum age of marriage, permitted widows to remarry (Hindus), and prohibited polygyny (Muslims) (Zevenbergen, 1980). Large numbers of Hindustanis migrated to the Netherlands in the years before and after idependence in 1975. The fear of becoming dominated by the Creoles (i.a. all people from African and mixed African/white descent) was the main motive behind this mass emigration to the Netherlands.

Marriage and Divorce Patterns about a Generation Ago

We interviewed the Hindustani women about their parental family. Most women grew up in a big family with seven children on average. Their fathers usually worked outside the agrarian sector; only a few were still farmers. Nearly all their mothers had to work too to augment the family's income. They mostly had unskilled jobs (growing rice or flowers, selling garden produce, etc.). Remarkably, more than half of the women themselves had lived in a female-headed family; their fathers had died during their youth or had divorced their mother. Two mothers were never married to the fathers of their children because of a difference in religion. Both fathers, however, were married to a woman of the same religion by whom they had children too. As already mentioned in the previous section, the parents attached much value to their children's education. The mothers in female-headed households particularly stressed the importance of a good education for girls. In short, the women grew up in Hindustani families in Surinam, which had acculturated to Dutch (colonial) culture to some degree. The families had adopted new values (for instance the importance of Dutch education for upward mobility) as well as maintained traditional Hindustani values (for instance Hindustani marriage ideology). Our second conclusion is that, whereas the parents transmitted the traditional Hindustani marriage and family values to their children, at the same time these children experienced a high degree of marriage instability in their day-to-day life.

Speckmann's study of Hindustani families in Surinam conducted about a generation ago confirms our conclusion on the discrepancy between marriage ideology and stability. With the help of trained Hindustani interviewers he interviewed 579 families from 1959 to 1961 in the districts of Nickerie and Saramacca and in Paramaribo. Nearly three quarters of the couples had been married according to traditional Hindu or Muslim rituals (so-called Asian marriages) compared with only eleven percent of the couples (mostly Christians) who had contracted a civil marriage. Sixteen percent of the couples were living in concubinage. This was mostly the case for women who had been married before. This is connected with the Hindu conviction that a marriage is eternally binding, especially for women. Sixty percent of the couples had lived with the husband's family for a couple of years (Table 1). About one third of the marriages had ended in a separation (divorce, abandonment or repudiation). Abandonment occurred more frequently in Hindus and repudiation exclusively in Muslims, although a high percentage of Muslim marriages in Paramaribo ended in desertion (37%). The respondents gave several reasons for the termination of the marriage such as adultery, conflicts within the family (in-laws), alcohol abuse, and physical violence (Table 1). Although these answers cannot be accepted at their face value, it seems that alcohol abuse and physical violence played only a minor role in the separation. The relatively high percentage of respondents who cited problems within the family as a reason for the termination of the marriage may be explained by the fact that more than 40% of couples ended their marriage within five years, thus in the period during which they were living in a joint family (cf. Jayawardena, 1960).

About three quarters of the households interviewed by Speckmann (1965) were nuclear families, less than 20% of the households were joint families and only 4% consisted of a single parent with children (Table 1). Speckmann's study shows that traditional marriage ideology and practices were still strong in the sixties, particularly in the districts. Nevertheless about one third of the marriages ended in separation. Most women returned to their family, remarried or entered a concubinage relationship. The percentage of single mothers living independently was very low at that time, particularly in rural areas.

Intergenerational Persistence and Change

Comparing the two studies on Hindustani in the Netherlands and in Surinam reveals that the discrepancy between marriage ideology and marriage instability we found in our research already existed about a generation ago, although in a changed form.

The high marriage instability of the Hindustani in the Netherlands appears not to be an acculturation phenomenon. Remarkable changes between the two generations, however, can be observed in the structure of the households, in the motives for ending a marriage, and the way the marriage is terminated. Whereas the percentage of single-parent families was very low in Surinam about a generation ago, about one third of the Hindustani households in the Netherlands currently consist of a mother and her children. The change in household structure is probably connected to the dispersion and decreasing social control of the Hindustani community and the increasing autonomy of the nuclear family. Hindustani women now more often decide to live independently with their children after divorce than was the case a generation ago. This decision may further be influenced by the fact that single mothers in the Netherlands are entitled to public housing and to welfare benefits, rights giving them the opportunity to become economically independent of their husbands. Hindustani men like to say that the Dutch welfare system encourages women to file for divorce in order to become independent. Although this system may facilitate a woman's decision to end her marriage, it does not explain the high degree of marriage instability which is primarily caused by marital problems.

The motives for ending a marriage also seem to have changed within the past 35 years. Whereas abandonment, adultery and conflicts with in-laws were the reasons most frequently given for ending a marriage in Surinam in the sixties, the Hindustani women interviewed in the Netherlands said they had been driven to divorce by their husbands' alcohol addiction, physical abuse and "outside wives." Some women said that they had been more tolerant of their husbands' "outside wife" than of his alcohol addiction and physical abuse. This change in motives for ending a marriage probably reflects a change in marital problems as well as an increasing assertivity of women vis-à-vis men. Although alcohol problems already existed about a generation ago in Surinam, as witnessed by the saying of some pandits that Surinam resembled a *Rum Radj* (a realm of rum) more than a *Ram Radj* (a realm of God) (Helman, 1978), the higher welfare of the Hindustani families in the Netherlands and the declining social control within the Hindustani community and families may have aggravated this problem. Another point to be stressed here is that Hindustani women have become aware of their vulnerable marital position in the previous generations and the need to strive for a better position in the family and community. The women in our research who grew up in a female-headed family reported that their mothers stressed the importance of a good education for girls. Despite their positive attitude towards education, many Hindustani women have not succeeded in achieving a high educational level in Surinam. The social security system in the Netherlands, moreover, offered them the opportunity to end their marriage when this became too problematic, and to become independent of their husband. The Hindustani mothers enrolled en masse in educational programs after their divorce.

Concluding Remarks

Our research on female-headed Hindustani families indicates the relevance of the study of acculturation processes at meso-level and of comparative intergenerational research between the countries of immigration and emigration. In-depth studies of acculturation at meso-level provide more insight into the interaction within families and ethnic communities and into the opportunities and constraints individuals experience in the acculturation process. Studying acculturation strategies should not only cover attitudes to behavioral shifts, but also include actual behavior. Although the Hindustani women in our research still had traditional attitudes toward marriage, they decided to file for divorce and even to live independently with their children in the Netherlands, resisting the social control of their family and ethnic community and accepting the opportunities provided by Dutch policy. Family conflicts after immigration have also been reported in other ethnic groups (Eldering & Borm, 1996b; Eldering & Knorth, 1996).

Comparative intergenerational research may help to assess whether phenomena are the result of acculturation or already existed in the country of origin. Thus the discrepancy between the traditional marriage ideology and the high degree of marriage instability, which we found in the Netherlands, already existed in Surinam about a generation ago. A point of difference between the two generations is the high percentage of female-headed Hindustani households in the Netherlands compared with a very low percentage of single mothers living independently in Surinam about a generation ago. The Dutch social security system not only makes it easier for women to end a marriage but also to live independently after divorce. Another relevant point of difference concerns education. The Hindustani mothers told us that although their families in Surinam had a positive attitude to Dutch education, many could not complete their secondary education. Not until after their divorce in the Netherlands were these women able to translate their positive attitudes into action and to enrol en masse in educational programs here.

Do East Indian immigrant groups living in other countries go through similar acculturation processes? Klass (1961) studied the acculturation of East Indians who came as indentured laborers to Trinidad. He hypothesizes that the British legal system in Trinidad, which did not recognize marriages contracted according Hindu rituals before 1946, has had a major influence on the marriage instability among Hindus in that colony. A similar explanation may apply to Hindustani in Surinam. In order to get more insight into the patterns of acculturation and the contextual factors influencing them, comparative research is needed between Hindustani groups which emigrated as indentured laborers from India to Western colonies (British Guiana, Dutch Surinam, British Trinidad etc.) about the turn of the 19th century (cf. Jayawardena, 1960; Klass, 1980; 1991). It would further be relevant to compare the acculturation processes of the Indian groups which departed as indentured laborers to Western (plantation) colonies with those in Indian groups which emigrated to Western industrial states at a later date (cf. Naidoo, 1994).

References

Berry, J. W. (1990). Psychology of acculturation: Understanding individuals moving between cultures. In R. Brislin (Ed.), *Applied cross-cultural psychology* (pp. 232-253). Newbury Park, London/New Delhi: Sage Publications.

Berry, J. W. (1997). Immigration, acculturation and adaptation. *Applied Psychology: An International Review, 46,* 5-68.

Berry, John W. (unpublished). Reply. Constructing and expanding a framework: Opportunities for developing acculturation research.

Eisenstadt, S. N. (1954). *The absorption of immigrants.* London: Routledge & Kegan Paul.

Eldering, L. (1995). Child rearing in bicultural settings: a culture-ecological approach. *Psychology in Developing Societies, 7,* 133-153.

Eldering, L., & Borm, J. A. (1996a). *Alleenstaande Hindostaanse moeders.* Utrecht: Uitgeverij Jan van Arkel.

Eldering, L., & Borm, J. A. (1996b). *Alleenstaande Marokkaanse moeders.* Utrecht: Uitgeverij Jan van Arkel.

Eldering, L., & Knorth, E. J. (1996). Immigrant youth and risk factors in their life. *Proceedings of the FICE Conference 1996.* Copenhagen: FICE.

Georgas, J., Berry, J. W., Shaw, A., Christakopoulo, S., & Mylonas, K. (1996). Acculturation of Greek family values. *Journal of Cross-Cultural Psychology, 27,* 329-338.

Gordon, M. M. (1964). *Assimilation in American life. The role of race, religion and national origins.* New York: Oxford University Press.

Helman, A. (1978). *Facetten van de Surinaamse samenleving.* Zutphen: De Walburg Pers.

Hooghiemstra, B. T. J., & Niphuis-Nell, M. (1995). *Sociale atlas van de vrouw. Deel 3: Allochtone vrouwen.* Rijswijk: Sociaal en Cultureel Planbureau.

Jayawardena, S. E. S. (1960). Marital stability in two Guyanese sugar estate communities. *Social and Economic Studies, 9,* 76-100.

Kakar, S. (1994). *The inner world: a psycho-analytic study of childhood and society in India.* Delhi/Oxford/New York: Oxford India Paperbacks (first print 1981).

Klass, M. (1961, reissued 1988). *East Indians in Trinidad. A study of cultural persistence.* Prospect Heights, IL: Waveland Press.

Klass, M. (1980). Ecology and family in two Caribbean East Indian communities. In S. Parmatma & E. Eames (Eds.), *The new ethnics. Asian Indians in the United States* (pp. 48-60). New York: Praeger.

Klass, M. (1991). *Singing with Sai Baba: The politics of revitalisation in Trinidad.* Boulder, San Francisco, Oxford: Westview Press.

Mungra, G. (1990). *Hindoestaanse gezinnen in Nederland.* Leiden: Rijksuniversiteit Leiden, Centrum voor Onderzoek van Maatschappelijke Tegenstellingen (dissertation).

Naidoo, J. C. (1994). *Research on South Asian women in Canada; Selected annotated bibliography with surname index 1972-1992.* Waterloo, Ontario: Wilfrid Laurier University.

Speckmann, J. D. (1965). *Marriage and kinship among the Indians in Surinam.* Assen: Van Gorcum.

SRS (1989). *Onderzoek naar de aard en omvang van alcoholproblematiek bij Surinamers in de gemeente 's-Gravenhage en randgemeenten: aanbevelingen voor een alcoholpreventie-beleid voor minderheden.* The Hague: Stichting Surinaams Regionaal Steunpunt.

Marginalization Among Blacks in South Africa

Dan Hocoy,
John F. Kennedy University
Orinda, CA, USA

ABSTRACT

The social policy of apartheid was hypothesized to have resulted in high levels of marginalization and lower mental health in Black South Africans. The extent to which this has occurred was examined in a 1995 study of 370 Black South Africans, employing both qualitative and quantitative research methods. An exceptionally high endorsement of marginalization (relative to other modes of acculturation) was found, and low mental health was significantly associated with it. The context of apartheid and the consequences on Black South Africans closely parallels that of the Aboriginal Peoples of Canada. In addition to marginalization, Blacks in this study exhibited resilience, determination, and defiance as a response to their oppression, and discovered confidence, pride, and identity in overcoming the difficulties of apartheid. Apartheid seems to have resulted in a duality of consequences for Black South Africans. It appears that apartheid resulted in psychological damage, but it also seems to have elicited responses of resilience, coping and strength. This duality was also found among women who bear the added discrimination of sexism; gender analyses revealed that apartheid has more devastating effects on women, and that they are at higher risk for marginalization than men.

Stonequist (1937), in his book *The Marginal Man*, introduced the notion of psychological "marginality", and posited that individuals caught between two conflicting social or cultural groups are prone to developing a "marginal personality", characterized by identity conflicts, insecurity, self-pity, and exaggerated sensitivity. Consistent with this original definition, marginalization is currently conceptualized as one of four modes of behaviour that results from acculturation, or continuous, first-hand contact between two distinct cultural groups (Redfield, Linton, & Herskovits, 1936). Marginalization involves a loss of cultural identity as well as the absence of positive relations with the dominant group (Berry, 1984) and of the four modes of acculturation, is generally associated with the most acculturative stress (Berry & Sam, 1997), that is, the (most) psychological, social and physical health problems emerging from acculturation (Berry, Kim, Minde, & Mok, 1987).

The prevailing framework of acculturation that accounts for attitudes towards the dominant group, the maintenance of cultural identity, and effects on mental health comes from J. W. Berry (1984). Three levels of acculturative processes are identified by Berry (1992a), all of which affect the impact of acculturation on the group and ultimately, the individual, and in the case of Black South Africans, may result in marginalization. The first level of acculturation pertains to the larger (dominant) society of South Africa, the second level to the relationship between the acculturating groups, and the third level to the individual. The first two of these levels of acculturation in South Africa is largely influenced by the former government policy of apartheid, an explanation of the acculturative influences on Black South Africans would be amiss without the consideration of apartheid.

Apartheid
"Apartheid" in the Afrikaans language means apartness or a state of separation, and refers to a series of laws that comprehensively governed all aspects of life and especially race relations for all South Africans during the years of 1948 to 1991. Some of the more historically signifi-cant acts of apartheid included the following. The Population Registration Act (1950) required that every person be designated under one of the racial categories [i.e., White, Coloured, Asian or Native/Bantu (Black)]. The Prohibition of Mixed Marriages Act (1949) and the Immorality Act (1950) made marriage and sexual relations between Whites and non-Whites illegal, The Group Areas Act (1950) made residential separation compulsory, which led to the eviction of 3,548,900 Blacks from their homes (Thompson, 1990, p. 194), to the establishment of Homelands, and the eventual emergence of townships. The Natives Act (1952) introduced a single reference (pass) book for all Africans as a means of controlling their influx and movement in cities. The Separate Amenities Act (1953) legalized separate facilities, as well as the inequality thereof, for the different race groups. It was not until 1991 that many of these acts were repealed, African political parties were unbanned, and most political prisoners released. However, the influence of apartheid continues to be prevalent and will likely be for years to come.

In terms of the first level of acculturation (i.e., the larger society), apartheid is a manifestation of national policy resulting in forced cultural segregation and the political and economic domination of European culture. On the second level of acculturating groups, the relationship between the groups, can be characterized as domination (or colonization) and exploitation by Whites, and resistance and resentment from Blacks. Blacks, denied electoral franchise under apartheid, have had little or no voice in their daily affairs or in the larger society, and often have found internal strife, ethnic or otherwise, (many times fuelled by apartheid forces) among themselves. On the third level of effects on and responses of the individual to these acculturative influences, various modes of adaptation have emerged, including marginalization.

Marginalization in South Africa

Evidence of marginalization among Black South Africans is abundant. The World Health Organization (WHO), the American Psychiatric Association, among many international health agencies, have concluded that apartheid "is a psychologically malignant situation", and damaging to the mental health of Black South Africans (WHO, 1983, p. 33). South African social scientists (e.g., Dawes, 1985; Foster, 1986; Whittaker, 1990) have long established the negative impact on the psychological development of Blacks, and especially in regards to racial identity. Apartheid has created feelings of "incompleteness" and "inferiority" among Blacks, and in general, has been "psychologically devastat(ing)" for the mental health of Black South Africans (Mohutsioa-Makhudu, 1989). Similarly, Simpson (1993, cited in Duncan & Rock, 1995) and Whittaker (1990) argue that the institutional racism of apartheid induces a host of race-related "disorders" or "conditions" among Blacks, including an extremely distorted and negative sense of self and anger towards their own group. Schlemmer (1976) found among 298 Black South Africans, 25% providing justification for apartheid by citing lack of education or skills in Blacks, or the natural superiority of White culture.

Although evidence of marginalization may be abundant, marginalization (as a strategy of acculturation) has never been formally measured among Black South Africans (Foster, personal communication, August 18, 1995). The purpose of this study was to examine levels of marginalization among Black South Africans relative to the other modes of acculturation (i.e., assimilation, integration, separation), and in comparison to other acculturating groups.

It was hypothesized that Black South Africans would exhibit high levels of marginalization (relative to the other modes of acculturation) and low levels of mental health.

Gender and Marginalization

There is abundant evidence suggesting that South African women may be at greater risk for marginalization. Research suggests that apartheid has had effects that are particularly damaging to women.

For instance, women were found to be experiencing considerable strain as a result of the migrant labour system (Gordon, 1994). Whittaker (1990) has identified "mamuphunyane", a form of hysteria afflicting Black women in the homelands whose husbands are migrant workers, as a disorder particular to women resulting from apartheid. The absence of husbands and traditional African custom were found to combine to place the responsibility of raising children exclusively on women. The discrimination and restrictions under apartheid also limit work for women, usually to servitude. Mohutsioa-Makhudu (1989) argues that apartheid was created to psychologically devastate the mental health of Black South Africans, and claim that nowhere is its effects worse than in the 800,000 Black female domestics in South Africa. Apartheid in South Africa may result in a greater incidence of rape. Rape is considered endemic in South Africa; Centre d'Information et de Documentation sur le Mozambique et l'Afrique Australe (CIDMAA, 1991) has estimated 370,000 rape cases a year. Although no formal hypotheses were made, the role of gender in marginalization was examined in this investigation.

Method

Both qualitative and quantitative research methods were used to assess the degree and nature of marginalization in Black South Africans. In terms of quantitative measures, variables previously demonstrated to be related to marginalization (e.g., Berry, 1992a; Berry & Sam, 1997) were contained in the questionnaire.

In terms of qualitative measures, Harari and Beaty (1990) found that traditional questionnaire and survey approaches generated superficial or inaccurate data for Blacks in South Africa, leading to misconceptions about Blacks. They warn of "the folly of relying solely on a questionnaire methodology in cross-cultural research" (p. 267) and strongly recommend that interviews be included with questionnaire methods. Consequently, interviews were included in this investigation. The particular method of interview stems from Outlaw's (1993) recommendation of the phenomenological approach of R. Lazarus and S. Folkman (1984) to understand the effects of racism on the stress and coping in Blacks. Consistency between the themes derived from qualitative analyses and findings of the quantitative analyses was considered a measure of the validity of any finding.

Quantitative Investigation

Participants
The sample consisted of 348 students, aged 18 years and over, of indigenous African descent, attending three South African technikons (i.e., Cape, Pretoria, and Vaal Triangle) across South Africa. The students of these technical schools (although generally younger) provided a representative sample of Black South African society.

Questionnaire

Self-Esteem. The 10-item Rosenberg (1965) Self-Esteem Scale was chosen to assess self-esteem in order to allow for comparisons with other racial groups (e.g., Phinney, Chavira, & Williamson, 1992) as well as other Black South Africans (e.g., Hirschowitz & Nell, 1985).

Mental Health. The mental health measure consisted of individual measures of anxiety, depression, and psychosomatic problems, which Berry (personal communication, November 3, 1994) identified as the most common mental health consequences for acculturation individuals. The combined mental health measure consisted of 60-items with anxiety, depression and psychosomatic problems weighted equally, that is, each contributing 20 items.

Anxiety. The 20-item A-Trait scale of the Spielberger State-Trait Anxiety Inventory (STAI; Spielberger, Gorsuch, & Lushene, 1970) was chosen to measure anxiety because of its proven cross-cultural applicability; it has been used extensively and successfully around the world, including African contexts (Spielberger & Diaz-Guerrero, 1976, 1983), allowing for culture-comparative analysis.

Depression. To measure depression, the 20-item Center for Epidemiologic Studies-Depressed Mood Scale (CES-D; Radloff, 1977) was selected because it was designed specifically to measure depression in the general population for epidemiological research, and its cross-cultural reliability, validity and factor structure has already been established on Black South Africans (e.g., Pretorius, 1991).

Psychosomatic Problems. To assess psychosomatic problems, the 20-item Cawte (1972) scale was employed; 10 items measure psychological symptoms and 10 measuring somatic symptoms associated with acculturative stress. The scale was derived from the Cornell Medical Index of Brodman, Erdman, Lorge, Gershenson and Wolff (1952). The Cawte scale has been widely used in studies of acculturative stress (e.g., Berry et al., 1987; Dona, 1993, Minde, 1985).

Mode of Acculturation. Mode of acculturation was measured by using a 20-item scale derived from Naidoo's (1994) adaptation of the Berry Acculturation Measure (Berry, Kim, Power, Young, & Bujaki, 1989) for Black and East Indian South Africans. The Berry Acculturation Measure has been used and shown validity with acculturating populations of various ethnic and racial groups worldwide (e.g., Kim, 1988).

Black Self-Perception. To measure Black self-perception or identification, the 15-item Racial Self-Perception Scale, developed and used in previous racial identity research (Hocoy, 1996) was administered. The reliability and validity of the scale has been established (Hocoy, 1993); its internal consistency in this study was 0.66.

Black Esteem. The 15-item Racial Esteem Scale, developed and used in previous racial identity research (Hocoy, 1996) was used to measure Black esteem. The reliability and validity of the scale has been established (Hocoy, 1993); its internal consistency in this study was 0.69.

Attitude Toward Whites. To assess attitude toward Whites, the 15-item Attitude Toward Racial Group Scale, developed from and used in previous racial identity research (Hocoy, 1993) was administered; its internal consistency in this study was 0.75.

Identification with Being Black or White. In addition to attitude toward both Blacks and Whites, personal identification with being Black or White was also measured, as previous marginalization research (e.g., Whittaker, 1990) has indicated this to be a relevant variable.

Perceived Racism. In order to measure perceived racism, the 18-item Perceived Racism Scale, developed from and used in previous racial identity research (Hocoy, 1993) was employed. The reliability and validity of the scale and has been established with a host of racial and ethnic groups worldwide (e.g., Ataca & Berry, 1997; Hocoy, 1994; Restoule, 1994).

Qualitative Investigation

Informants
The informants for the qualitative portion of the study consisted of 7 women and 8 men, aged 18 to 54, all of whom were Black (i.e., both parents were of indigenous African heritage), except in the case of one woman and one man, for whom one parent was Coloured. Informants were drawn from the technikons, and selected so as to constitute a fairly diverse cross-section of society.

Procedure
The particular procedures used in this study conform to the phenomenological techniques recommended by Giorgi (1983), Kruger (1982), Kvale (1989), and Spinelli (1989). Subjects were asked, "How have you experienced discrimination, and what are some of the effects on your life?" Each interview was audiotaped, reviewed, transcribed, and analyzed for common themes among informants. The themes were then compared with findings from the quantitative analyses.

Table 1. Mean Endorsement of Modes of Acculturation (N = 348)

Integration	5.69
Marginalization	4.44
Separation	4.18
Assimilation	2.50
(Minimum = 1; Maximum = 7)	

Results

Quantitative Findings

Modes of Acculturation and Mental Health
In terms of mode of acculturation of choice for Black South Africans, integration, which has consistently been found to be the most preferred mode of acculturation (e.g., Berry & Sam, 1997), was found to have a significantly (i.e., $p < .01$) higher endorsement than any other mode of acculturation scale. Marginalization had the second highest endorsement, followed by separation and assimilation. See Table 1. The integration mode of acculturation is also consistently associated with the highest mental health levels (Berry, personal communication, January 21, 1995) and was found here to be the only scale to correlate positively with both mental health ($p < .01$), and self-esteem ($p < .01$). The marginalization mode of acculturation is consistently associated with the lowest mental health, and was found here to correlate negatively with both mental health ($p < .01$) and self-esteem ($p < .01$). In terms of mental health, assimilation and separation modes of acculturation are also consistently found to lie between integration and marginalization, the order dependent on cultural group. In this case, separation was associated with higher mental health than assimilation, as is found with Native Peoples of Canada (Berry, personal communication, April 24, 1996).
Integration. The integration mode of acculturation, which is defined as the "maintenance of the cultural integrity of the group as well as...becom(ing) an integral part of a larger societal framework" (p. 18, Berry, 1992a), consistent with theoretical expectations, was significantly correlated with high self-esteem ($N = 348$ for all correlations; $r = 0.25$; $p < .01$), high mental health ($r = 0.22$; $p < .01$), as well as low

anxiety ($r = 0.16$; $p < 0.01$), low depression ($r = 0.22$; $p < .01$), and low psychosomatic symptomatology ($r = 0.15$; $p < 0.01$).

Marginalization. The marginalization mode of acculturation, which is defined as "los(ing) cultural and psychological contact with both... traditional culture and the larger society" and characterized by feelings of alienation, loss of identity and acculturative stress (p. 19, Berry, 1992a), also consistent with theoretical expectations, was significantly correlated with low self-esteem ($r = 0.28$; $p < .01$), low mental health ($r = 0.37$; $p < 0.01$) as well as high anxiety ($r = 0.30$; $p < 0.01$), high depression ($r = 0.30$; $p < .01$), high psychosomatic symptomatology ($r = 0.30$; $p < .01$), and high perceived racism ($r = 0.21$; $p < 0.01$).

Separation. The separation mode of acculturation, which is defined as desiring "no substantial relations with the larger society, accompanied by a maintenance of (racial) identity and traditions" (p. 19, Berry, 1992a), consistent with theoretical expectations, was significantly correlated with high Black self-perception ($r = 0.28$; $p < 0.01$), high Black esteem ($r = 0.14$; $p < 0.05$), low identification with being White ($r = 0.18$; $p < .01$), negative attitude toward Whites ($r = 0.21$; $p < 0.01$), and high perceived racism ($r = 0.37$; $p < 0.01$), and with being a man (gender) ($r = 0.13$; $p < .05$).

Assimilation. The assimilation mode of acculturation, which is defined as "relinquishing one's cultural identity and moving into the larger (White) society" (p. 18, Berry, 1992a), was significantly correlated with identification with being White ($r = 0.19$; $p < .01$), low self-esteem ($r = 0.36$; $p < .01$), low mental health ($r = 0.12$; $p < 0.05$), low Black self-perception ($r = 0.12$; $p < 0.05$), low Black esteem ($r = 0.17$; $p < 0.01$), positive attitude toward Whites ($r = 0.21$; $p < 0.01$), and low perceived racism ($r = 0.13$; $p < 0.05$). Table 2 presents the correlations among the primary variables in the study (see Table 2).

Qualitative Findings

Themes revealed in the qualitative analyses provided support for findings of the quantitative analyses. For instance, the negative correlations between perceived racism and self-esteem, mental health, Black esteem, attitude toward Whites, and positive correlation between perceived racism and Black self-perception were reflected in the testimonies of those interviewed. Heightened racial self-identification, hatred toward Whites, challenges to self-esteem and Black esteem, and negative mental health consequences, as a result of racism and apartheid, were all themes that emerged from the aggregate analysis of the transcribed data.

Themes generally corresponded to a duality in the themes, one category concerning the effects of apartheid and indications of marginalization, and the second concerning resilience, coping and strength. Themes

Table 2. *Correlations Among Primary Variables in Study*

	MH	BSP	BE	ATW	PR	INT	SEP	ASS	MAR
SE	.46***	-.01	.34***	-.04	-.15**	.25**	.01	-.36**	-.28**
MH		-.08	.26**	.01	-.27**	.22**	.10	-.12*	-.37**
BSP			.16**	-.21**	.19**	-.09	.28**	-.12*	.05
BE				-.01	-.21**	.08	.14*	-.18**	-.08
ATW					-.29 **	.01	-.21**	.21**	-.00
PR						-.01	.37**	-.13	.21**
INT							.01	-.13*	.02
SEP								-.10	.18**
ASS									.14*

Abbreviations: SE = Self-esteem, MH = Mental health, BSP = Black self-perception, BE = Black esteem, ATW = Attitude towards Whites, PR = Perceived racism, INT = Integration, SEP = Separation, ASS = Assimilation, MAR = Marginalization.

*$p < .05$. **$p < .01$.

concerning marginalization included experiencing anxiety and fear, challenges to one's self-esteem, symptoms of depression, physiological problems, negative self or race attributions, socio-economic restrictions, racial inequities, personal loss, and pressures from the larger society to reject their own culture in order to succeed. Currents found in these themes included: interpersonal conflict and aggression, homicide, suicide, and substance abuse.

Themes concerning resilience included possessing high Black esteem, discovering one's own resilience, determination and defiance, employing various coping mechanisms, receiving support, heritage and inspiration from various sources, and making positive self and race attributions in the face of apartheid. Informants declared that they felt "stronger" and "more confident" as a result of overcoming the obstacles apartheid presented, and more resilient as a direct result of living in apartheid. Apartheid allowed informants to witness their own strength, capabilities, versatility, and ultimately their own worth. Many articulated that apartheid stimulated their personal "maturation" and formation of their racial identity, and witnessing their resilience allowed for belief and pride in themselves.

Gender and Marginalization
Quantitative analyses suggested that women are at more risk to be marginalized by apartheid. Compared to men, being a woman was associated with lower self-esteem ($p < .01$), lower Black self-perception ($p < .01$), lower Black esteem ($p < .01$), lower identification with being Black ($p < .05$), greater identification with being White ($p < .05$), perceiving less racism ($p < .01$).

Qualitative analysis revealed that women experience a "double discrimination" in apartheid, one of sexism as well as racism, and from not only Whites but other Africans as well. The processes a woman experiences, although similar to man's, seems to be of an entire magnitude greater. A woman experiences greater socio-economic restrictions on her life, as a result of strict gender roles in patriarchical African traditions, and greater challenges to her self-esteem. However, women in this study also experienced a greater sense of their own power and resilience as a result of having overcome barriers related to gender, in addition to those related to race. Women informants felt that they had to liberate themselves, and consequently, were forced to examine, discover and believe in themselves. The double discrimination provided them with double motivation to prove themselves. These women also felt that having to overcome additional barriers in life resulted in them, a greater strength, courage and resilience.

Discussion

Integration, consistent with acculturation research (Berry & Sam, 1997) was found to be the preferred mode of acculturation. However, contrary to acculturation research, marginalization was the second most highly endorsed mode of acculturation. Marginalization is typically the least favoured mode of acculturation (Berry, personal communication, August 8, 1996). Marginalization was also found to be significantly associated with the lowest mental health, which is consistent with the acculturation literature (Berry & Sam, 1997). This high endorsement of marginalization among Black South Africans and the low mental health associated with it attests to the exceptional degree of oppression faced by Blacks under apartheid. In terms of mental health, between integration and marginalization, was separation and assimilation, with separation was associated with higher mental health than assimilation. This pattern parallels that of Canadian Aboriginal peoples (Berry, personal communication, April 24, 1996). The qualitative investigation also found similarities with Aboriginals in Canada.

The process of acculturation in Black South Africans was found to result in interpersonal conflict and aggression, homicide, suicide, substance abuse, as well as a variety of psychosocial and psychosomatic health problems. These outcomes are identical to those found in Canadian Aboriginal communities (Berry, 1990; Berry & Hart Hansen, 1985).

Parallels to Aboriginal Peoples of Canada
It is not surprising that acculturation outcomes found with Blacks in South Africa resemble those of Native Peoples of Canada, the situation of Blacks in South Africa closely parallels that of the Aboriginals in Canada. Both are the indigenous peoples of their respective lands, were subsequently colonized by foreign peoples, exploited for their knowledge or labour, indoctrinated with a European education and religion, had their lands taken away, and confined in reservations or homelands, and had their languages, spirituality, and culture repressed. Another parallel is the importance of land ownership or control in cultural identity and self-esteem (e.g., Berry, 1992b). Qualitative analyses found African identity to be threatened and eroded by culturally repressive government measures. Similarly, poverty, racism and insensitive government policies were identified by Aboriginal people as threats to Aboriginal identity as well as human dignity (Berry, 1994).

Gender and Marginalization
Gender analyses of both qualitative and quantitative data clearly indicate that women are at higher risk to be marginalized. Women suffer a triple

oppression in South Africa, being Black, working-class and women (Haffajee, 1995). Women, both traditionally and currently "remain chained to the lowest end of the job market, to the most poorly paid and insecure jobs, to the enslavement of domestic labour in White homes (approximately 800,000), to back-breaking roles of tilling the land and tending the children, the humiliations and violence of their male compatriots", CIDMAA, 1992, p. 5). Women also experience the constraints of African tradition, which burdens women with domestic duties in addition to paid employment, and often bear the brunt of men's frustration (the reason cited for half of the divorce cases in 1993 was domestic violence, cited in Haffajee, 1995).

However, results also revealed that a duality exists for South African women. On the one hand, South African women seem to exhibit the mark of oppression and internalize apartheid ideology to a greater degree. On the other hand, South African women also seemed to stronger, more resilient, defiant, motivated, more racially aware and gender conscious.

Resistance
Qualitative findings found a duality exists in response to apartheid in South Africa. In addition to marginalization, Blacks in this study exhibited resilience, determination, defiance, and courage in response to their oppression. As well, overcoming the difficulties of apartheid resulted in confidence, character, pride, identity and strength. Similar findings are purported in acculturation studies as well. Berry (1992b) writes that some individuals change psychologically in an adaptive fashion rather than necessarily in a maladaptive way, and that "acculturation sometimes enhances one's life chances and mental health" (p. 9, Berry, 1992a). Similarly, there have been findings of equal or higher self-esteem in Blacks, (e.g., Rosenberg, 1979; Stone, 1981) as well as themes of protest, resistance to assimilation (Pettigrew, 1964), resilience and strength in overwhelming oppression (Coles, 1964) and "Black rage" against continued discrimination (Grier & Cobb, 1968). More recently, Parham and Austin (1994) argue for the recognition of the nigrescence concept (i.e., that Blacks have not universally assimilated into European American culture). In addition, Haw (1991) has found African Americans, rather than capitulating to dominant culture ideology, construct their own, one in which affirms their racial heritage is affirmed. Similarly, Duncan and Rock (1995) assert that South African Blacks are not passive victims of apartheid, but rather active agents in shaping their reality.

Duality

The findings from this study reflect that of acculturation research, and the general literature, in that they demonstrate the psychological "damage" related to marginalization, but at the same time, indicate buffering mechanisms, and positive developments that emerge from the individual as a result of oppression. It seems that these two tendencies are not mutually exclusive and that there exists a duality with regard to the effects of apartheid.

This duality was also found among women, who bear the added discrimination of sexism; as reflected in the qualitative analyses, the greater oppression against women seemed to be met with an equally greater degree of resilience. There appears to be some basic psychological process that summons and raises one's resources and defenses to meet the level of one's oppression.

References

Ataca, B., & Berry, J. W. (1997, July). *Discrimination, religious attachment, acculturation attitudes, and immigrant adaptation*. Poster presented at the Fifth European Congress of Psychology, Dublin, Ireland.

Berry, J. W. (1984). Cultural relations in plural societies: Alternatives and their sociological implications. In N. Miller & M. Brewer (Eds.), *Groups in contact*. New York: Academic.

Berry, J. W. (1990). *Body and soul: Physical, social and psychological health contrasts among Aboriginal Peoples in Canada, Greenland and Alaska*. Paper presented to 8th International Congress on Circumpolar Health, Whitehorse.

Berry, J. W. (1992a). Paper prepared for the Royal Commission on Aboriginal Peoples, Ottawa.

Berry, J. W. (1992b). Draft report submitted to the Moose River/James Bay Coalition.

Berry, J. W. (1994). Report prepared for the Royal Commission on Aboriginal Peoples, Urban Perspectives Research.

Berry, J. W., & Hart Hansen, J. P. (1985). Problems of family health in circumpolar regions. *Arctic Medical Research, 40*, 7-20.

Berry, J. W., & Sam, D. (1997). Acculturation and adaptation. In J. W. Berry, M. Segall, & C. Kagitcibasi (Eds.), *Handbook of cross-cultural psychology* (Volume 3). Needham Heights, MA: Allyn and Bacon.

Berry, J. W., Kim, U., Minde, T., & Mok, D. (1987). Comparative studies of acculturative stress. *International Migration Review, 21*, 491-511.

Berry, J. W., Kim, U., Power, S., Young, M., & Bujaki, M. (1989). Acculturation attitudes in plural societies. *Applied Psychology: An International Review, 38,* 185-206.

Brodman, K., Erdmann, A. J., Lorge, E., Gershenson, C. P., & Wolff, H. G. (1952). The Cornell Medical Index Health Questionnaire. *Journal of Clinical Psychology, 8,* 119-124.

Cawte, J. (1972). *Cruel, poor and brutal nations.* Honolulu: University of Hawaii Press.

Centre d'Information et de Documentation sur le Mozambique et l'Afrique Australe. (1991). *Fighting for their rights.* Montreal: Author.

Coles, R. (1964). *Children of crisis.* Boston: Atlantic Monthly.

Dawes, A. (1985). Politics and Mental Health: The position of clinical psychology in South Africa. *South African Journal of Psychology, 15,* 55-61.

Dona, G. (1993). *Acculturation, coping, and mental health of Guatemalan refugees living in settlements in Mexico.* Unpublished Ph.D. thesis. Queen's University, Kingston, ON, Canada.

Duncan, N., & Rock, B. (1995). *Inquiry into the effects of public violence on children* (preliminary report). Cape Town: Commission of Inquiry Regarding the Prevention of Public Violence and Intimidation. (GPS Publication No. 003-0198).

Foster, D. (1986). The development of racial orientation in children: A review of South African literature. In S. Burman & P. Reynolds (Eds.), *Growing up in a divided society: The context of childhood in South Africa.* Johannesburg: Raven Press.

Giorgi, A. (1983). Concerning the possibility of phenomenological research. *Journal of Phenomenological Psychology, 14,* 23-29.

Gordon, E. B. (1994). The plight of the women of Lesotho: Reconsideration with the decline of apartheid? *Journal of Black Studies, 24,* 435-446.

Grier, W. H., & Cobb, P. M. (1968). *Black rage.* New York: Basic Books.

Haffajee, F. (1995, March). The Sisterly Republic. *The New Internationalist, 265,* 11-13.

Harari, O., & Beaty, D. (1990). The folly of relying solely on a questionnaire methodology in cross-cultural research. *Journal of Managerial Issues, 2,* 267-281.

Haw, K. F. (1991). Interactions of gender and race - a problem for teachers? A review of the emerging literature. *Educational Research, 33,* 12-21.

Hocoy, D. (1993). *Ethnic identity among Chinese in Canada: Its relationship to self-esteem.* Unpublished master's thesis. Queen's University, Kingston, ON, Canada.

Hocoy, D. (1994, July). *Ethnic identity among Chinese in Canada: Its relationship to self-esteem.* Paper presented at the 23rd International Congress of Applied Psychology, Madrid, Spain.

Hocoy, D. (1996). Empirical distinctiveness between cognitive and affective elements of ethnic identity and scales for their measurement. In H. Grad, A. Blanco, & J. Georgas (Eds.), *Key issues in cross-cultural psychology.* Lisse: Swets & Zeitlinger Publishers.

Hirschowitz, R., & Nell, V. (1985). The need for power and fear of assertiveness in English-speaking South African female graduates. *Journal of Psychology, 119,* 603-612.

Kim, U. (1988). *Acculturation of Korean immigrants to Canada: Psychological, demographic and behavioural profiles of emigrating Koreans, non-emigrating Koreans, and Korean-Canadians.* Unpublished Ph.D. thesis, Psychology Dept., Queen's University, Kingston, Canada.

Kruger, D. (1982). *An introduction into phenomenological psychology.* Pittsburg: Duquesne University Press.

Kvale, S. (1989). The primacy of the interview. *Methods* (Spring 1989 Annual Edition).

Lazarus, R. S., & Folkman, S. (1984). *Stress, appraisal and coping.* New York: Springer

Minde, T. (1985). *Foreign student adaptation at Queen's University.* Unpublished honours thesis, Queen's University, Kingston, ON, Canada.

Mohutsioa-Makhudu, Y. N. (1989). The psychological effects of apartheid on the mental health of Black South African women domestics. *Journal of Multicultural Counseling and Development, 17,* 134-142.

Naidoo, J. (1994). [Modes of acculturation in Black and Indian South Africans]. Unpublished raw data.

Parham, T. A., & Austin, N. L. (1994). Career development and African Americans: A contextual reappraisal using the nigrescence construct. *Journal of Vocational Behavior, 44,* 139-154.

Pettigrew, T. F. (1964). *A profile of the American Negro.* Princeton: Van Nostrand.

Phinney, J. S., Chavira, V., & Williamson, L. (1992). Acculturation attitudes and self-esteem among high school and college students. *Youth and Society, 23,* 299-312.

Pretorius, T. B. (1991). Assessing the problem-solving appraisal of Black South African students. *International Journal of Psychology, 28,* 861-870.

Radloff, L. S. (1977). The CES-D scale: A self-report depression scale for research in the general population. *Applied Psychological Measurement, 1,* 385-401.

Redfield, R., Linton, R., & Herskovits, M. J. (1936). Memorandum on the study of acculturation. *American Anthropologist, 38,* 149-152.

Restoule, B. (1994). *Cultural identity of Ojibwa Youth: The relationship of acculturation, discrimination and multiculturalism to physical and mental health.* Unpublished master's thesis, Queen's University, Kingston, ON, Canada.

Rosenberg, M. (1965). *Society and the adolescent self-image.* Princeton: Princeton University Press.

Rosenberg, M. (1979). *Conceiving the self.* New York: Basic Books.

Schlemmer, L. (1976). Political adaptation and reaction among urban Africans in South Africa. *Social Dynamics, 2,* 3-18.

Spinelli, E. (1989). *The interpreted world.* London: Sage Publications.

Spielberger, C. D., & Gorsuch, R. L., & Lushene, R. E. (1970). *State-trait anxiety inventory.* Palo Alto, CA: Consulting Psychologists Press.

Spielberger, C. D., & Diaz-Guerrero, R. (1976). *Cross-cultural anxiety (Vol. 1).* New York: Hemisphere Publishing Corporation.

Spielberger, C. D., & Diaz-Guerrero, R. (1983). *Cross-cultural anxiety (Vol. 2).* New York: Hemisphere Publishing Corporation.

Stone, M. (1981). *The education of the black child in Britain.* London: Fontana.

Stonequist, E. V. (1937). *The marginal man.* New York: Scribners.

Thompson, L. (1990). *A history of South Africa.* Westford, MA: Murray Printing Co.

Whittaker, S. R. (1990). Education for oppression: The case of psychology in Azania/South Africa. *Psychology Quarterly, 1,* 5-14.

World Health Organization. (1983). *Apartheid and health.* Geneva: Author.

Loneliness among Second Generation Migrants

Félix Neto
University of Porto, Portugal

ABSTRACT

This paper examines the relationship between loneliness and some psychosocial variables among Portuguese youth born in France. The study sample consisted of 109 Portuguese second generation migrants living in Paris (34% were male and 66% female). The following instruments were administered to all subjects: the Revised UCLA Loneliness Scale, the Acculturation Attitudes Scales, the Acculturative Experience Scale, the Cultural Maintenance Scale, the Acculturative Stress Scale, the Social Anxiety Scale, the Satisfaction with Life Scale, as well as a background inventory. The loneliness score of second generation migrants is comparable to that of Portuguese adolescents living in Portugal. No gender, age, religion participation and ethnic identity differences were found, but there was significant effect on loneliness with acculturation attitudes. Youngsters whose attitudes in relation to acculturation were favorable to integration showed lower loneliness than those who were favorable to assimilation and separation. Loneliness showed negative correlation with French acculturation experience and life satisfaction, and positive with acculturative stress and social anxiety. Results supported situational and characterological explanations of loneliness.

The importance for cross-cultural research of various human experiences is well established. Spielberger and Diaz-Guerrero (1976) indicated that, given the unique qualities of certain emotional states (e.g., loneliness, anxiety, stress), and the fact that everyone experiences these emotional states, cross-cultural research on emotions would seem to provide an excellent approach for establishing general laws about human experience and behavior. However cross-cultural research on loneliness (Jones, Carpenter, & Quintana, 1985) or on adolescent loneliness (Ostrov & Offer, 1981; Brennan, 1982) is scarce. An area which has received almost no attention is loneliness within the migrant experience. This is particularly striking given that loneliness has been commonly mentioned as a consequence of cross-cultural transitions, and is very present in descriptions of "culture shock". Indeed, second generation migrants have virtually been ignored in empirical studies of loneliness. This paper, therefore, will focus on ordinary loneliness and on some of the potential determinants of the migrant experience.

The loneliness of the human being is a condition that is "widely distributed and severely distressing" (Weiss, 1973). Loneliness is an inescapable fact of life and knows no boundaries. Young and old, married and unmarried, rich and poor, educated and illiterate, healthy and unhealthy, extroverts and introverts - everybody eventually experiences loneliness in some form, at some point in one's life. However, loneliness was described by Seligman (1983) as one of the most poorly understood of all psychological phenomena. Loneliness is typically defined as "the unpleasant experience that occurs when a person's network of social relationships is deficient in some important way, either qualitatively or quantatively" (Perlman & Peplau, 1981, p. 31). Such a deficit occurs when a subject's interpersonal needs cannot be satisfied within his or her social network. As a result of these unmet needs, the subject experiences a variety of aversive affective states. Feelings of loneliness are often situationally determined and tend to be short lived. However, some people experience loneliness in many different settings and it occurs so frequently that it comes to resemble an enduring personality trait. Social scientists have increasingly come to emphasise that loneliness is a subjective experience and is not synonymous with objective social isolation. "People can be alone without being lonely, or lonely in a crowd" (Peplau & Perlman, 1982, p. 3). With this important distinction in mind, psychologists have increasingly focused attention upon the subjective experience of being alone. As such it is an index of dissatisfaction with one's relationships and is not synonymous with solitude or any particular form of relational status (e.g., married vs. single).

An understanding of factors that contribute to loneliness is important for various reasons, including its connection with both physical illness and mental health problems. Weiss (1973) identified two types of loneliness, emotional loneliness and social loneliness, and suggested that the former results from the loss or lack of an intimate tie (usually with spouse, lover, parent, or child), whereas the latter results from the lack of a network of involvements with peers, fellow workers, neighbors or friends.

Theoretical statements about loneliness have emphasized the causal influence of both internal and external factors. In his early conceptualization, for example, Weiss (1973) attributed the origins of loneliness to a combination of personal vulnerabilities (e.g., social anxiety, shyness, etc.) and interpersonal disruptions (e.g., divorce, geographical mobility). Evidence advanced in support of the personal vulnerability side of this equation suggests the importance of social skill deficiencies (e.g., Jones, 1982). In the model of loneliness outlined by Peplau and Perlman (1982), characteristics of individuals and situations, as well as cultural values and norms, are seen as predisposing factors affecting both desired and actual social relations. Situational influences have been discussed (Cheek & Busch, 1981), with moving to a new city commonly mentioned as cause of loneliness. The negative impact of life changes often associated with shifting residence can however be diminished by social support. While everybody in cross-cultural contact is likely to be at risk, certain characteristics or circumstances may increase loneliness, including being young (Fisher & Philipps, 1982).

To date only a limited number of studies have empirically examined the nature of loneliness in adolescent populations (Brage, Meredith & Woodard; Brennan, 1982; Moore & Schultz, 1983; Ostrov & Offer, 1981). Much of the available data on loneliness concerns college students. However, loneliness is especially relevant to adolescence. According to Woodward (1988), adolescence is frequently characterized by alienation, solitude, loneliness and distress. Gaev (1976) said that feelings of loneliness and isolation are usually most intense in adolescence. Further, Ostrov and Offer (1981) pointed out during adolescence the young person develops the ability to reflect intellectually about a whole new range of possibilities regarding values and life choices. During this time, it becomes clear that some day the adolescent will have to leave his/her parents and separate from them psychologically. Although it is difficult to integrate findings from studies with different approaches in sampling, in conceptualization and operational measures of loneliness, the evidence, particularly from the large scale studies (Ostrov & Offer, 1981), suggests that about 15 to 20% of the adolescent population experience painful levels of loneliness, with over 50% of youth experiencing recurrent feelings of loneliness. The importance of loneliness in the study of affective disorders among adolescents cannot be overemphasized (Brage et al., 1993). It has been linked to drug abuse and alcoholism, adolescent delinquency, and suicide (Trout, 1980).

The focus of the present paper is to examine the loneliness of young Portuguese living in France, a country that received the greatest number of Portuguese since the 60s (Mullet & Neto, 1991; Neto, 1993a). Although the community reached a certain importance at the end of First World War, the great migratory flux to France started in the 60s. And in 1963, legal migration to France overtook that to Brazil (15,223 against 11,281), marking the end of a trend that had gone on for centuries.

The purpose of this exploratory investigation was two-fold. The first objective was to examine whether migration had an effect on loneliness. One basic question about bicultural individuals is whether they are confused outsiders or special individuals with a broader understanding. The "marginal man" conceptualization (Park, 1928; Stonequist, 1961;

Wright & Wright, 1972) is still guiding research. Park's view was that, with migration and the loosening of bonds to his original culture, the marginal man —a person at the edge of two cultures— becomes "the individual with the keener intelligence, the wider horizon, the more detached and rational viewpoint" (Park, 1950, pp. 375-376). In contrast, Stonequist (1961) viewed the marginal man as a person caught between two cultures, never fitting in. Until recently, the dominant western view of the multiethnic person was consistent with that of Stonequist. Multiethnic people have been portrayed as troubled and anxious outsiders who lack a clear identity. However, the results of recent empirical research have indicated that multiethnic individuals are at no psychological disadvantage in comparison to monoethnic individuals. Researchers have consistently found no differences between self-esteem of multiethnic and monoethnic groups (Phinney & Alipuria, 1996). A recent study has shown that young Portuguese living in France did not differ on satisfaction with life from young Portuguese who had never migrated and were still living in Portugal (Neto, 1995). The present study compares loneliness of young Portuguese living in France to that of young Portuguese living in Portugal, expecting no difference between the two groups.

The second aim was to examine acculturation and personality predictors of loneliness. Acculturation represents currently one of the major areas of investigation in cross-cultural psychology (Berry, Poortinga, Segall, & Dasen, 1992). Acculturation has been defined as a culture change that results from continuous, first hand contact between two distinct cultural groups (Redfield, Linton, & Herskovits, 1936).

Berry and his colleagues (e.g., Berry et al., 1989) have developed a two-dimensional model of acculturation, providing a framework for the study of acculturation attitudes. He suggests that two critical issues determine the type of acculturation: (a) the extent to which individuals consider it of value to identify with and maintain the cultural characteristics of their own ethnic groups, and (b) the importance one attributes to maintaining positive relationships with the larger society and other ethnic groups.

On the basis of this model, there are four possible ways in which ethnic group members can participate in a culturally diverse society. Assimilation is the outcome when ethnic group members choose to identify solely with the culture of the dominant society and to relinquish all ties to their ethnic culture. Integration is characterized by strong identification and involvement with both the dominant society's culture and the traditional ethnic culture. Separation involves exclusive focus on the cultural values and practices of the ethnic group and little or no interaction with the dominant society. Marginality is defined by the absence or loss of one's culture of origin and the lack of involvement with the dominant society. The literature generally suggests that among the four acculturation options, integration must be the most adaptative (Berry et al., 1989; Neto, 1994). Based on Berry's model, we hypothesised that individuals who adopt an integration mode will show lower loneliness than those who chose an assimilation or separation mode; individuals who adopt a marginalization mode will show higher levels of loneliness than individual in the three other modes.

During accculturation individuals are confronted not only with different attitudinal options but also with new lifestyles. Individuals holding different attitudes engage in different levels of cultural maintenance and of contact with the host society (Dona & Berry, 1994). There are some indications that lonely individuals have less contact than do individuals who are not lonely. Among adolescents, loneliness has been associated with less participation in the social and extracurricular school activities, less time spent with peers and parents, lower dating frequency, more time spent alone and less frequent membership in social organizations and clubs (Brennan, 1982). On the other hand, several studies have failed to find a relationship between loneliness and social contact or activities. Other studies have indicated that satisfaction with contact is more important than actual frequency (Jones, 1982). Because of conflicting evidence between loneliness and social contact, no prediction was made regarding its relationship to French acculturative experience and Portuguese cultural maintenance.

As we expect acculturation and personality factors to be predictors of loneliness, we will explore its relationship to personality constructs, such as life satisfaction, social anxiety and acculturative stress. Previous research suggests that loneliness is associated with different affective states and well-being (Fisher & Philips, 1982; Neto, 1992a; Paloutizian & Ellison, 1982; Russell, Peplau, & Ferguson, 1978). We thus predict that loneliness will be associated positively with acculturative stress and social anxiety, and negatively with life satisfaction.

Method

Sample
The sample consisted of 109 Portuguese youngsters living in Paris and born in France, of Portuguese parents (37 boys and 72 girls). The age of the subjects ranged between 15 and 18 years ($M = 16.7$, $SD = 1.2$). According to the assessment method of Lautrey (1980; Neto, 1986), a joint function of parental occupation and education, their socioeconomic level was low.

Instruments

The participants were presented with a questionnaire including the following:

a) The Portuguese version of the *Revised UCLA Loneliness Scale* (Russel, Peplau and Cutrona, 1980) has been described in Neto (1992a, 1992b). This is a 18-item questionnaire which nine of the questions were reverse scored. The subject is asked to indicate how often she or he feels that way (never/rarely/sometimes/often).

b) *Acculturation attitudes scales.* French or Portuguese acculturation attitudes were assessed on fourteen topics like custom, language, marriage, parties, etc. Two items were developed for each topic, one reflecting preferences for French society, the other for Portuguese culture. The items were randomly ordered in the questionnaire and the answers to each item were given on a 5-point Likert scale, ranging from strong disagreement (1) to strong agreement (5).

c) Acculturation experience and cultural maintenance were assessed with indicators proposed by Berry, Trimble and Olmedo (1986), by Donà and Berry (1994) and by Neto (1986). Respondents were asked to rate their degree of involvement on a 4-point scale ranging from never (1) to often (4), in each of the following activities: newspaper reading, television, radio, food preference, language, club membership, degree of interaction with neighors and friends, music preference and dreams. These measures were used to assess the degree of cultural maintenance and the amount of acculturative experience with French society.

d) The *Acculturative Stress Scale* of Cawte (Cawte, Bianchi, & Kiloh, 1968; Berry & Annis, 1974; Neto, 1994) consists of 10 somatic symptoms and 10 psychological symptoms, with dichotomous answers (Yes/No).

e) The Social Anxiety subscale contains 6 items from the *Self-Consciousness Scale* (Fenigstein, Scheier, & Buss, 1975). These items were answered on a 5-point scale. The range of this scale extends from 0 to 24. The reliability and factorial validity of the scale has been demonstrated for a Portuguese population (Neto, 1989).

f) The *Life Satisfaction Scale* (Diener, Emmons, Larsen, & Griffin, 1985) includes five items, which subjects were asked to answer on a seven point scale. The range of the total scale extends from 5 (low satisfaction) to 35 (high satisfaction). Reliability and validity has also been demonstrated for a Portuguese population (Neto, 1993b, 1997).

g) Finally, subjects were asked information about socio-demographic characteristics, ethnic identity, friends and difficulties experienced in France in different settings.

Table 1. Means, Standard Deviations and Reliabilities

Scales	*M*	*SD*	Cronbach α	# items
Loneliness	33.3	6.5	0.80	18
French acculturative experience	34.1	3.6	0.67	10
Portuguese cultural maintenance	26.8	5.2	0.80	10
French acculturative attitudes	50.1	7.9	0.86	14
Portuguese acculturative attittudes	51.5	7.5	0.81	14
Acculturative stress	6.8	3.3	0.69	20
Social anxiety	13.2	4.1	0.69	6
Satisfaction with life	22.7	5.5	0.78	5

Results

Scale means, standard deviations and reliabilities are reported in Table 1. Even though Cronbach alphas are not equally high, the eight scales are retained in their present format. The Loneliness Scale internal consistency (.80) is very close to the data reported on another adolescent population (Neto, 1992a).

The total loneliness score (33.3) of the Portuguese version of the *Revised UCLA Loneliness Scale* is lower than the scores found on a Portuguese college population (36.7 - Neto, 1989a) and on a teacher population (35.2 - Neto, 1992b), but comparable to the mean for Portuguese adolescents from a low socioeconomic level living in urban areas, in Portugal (32.8 - Neto, 1992a).

A number of specific questions were treated as independent variables, while sum scores on loneliness was a dependent variable. One-way analyses of variance were then performed.

Gender. There were no gender differences ($M = 32.9$ for girls and 34.1 for boys: $F(1, 107) = .76, p > .05$), as in Neto's study (1992a). These results are quite consistent with the analysis on gender differences presented by Boris and Perlman (1985).

Religious participation. There was no significant effect of religious participation. Whether practicing or not, Catholics did not differ on their loneliness score.

Ethnic identity. There was no significant effect of ethnic identity: subjects considering themselves Portuguese, French or both did not differ on loneliness either.

Acculturation attitudes. Acculturation attitudes were assessed with a scale on attitudes toward French culture and another towards Portuguese culture. Answers were dichotomized (Donà & Berry, 1994) rather than considering them continuous. Theoretical and statistical considerations led Donà and Berry (1994) to select a midpoint categorization. The cross-tabulation of the two French Attitude categories with the two Portuguese categories resulted thus in four types of respondents. Responses below or equal to the midpoint on both scales categorized individuals in the Marginalization mode. Responses above the midpoint on both scales classified individuals in the Integration mode. Responses below or equal to the midpoint on Portuguese attitudes and above the midpoint on French attitudes classified individuals in the Assimilation mode. The opposite answers categorized respondents in the Separation mode. Twelve respondents were thus classified in the Assimilation category, twelve in the Separation category, eighty-three in the Integration category, and two respondents were classified in the Marginalized category. Due to the very few respondents in the Marginalized category, analyses reported here were performed only with the others three modes of acculturation. In addition, due to the small numbers, results for Assimilation and Separation will have to be considered with caution. In order to test the hypothesis concerning the relationship of loneliness to acculturation attitudes, Separation and Assimilation were thus compared to Integration. Significant differences were found on the loneliness scale ($F(1, 105) = 6.48$, $p < .05$) with individuals in an Integration mode showing less loneliness ($M = 32.3$) than respondents in the other two categories ($M = 35.8$).

As can be seen in Table 2, correlations between loneliness and French acculturative experience and life satisfaction were significant and negative; correlations with social anxiety and acculturative stress were also significant, but positive. The correlation between loneliness and Portuguese culture maintenance was not significant. Multiple regression predictors of loneliness were: gender, religious participation, ethnic identity, acculturation attitudes (Integration versus Assimilation and Separation), French acculturative experience, Portuguese cultural maintenance, acculturative stress, social anxiety and life satisfaction (Table 3). Four significant and independent predictors emerged (French acculturative experience, life satisfaction, acculturation attitudes and social anxiety), accounting for 30% of the variance.

Table 2. *Correlations Between Loneliness and Other Variables*

Variables	Loneliness
Acculturative stress	.22**
French acculturative experience	-.36***
Portuguese cultural experience	-.03
Satisfaction with life	-.28**
Social anxiety	-.24**

$*p < .05; **p < .01; ***p < .001.$

Table 3. *Stepwise Regression of Psychosocial Variables on Loneliness*

Variables	Multiple R	R^2	Beta	t
French acculturative stress	.38	.15	-.38	-4.25***
Satisfaction with life	.47	.22	-.28	-3.19**
Acculturation atitudes	.52	.27	-.21	-2.47*
Social anxiety	.55	.29	.18	2.16*

$*p < .05; **p < .01; ***p < .001.$

Discussion

As a cross-sectional convenience sample was used, the findings presented here are tentative and should be interpreted with caution. However, the results show the wide array of situational and personality variables which loneliness is related to.

Loneliness is a complex phenomenon, meaning different things to different people. Like all complex emotions, loneliness is caused by an interaction of personal dispositions and situational forces. Consistent with the results of several recent studies (e.g., Grove, 1991; Neto, 1995; Phinney & Alipuria, 1996), we found multiethnic young people were not at a psychological disadvantage because of their mixed background. The loneliness measure did not indicate any difference between young

Portuguese living in France or in their home couuntry, in terms of psychological well-being.

Loneliness could be a major problem in the host country for first generation immigrants. For example, Mullet and Neto (1991) found homesickness, language and loneliness were major difficulties in France among immigrants. These three factors were mentioned in this same order, in a diachronic study about social representations of migration among young people living in Portugal (Neto, 1993a). But the picture emerging from the present study is quite different. Adolescents mentioned homesickness (48%), separation from family (43%) and climate (36%) as major difficulties. The three lowest difficulties were language (14%), loneliness (13%) and eating habits (9%). Thus the notion that geographic mobility of parents is a primary cause of loneliness in their children appears to be incorrect.

Explaining these data is not easy. We found similar results about life satisfaction, i.e., no differences between young Portuguese living abroad or in Portugal (Neto, 1995). Thus, if we consider loneliness as an indicator of low quality of life, the picture is consonant. However, more research is needed to explain these results. An avenue that deserves exploration is the child-rearing practices from first generation immigrants. Did the Portuguese adolescents grow up with supportive parents? Brennan (1982) has shown lonely adolescents report a complex pattern of negative and nonsupportive relationships with their parents. Some findings also suggest that chronic "anxiety" leaves a person more vulnerable to situational pressures that can cause loneliness (Rubenstein & Shaver, 1981).

The loneliness experienced by second generation migrants is not necessarily associated with sociodemographic characteristics such as gender, religion or ethnic identity. These findings are in agreement with Williams' data on adolescents (1983). Our results also shed some light into the selective importance of social contacts second generation immigrants have with people of their home country versus contacts with the host society. Those who reported more French acculturative experience were less lonely. However, Portuguese cultural maintenance didn't influence loneliness, since attending church, very often an occasion to meet compatriots, didn't have an impact on loneliness. In sum, lonely adolescents have fewer social ties with members from the host society.

Acculturation attitudes play an important part in the experience of loneliness. Adolescents who had adopted Integration attitudes reported less loneliness than those who had chosen Assimilation or Separation. The subjective conditions that favour Integration attitudes in a pluralistic society should be promoted so as to reduce the potential feelings of loneliness among second generation immigrants.

In the present study, loneliness was significantly related to second generation adolescent acculturative stress. Rubenstein and Shaver (1982) have also shown that lonely people report more psychosomatic symptoms, such as headaches, poor appetite and tiredness. There was a significant negative relation between loneliness and satisfaction with life. We can consider loneliness as an important indicator of poor quality of life. Paloutzian and Ellison (1982) also found a substantial association between loneliness and existential well-being among college students. In addition, loneliness was related to social anxiety, which could interfere with the ability to initiate social contacts. This is in agreement with other findings with adolescents (Moore & Schultz, 1983) and college students (Jones, 1982).

In summary, our results showed the expected association between loneliness and psychological maladjustment. Overall, French acculturative experience, acculturation attitudes and personality factors (life satisfaction and social anxiety) were the strongest predictors of loneliness. Results therefore supported situational and characterological explanations of loneliness.

Longitudinal data are required to explain the interactions between developmental changes and personal and social factors linked to adolescent second generation migrant loneliness. Such research would have important implications for the development of intervention strategies geared to the specific stage and type of loneliness of the second generation migrants. Future research should also address the generational effect of migration upon loneliness, not only for adolescents but for other age groups as well.

References

Berry, J. W., Kim, U., Power, S., Young, M., & Bujaki, M. (1989). Acculturation attitudes in plural societies. *Applied Psychology: An International Review, 38,* 185-206.

Berry, J. W., Poortinga, Y. H., Segall, M. H., & Dasen, P. R. (1992). *Cross-cultural psychology: Research and applications.* New York. Cambridge University Press.

Berry, J. W., Trimble, J. E., & Olmedo, E. L. (1986). Assessment of acculturation. In W. J. Lonner & J. W. Berry (Eds.), *Field methods in cross-cultural research: Vol. 2 Methodology.* Boston: Allyn and Bacon.

Berry, J., & Annis, R. (1974). Acculturative stress. *Journal of Cross-Cultural Psychology, 5,* 382-406.

Borys, S., & Perlman, D. (1985). Gender differences in loneliness. *Personality and Social Psychology Bulletin, 11,* 63-74.

Brage, D., Meredith, W., & Woodard, J. (1993). Correlates of loneliness among midwestern adolescents. *Adolescence, 28,* 685-693.

Brennan, T. (1982). Loneliness at adolescence. In L. Peplau & D. Perlman (Eds.), *Loneliness: A sourcebook of current theory, research and therapy.* New York: Wiley-Interscience.

Cawte, J., Bianchi, G., & Kiloh, L. (1968). Personal disconfort in Australian Aborigines. *Australian and New Zealand Journal of Psychiatry, 2,* 69-79.

Cheek, J. M., & Bush, C. M. (1981). The influence of shyness on loneliness in a new situation. *Personality and Social Psychology Bulletin, 7,* 572-577.

Diener, E., Emmons, R., Larsen, R., & Griffin, S. (1985). The satisfaction with life scale. *Journal of Personality Assessment, 49,* 1, 71-75.

Donà, G., & Berry, J. W. (1994). Acculturation attitudes and acculturative stress of central American refugees. *International Journal of Psychology, 29,* 57-70.

Fenigstein, A., Scheier, M., & Buss, A. (1975). Public and private self-consciousness: Assessment and theory. *Journal of Consulting and Clinical Psychology, 43,* 522-527.

Fisher, C., & Phillips, S. (1982). Who is alone? Social characteristics of people with small networks. In L. Peplau & D. Perlman (Eds.), *Loneliness: A sourcebook of current theory, research and therapy.* New York: Wiley-Interscience.

Gaev, D. M. (1976). *The psychology of loneliness.* Chicago: Adams Press.

Grove, K. (1991). Identity development in interracial Asian/White late adolescents: Must it be so problematic? *Journal of Youth and Adolescence, 20,* 617-628.

Jones, W. H. (1982). Loneliness and social contact. *Journal of Social Psychology, 113,* 295-296.

Jones, W. H., Carpenter, B. N., & Quintana, D. (1985). Personality and interpersonal predictors of loneliness in two cultures. *Journal of Personality and Social Psychology, 48,* 1503-1511.

Moore, D., & Schultz, N. (1983). Loneliness at adolescence: Correlates, attributions, and coping. *Journal of Youth and Adolescence, 12,* 95-100.

Mullet, E., & Neto, F. (1991). Intention to migrate, job opportunities and aspiration for better pay: An informational integration approach. *International Journal of Psychology, 26,* 95-113.

Neto, F. (1989). L'évaluation de la conscience de soi: Réplication portugaise. In J. Retschitzky, M. Bossel-Lagos, & P. Dasen (Eds.), *La recherche interculturelle* (Vol. 1). Paris: L'Harmattan.

Neto, F. (1992a). Loneliness among Portuguese adolescents. *Social Behavior and Personality, 20,* 15-22.

Neto, F. (1992b). *Solidão, embaraço e amor.* Porto: Centro de Psicologia Social.

Neto, F. (1993a). *Psicologia da migração portuguesa.* Lisboa: Universidade Aberta.

Neto, F. (1993b). Satisfaction with life scale: Psychometric properties in an adolescent sample. *Journal of Youth and Adolescence, 22,* 125-134.

Neto, F. (1994). Le stress d'acculturation chez des jeunes d'origine portugaise en France. *Enfance, 1,* 83-94.

Neto, F. (1995). Predictors of satisfaction with life among Portuguese second generation. *Social Indicators Research, 35,* 93-116.

Neto, F. (1997). *Estudos de Psicologia Intercultural: Nós e outros.* Lisboa: Fundação Calouste Gulbenkian, Junta Nacional de Investigação Científica.

Ostrov, E., & Offer, D. (1981). Loneliness and the adolescent. In J. Hartog, J. Audy, & Y. Cohen (Eds.), *The anatomy of loneliness.* New York: International Universities Press.

Paloutzian, R., & Ellison, C. (1982). Loneliness, spiritual well-being and the quality of life. In L. Peplau & D. Perlman (Eds.). *Loneliness: A sourcebook of current theory, research and therapy.* New York: Wiley-Interscience.

Park, R. E. (1928). Human migration and the marginal man. *The American Journal of Sociology, 33,* 881-893.

Park, R. E. (1950). *Race and culture.* Glencoe, IL: Free Press.

Peplau, L. A., & Perlman, D. (1982). Perspectives on loneliness. In L. A. Peplau & D. Perlman (Eds.), *Loneliness: A sourcebook of current theory, research and therapy.* Wiley-Interscience: New York.

Perlman, D., & Peplau, L. (1981). Toward a social psychology of loneliness. In S. Duck & R. Gilmour (Eds.), *Personal relationship 3: Personal relationships in disorder.* London: Academic Press.

Phinney, J., & Alipuria, L. (1996). At the interface of cultures: Multiethnic/multiracial high school and college students. *The Journal of Social Psychology, 136,* 139-158.

Pittel, S. (1971). Developemental factors in adolescent drug use: A study of psychedelic drug users. *Journal of The American Academy of Child Psychiatry, 10,* 640-660.

Redfield, R., Linton, R., & Herskovits, M. (1936). Memorandum on the study of acculturation. *American Psychologist, 38,* 149-152.

Rubenstein, C. M., & Shaver, P. (1982). The expression of loneliness. In L. Peplau, & D. Perlman (Eds.), *Loneliness: A sourcebook of current theory, research and therapy.* New York: Wiley-Interscience.

Rubenstein, C., & Shaver, P. (1981). Loneliness in two northeastern cities. In J. Hartog, J., Audy, & Y. Cohen (Eds.), *The anatomy of loneliness*. New York: International Universities Press.

Russel, D., Peplau, L., & Cutrona, C. (1980). The revised UCLA Loneliness Scale: Concurrent and discriminant validity evidence. *Journal of Personality and Social Psychology, 39,* 472-480.

Russel, D., Peplau, L., & Ferguson, M. (1978). Developing a measure of loneliness. *Journal of Personality Assessment, 42,* 290-294.

Seligman, A. G. (1983). The presentation of loneliness as a separate diagnostic category and its disengagement from depression. *Psychotherapy in Private Practice, 1,* 33-37.

Spielberger, C. D., & Diaz-Guerrero, R. (Eds.) (1976). *Cross-cultural anxiety*. New York: Wiley.

Stonequist, E. V. (1961). *The marginal man: A study in personality and culture conflict*. New York: Russell & Russell.

Weiss, R. S. (1973). *Loneliness: The experience of emotional and social isolation*. Cambridge, MA: MIT Press.

Williams, E., G. (1983). Adolescent loneliness. *Adolescence*, vol. XVIII, n°69, 51-66.

Woodward, J. (1988). *The solitude of loneliness*. Lexington, MA: Lexington Books.

Wright, R. D., & Wright, N. (1972). A plea for a further refinement of the marginal man theory. *Phylon, 33,* 361-368.

Psychological and Sociocultural Adjustment of Filipina Domestic Workers in Singapore

Colleen A. Ward, Weining C. Chang & Susan Lopez-Nerney
National University of Singapore, Singapore

ABSTRACT

The research extended the investigation of psychological (depression) and sociocultural (social difficulty) adjustment problems of sojourners to a sample of 191 Filipina domestic workers in Singapore. Work conditions (salary and schedule), locus of control (achievement and affiliation), cultural identity, co-national relations, discrepancies between life satisfaction in the Singapore and the Philippines, and sociocultural adaptation were examined as predictors of psychological adjustment. Multiple regression indicated that poor work conditions, weak identification as Filipino, small discrepancy between life satisfaction in Singapore and the Philippines, and social difficulty were significantly associated with a higher level of depression ($r^2 = .30$). A second regression analysis examined language ability and education, length of residence in Singapore, host national relations, and psychological adjustment as predictors of sociocultural adaptation. Poor knowledge-based resources (English language ability and level of education), low satisfaction with host national contact, and depression were significant predictors of social difficulty ($r^2 = .15$). The results are interpreted in terms of stress and coping and culture learning approaches to sojourner adjustment.

The international migration of domestic workers has become a rapidly increasing phenomenon in the last two decades. It has been estimated that there are at least 1.4 million women working in domestic service in Southeast Asia (Singapore, Malaysia, Brunei and Hong Kong) and parts of the Middle East (Bahrain, Oman, Kuwait and Saudi Arabia). Although Sri Lanka and Indonesia are large exporters of female domestic labor in the Asian region, the Philippines is the major source of the "maid trade" (Heyzer & Wee, 1992). More than 275,000 Filipina women are currently working abroad as domestic helpers (Asian Pacific Development Center, 1992), and approximately 60,000 of these are employed in Singapore (Wong, 1995).

The psychological and social adaptation of Filipina domestic workers is pertinent to policy makers as well as psychologists as the topic spans applied and theoretical domains and raises both practical and conceptual issues. Domestic laborers in Singapore make a significant contribution to the nation's socioeconomic development by providing support to middle income families and permitting skilled and professional women to remain in the local workforce. Indeed, the Singaporean government has recognized the pressing need for imported domestic support as a means of propping up the skilled component of the indigenous workforce in a country where the demand for labor exceeds the overall supply. Given the contention that "foreign labor is a resource that should be protected and recognized as a valuable contribution to the maintenance and reproduction of society and economic productivity" (Heyzer & Wee, 1992, p. 17), empirical research concerning the factors which facilitate psychological and sociocultural adjustment of this group should prove practical and useful.

The study of foreign laborers in domestic employment also has the potential to contribute to the conceptual development of theory and research on acculturation. Domestic laborers provide a striking contrast to the more frequently surveyed samples of foreign students and international business people. In contrast to the socioeconomic profiles of other sojourning groups, the international migration of domestic helpers represents a downwardly mobile brain drain. The majority of maids in Singapore, for example, are overqualified for their positions; at least 50% have a secondary school background and 43% have college degrees (Asia Pacific Development Center, 1992). Domestic helpers also differ from other groups in transition in that their daily routines are almost completely circumscribed by their employment conditions. Their main operating environment, both home and work, exists exclusively within a group of strangers from another culture. Pre-existing social and family ties are extensively disrupted, and support from co-nationals may be limited by terms of employment and amount of free time granted. Unlike foreign students or corporate employees, this group of sojourners is also handicapped by lack of a formal institution or agency, such as a school or multi-national corporation, to provide both peer contact and practical assistance in adapting to a new cultural milieu. These combined factors are likely to promote a strong sense of social and cultural isolation. For all of these reasons an empirical investigation based on a sample of Filipina domestic workers in Singapore may provide a valuable extension to current work on psychological and sociocultural adjustment of sojourners and test the external validity of current theory and research.

While there are a variety of theoretical approaches for the investigation of cross-cultural adjustment of Filipina domestics in Singapore, this research relies on the bipartite framework advanced by Ward and colleagues for the study of acculturation and adaptation (Ward, 1996). The framework distinguishes two adjustive outcomes —psychological and sociocultural— and blends stress and coping with social learning approaches to the study of culture contact and change. In this context psychological adjustment is defined in terms of psychological and emotional well-being and satisfaction, operationalized in terms of depression and/or global mood disturbance, and interpreted in terms of extant theory and research on stress, coping and adjustment (e.g., Berry, 1997; Lazarus & Folkman, 1984). Sociocultural adaptation, by contrast, is viewed in relation to behavioral competence, operationalized in terms of social difficulty, and considered within the culture learning paradigm (e.g., Brislin, 1981; Furnham & Bochner, 1986). An emerging program of research has indicated that psychological and sociocultural adjustment are inter-related but that they are largely predicted by different types of variables (Searle & Ward, 1990; Ward & Kennedy, 1992, 1993a,b) and that they show different patterns of variation over time (Ward & Kennedy, 1996a,b; Ward, Okura, Kennedy, & Kojima, in press). The main findings have suggested that personality, social support and life change variables are more predictive of psychological adjustment while length of residence in host culture, culture-specific knowledge and contact with host nationals appear to relate more strongly to sociocultural adaptation.

In line with past research and contemporary theory on stress and coping, this study explores the relationship between personality, cognitive and social support variables in relation to psychological adjustment of Filipina domestic workers in Singapore. These include locus of control, cultural identity, and relationship satisfaction with co-nationals. In addition, work conditions and the discrepancy between life satisfaction in the Philippines and in Singapore are also investigated in relationship to psychological well-being.

Locus of control has been widely recognized as a major determinant of psychological health and illness. Clinical and social psychological studies have demonstrated that an external locus of control is associated with psychological dysfunction and distress, and these findings have been consistently replicated in studies of sojourners and immigrants (Dyal, Rybensky, & Somers, 1988; Hung, 1974; Kuo, Gray, & Lin, 1976; Searle & Ward, 1990; Ward & Kennedy, 1992, 1993a). Along these lines it is predicted that external locus of control will be linked to more depressive symptoms in Filipina domestic workers.

Personality variables are not the only salient predictors of psychological well-being in acculturating individuals. Berry and Blondell (1982) have contended that links to one's ethnic community are also crucial for mental health. Of course these links may be forged in a number of ways. One way is via the development of ethno-cultural identity. Our own research, for example, has indicated that sojourners who maintain a strong co-national identity experience fewer psychological adjustment problems (Ward & Kennedy, 1994). A second method is through extensive and satisfying co-national contact. A number of studies have suggested that co-national relations are the most salient and powerful source of social support for sojourners and immigrants (e.g., Berry, Kim, Minde, & Mok, 1987; Sykes & Eden, 1987; Ward & Kennedy, 1993a; Ying & Liese, 1991). Consequently, it is predicted that a stronger Filipina identity and greater satisfaction with co-national relations will be associated with lower levels of psychological distress.

In many instances work conditions may also directly impact on psychological well-being (Church, 1982). Work-related variables such as income and occupation have been shown to affect immigrants' psychological adjustment (Aycan & Berry, 1994), and job satisfaction has been found to relate negatively to acculturative stress in sojourners (Lance & Richardson, 1988; Kealey, 1989; Pilcher, 1994). As such, it is hypothesized that favorable work conditions will be inversely related to symptoms of depression. Finally, the level and fluctuation of general life satisfaction is likely to influence psychological adjustment of acculturating individuals as documented by the significant negative relationship reported between life satisfaction and indices of psychological and psychosomatic stress (Kealey, 1989). This study, however, considers the discrepancy between previous and current life satisfaction. In this context it is hypothesized that reported improvement in satisfaction between life in the Philippines and life in Singapore would be associated with less psychological distress and lower levels of depression.

In contrast to the stress and coping approach to psychological adjustment sociocultural adaptation is examined from a culture learning perspective with emphasis on knowledge-based resources such as education and English language fluency, length of stay in Singapore, and satisfaction with host national contact as potential predictive variables. Consistent with this perspective on cross-cultural adaptation, research has demonstrated that both the acquisition of culture-specific knowledge (Armes & Ward, 1989; Torbiorn, 1982) and the development of culture-specific behavioral competencies increase over time (Ward, 1996). This has been reliably observed in both cross-sectional (Celano & Tyler, 1991) and longitudinal research (Ward & Kennedy, 1996a,b; Ward et al., in press). Therefore, it is predicted that sociocultural difficulties will be negatively related to length of residence in the host culture.

Both education and language fluency are likely to function as resources during the cross-cultural adjustment process (Berry, 1997). Indeed, empirical research has documented that language ability is positively related to sociocultural adaptation and that those fluent in the host culture language experience fewer social difficulties (Chen, 1992; Sano, 1990; Ward & Kennedy, 1993b). Language fluency is also associated with increased interaction with host nationals (Gullahorn &

Gullahorn, 1966) which may exert additional positive influences on sociocultural adaptation by expanding available networks for culture learning. Our own research and that of others have demonstrated that sojourners who have more extensive interactions with host nationals and those who are more satisfied with these relationships experience less sociocultural adjustment problems (Church, 1982; Searle & Ward, 1990; Ward & Kennedy, 1993b). Given these findings, it is hypothesized that knowledge-based resources, such as education and language fluency, and satisfaction with host national contact will be negatively associated with sociocultural adaptation problems.

In summary, the research hypotheses are:

1) An external locus of control, weaker identification as Filipino, less satisfaction with co-national interactions, less improvement in life satisfaction after relocation to Singapore and greater sociocultural adaptation problems will predict higher levels of depression (psychological adjustment problems).

2) Knowledge-based resources (English language ability and level of education), shorter length of residence in Singapore, less satisfaction with host national relations, and higher levels of depression will predict greater social difficulty (sociocultural adaptation problems).

Method

Participants
One hundred and ninety-one Filipina women, employed as domestic helpers in Singapore, participated in the research. Ages ranged from 19-48 years ($M = 28.6$ years, $SD = 5.3$). The majority of the women were single ($N = 141$, 74%) with 20% ($N = 38$) married and the remainder separated, divorced or widowed. Of those previously or currently married, the majority had children (89%), and their husbands came primarily from production, transportation, service and farm-related occupations. The women themselves were generally well educated with 88 (46%) having university degrees, 38 (20%) vocational and technical qualifications and 58 (30%) having secondary education. The respondents originated from various parts of the Philippines, with Ilocano (38%) and Tagalog (27%) being the main dialects; however, the sample also included Cebuano, Ilonggo, Pangasinan and other dialect-speakers. The Filipinas were generally fluent in English with only 3% regarding their English ability as poor. In addition, 12.6% ($N = 24$) of the sample spoke a local (Singaporean) language or dialect.

A small portion of the sample ($N = 18$, 9.4%) had previously worked abroad as domestic helpers; however, for the majority (89%) of respondents Singapore was the first country of overseas employment. Length of stay in Singapore varied from one month to 9.5 years ($M = 33.0$ months, $SD = 22.9$). Salaries ranged from S\$ 230-900 or approximately US\$ 160-630 ($M = $ S\$ 322, $SD = $ S\$ 78.71).

Materials

The questionnaire included demographic information, personality and cognitive variables (locus of control and cultural identity), measures of life satisfaction and interpersonal relations, and assessments of sojourner adjustment (psychological and sociocultural adaptation). The survey was constructed in English, translated into Tagalog by the third author, and back-translated to English by another Tagalog-English bilingual. Both English and Tagalog versions were used in the research.

Demographics. Participants provided demographic information about length of residence in Singapore, level of education, and current work conditions (salary, hours worked per day, number of days off per month). They also rated their English language ability on a four point scale (endpoints: poor/excellent).

Locus of Control. The Multidimensional-Multiattributional Causality Scale (MMCS; Lefcourt, Von Baeyer, Ware, & Cox, 1979) was employed for the assessment of locus of control. The instrument includes two sets of 24-item Likert scales for the measurement of achievement and affiliation domains, respectively. In each case 12 internal and 12 external items are counterbalanced for success and failure attributions.

Participants respond to each set of 24 statements on 5-point agree/disagree scales. The authors have specified that the MMCS may be scored as a whole or broken into subscales. In the first instance, 24 items may be scored for externality (range 0-96). Alternatively, internal and external subscales (0-48) may be scored separately.

Cultural identity. The construction of this measurement was originally inspired by Tajfel's theory of social identity. Participants rely on 7-point bipolar scales to respond to questions about in- and outgroup membership and identity. The original 12-item version of this author-devised scale was used in Ward and Searle's (1991) study of sojourner adjustment. The current version contains 10 items; scores range from 0-60 with higher scores representing a stronger cultural identity.[1]

Interpersonal relations. Participants were asked to rate their satisfaction with the quality and quantity of interactions with Filipinos and

---

1   The scale was referred to as a measure of social identity in the earlier study. As the emerging program of research has focused on identity issues within acculturating groups, this measure is currently referred to as cultural identity.

Singaporeans. Ratings were made on 5-point scales (endpoints: not at all satisfied/very satisfied).

Life satisfaction. Participants rated prior life satisfaction in the Philippines and current life satisfaction in Singapore. Ratings were made on 5-point scales (endpoints: not at all satisfying/very satisfying).

Psychological Adjustment. In line with our previous research the Zung Self-Rating Depression Scale (ZSDS; Zung, 1965) was used as the measurement of psychological adjustment. Participants rely on 4-point rating scales (endpoints: a little of the time/most of the time) to respond to 20 statements that cover affective, physiological and psychological components of depression. Scores range from 0-60 with higher scores indicative of greater depression. The ZSDS has been used extensively in cross-cultural research (e.g., Zung, 1969), including work with Filipino participants (Lester, Castromayor & Icli, 1991).

Sociocultural Adaptation. This author-devised instrument concerns the skills that are required to cope with everyday living situations in a new culture. The scale development was based on work by Furnham and Bochner (1982) with the Social Situations Questionnaire; however, unlike the earlier instrument, the reference points for social difficulty are not framed in affective terms (e.g., fear, anxiety). Participants use 5-point rating scales (end points: no difficulty/extreme difficulty) to assess the amount of social difficulty experienced in a range of situations. The version of the Sociocultural Adaptation Scale (SAS) used in this research contains 23 items. Scores range from 0-92, with higher scores indicating greater social difficulty, and consequently, more sociocultural adaptation problems. The scale has previously proven reliable and valid in a series of studies on cross-cultural sojourner adjustment (e.g., Ward & Kennedy, 1993a,b, 1994).

Procedure

Data collectors were recruited from known Filipina domestic helpers who agreed to distribute questionnaires among the Filipina community. Personal contacts were used as well as organized groups, such as church congregations. Of the 260 questionnaires which were distributed, 201 (77.3%) were returned to the research assistants who were paid S$ 5 (US$ 3.50) per completed questionnaire. Ten of the questionnaires were discarded as they were incomplete, resulting in a final sample of 191 respondents.

Participation in the research was anonymous and voluntary, and participants were allowed to complete the questionnaire in either English or Tagalog.

Results

Preliminary Analyses

Preliminary analysis indicated that the cultural identity (α = .70), psychological adjustment (ZSDS α = .72) and sociocultural adaptation (SAS α =.85) measures were internally consistent. The MMCS locus of control measures, however, proved problematic.

Analysis indicated that the MMCS could not be scored as a unidimensional measurement of externality. After item reversals for unidimensional scoring the alphas were unacceptably low (.31 - .41) and far below the .58 - .81 range cited by Lefcourt et al. (1979). Additional analyses indicated that the internal and external subscales were positively rather than negatively correlated: r = .53 (p < .001) for affiliation, and r = .50 (p < .001) for achievement.

In contrast, the reliability figures for the separate internal and external subscales of the Achievement and Affiliation instruments were more substantial (α = .67 - .78) and within the range cited by Lefcourt and associates for these measurements. Item-total correlations ranged from .12 to .60 with mean correlations of .31 for internal achievement, .42 for external achievement, and .36 for both internal and external affiliation. In this event the separate assessment of the internal and external subscales for both the affiliation and achievement domains was considered for inclusion in the subsequent regression analysis. However, given that: a) there were significant correlations (r's > .50) between the internal and external measurements of both affiliation and achievement, b) zero order correlations revealed only the external subscales related to psychological adjustment, and c) the external subscales of the achievement and affiliation measurements were also significantly correlated (r = .63), the two external subscales were combined (α = .84). This provided a broad measurement of external locus of control and circumvented potential problems of multicollinearity for the planned regression analysis.

Along similar lines the education and English language ability variables (r = .41) were collapsed into one variable representing knowledge-based resources. Likewise, salary, hours of work, and days off measures were standardized and collapsed into a broader work conditions variable. Satisfaction with quality and quantity of interactions with co-nationals (r =.73) was scored as a single variable as was its host national relations parallel (r = .84). Finally, a discrepancy score was calculated for previous and current life satisfaction. Retrospective Philippines-based ratings were subtracted from current Singapore-based ratings so that higher scores represent increased life satisfaction.

Table 1. Pearson Correlations Coefficients among Predictor Variables

	1	2	3	4	5	6	7	8
1. External locus of control	--	.17	-.02	.07	-.14	.23	.19*	.12
2. Cultural identity		--	-.14	.04	.02	.12	.04	-.06
3. Satisfaction with host national relation			--	.22**	.10	.17	.04	.12
4. Satisfaction with co-national relations				--	-.06	.00	.03	.13
5. Increased life satisfaction					--	.12	-.06	.04
6. Work conditions						--	.12	.36**
7. Knowledge-based resources							--	.12
8. Length of residence								--

*p < .01; **p < .001.

The zero order correlations amongst the predictor variables are presented in Table 1. Correlation coefficients are generally low, and there is no evidence of multicollinearity. In addition and as expected, the correlation between the psychological and sociocultural adjustment was significant ($r = .27$, $p < .001$).

Regression Analyses

In line with the first hypotheses, locus of control, cultural identity, co-national relations, work conditions, improved life satisfaction, and sociocultural adjustment were examined as predictors of psychological adjustment (depression). A standard multiple regression with simultaneous entry of the predictor variables was used for this analysis. The results revealed that these variables accounted for 30% of the variance in psychological adjustment; $F(6, 136) = 9.61$, $p < .001$. As can be seen in Table 2, however, only four of the six variables emerged as significant predictors. More specifically, depression was predicted by small improvements in life satisfaction, greater social difficulties, weak Filipina identity, and poor work conditions. Locus of control and satisfaction with co-national relations did not significantly relate to psychological adjustment.

In line with the second hypothesis, length of residence in Singapore, knowledge-based resources, relations with host nationals, and psychological adjustment were investigated as predictors of sociocultural adaptation (social difficulty). Regression analysis revealed that these variables accounted for only 15% of the variance in the adaptation outcome; $F(4, 183) = 8.20$, $p < .001$. More specifically, social difficulty was predicted by a high incidence of depressive symptoms, low satisfaction with host national interactions and limited educational and linguistic resources. Contrary to the second hypothesis, however, length of stay in Singapore, did not significantly relate to sociocultural adaptation (see Table 3).

Discussion

The research considered the psychological and sociocultural adaptation of Filipina domestic workers in Singapore. Congruent with studies of other sojourner groups, the findings revealed that improved life satisfaction, strong cultural identity, low incidence of social difficulties and favorable work conditions were significant predictors of psychological adjustment; in contrast, depression, satisfaction with host national contact, and

Table 2. Predictors of Depression

Predictor variables	Beta	$p <$
Improved life satisfaction	-.28	.001
Cultural identity	-.26	.001
Social difficulty	.23	.003
Work conditions	-.15	.05
Co-national relations	.06	n.s.
External locus of control	-.09	n.s.

Table 3. Predictors of Social Difficulty

Predictor variables	Beta	$p <$
Depression	.24	.001
Host-national relations	-.20	.004
Knowledge-based resources	-.16	.025
Length of residence	-.08	n.s.

cognitive resources such as education and language ability significantly affected sociocultural adaptation. Although only a modest proportion of the variance in the adjustive outcomes was explained by these variables, the results are compatible with the conceptual and empirical distinction of psychological and sociocultural dimensions of adjustment and the theoretical framework employed by Ward and colleagues for the study of cross-cultural transition and adaptation.

Previous investigations have indicated that psychological adjustment during cross-cultural relocation can be meaningfully interpreted within a stress and coping framework. Consequently, factors which are generally associated with adaptive psychological responses to stress are also likely to predict psychological adjustment during the acculturation process. Indeed, social psychological, organizational and clinical studies have consistently reported a) a link between social skills deficits and depression (e.g., Haley, 1985); b) an association between the reported experience of positive and pleasurable life events and lower levels of depression (e.g., MacPhillamy & Lewinsohn, 1974); and c) a strong connection between work and life satisfaction (e.g., Keon & McDonald, 1982; Schmitt & Bedeian, 1982). The same patterns have been observed in this research where increased sociocultural competence, improvements in life satisfaction, and more favorable work conditions were associated with lower levels of depression.

In addition to these general correlates and predictors of psychological well-being, there are also factors which are more specifically embedded in acculturation-based stress and coping processes. Cultural identity appears to be one of these factors. Although research findings have been somewhat controversial on this count, studies by both Berry and Kim (1988) and Ward and Kennedy (1994) have noted the positive benefits of identification with and maintenance of original cultural heritage. Our findings on co-national identity of Filipina domestics in Singapore are in accordance with results of these previous studies. Satisfaction with the quality and quantity of co-national relations, however, failed to predict psychological adjustment of Filipina domestics. Although sojourner research has frequently demonstrated that co-nationals provide the most salient and important source of social support (Sykes & Eden, 1987; Ying & Liese, 1991), there are other valuable channels to meet these needs (Church, 1982). It may be the case that these Filipina maids have little real time to interact with individuals outside of their domestic setting, and that they may be forced to rely on alternative avenues for necessary assistance and support.

Locus of control also failed to predict the psychological well-being. We believe that this may be accounted for by measurement problems. In this research there were apparent difficulties with the Multidimensional-Multiattributional Causality Scale. Locus of control could not be scored as a unidimensional construct, and there were positive correlations between the internal and external subscales in both the achievement and affiliation domains. As our previous research, which has been based on modifications of Rotter's (1966) Locus of Control scale, has consistently demonstrated a relationship between external locus of control and psychological distress (e.g., Searle & Ward, 1990; Ward & Kennedy, 1992, 1993a), it is likely that Lefcourt et al.'s (1979) MMCS was responsible for the unanticipated outcome.

In contrast to psychological adjustment during cross-cultural transition, sociocultural adaptation was considered within a culture learning framework. As this perspective highlights the significance of learning-related variables in the acquisition of social skills (Furnham & Bochner, 1986), it was not surprising that cognitive resources such as level of education and language fluency were associated with a lower level of social difficulties. These knowledge-based assets are likely to facilitate enhanced work performance, which forms a major component of the domestic helper's experience abroad, as well as the development of more general, but necessary, culture-specific skills. Proponents of the culture learning approach have also argued that increased interaction with host nationals, who act as expert cultural informants, is likely to enhance behavioral competence in a new cultural milieu (Furnham & Bochner, 1982). Along these lines, satisfaction with the quality and quantity of interactions with host nationals was associated with fewer social difficulties in this sample.

Contrary to expectation, however, length of stay in Singapore was unrelated to sociocultural adjustment. We believe that this may be dependent upon the duration of residence in Singapore for the Filipina domestic helpers in this sample. Longitudinal research has suggested that sociocultural adjustment problems decrease rapidly in the first months of relocation and then tend to level (Ward & Kennedy, 1996a; Ward et al., in press). Although the range of residence of the Filipina domestic helpers in this study varied from one month to over 9 years, mean length of stay was 33 months. It may be the case, then, that this cross-sectional sample did not provide sufficient variance in sociocultural adaptation across the longer periods of residence in Singapore. We suggest that the precise relationship between length of residence and sociocultural adaptation should be further investigated in longitudinal studies.

On the whole the findings attest to good external validity of theory and research on cross-cultural transition and adaptation. Research with Filipina domestics in Singapore reiterated the usefulness of the stress and coping approach to the study of psychological adjustment of sojourners and a social learning approach to the parallel investigation of socio-cultural adaptation. However, it is also important to note that only a small to modest proportion of the variance in adjustive outcomes was accounted for in this sample. This suggests the presence of salient and sample-specific factors which affect the psychological and sociocultural adjustment of Filipina domestic workers in Singapore, in addition to the general and acculturation-related variables examined in this research. Gonzalez' (1995) discussion of the patterns and trends of the Philippine labor diaspora supports this contention. He makes reference not only to the general problems experienced by sojourning laborers such as emotional stress, social challenges and culture shock, but also comments upon the particular problems and vulnerabilities of Filipina domestic workers abroad. Noting that female overseas contract workers were responsible for 83% of the complaints monitored by the Philippines Overseas Workers Welfare Administration, Gonzalez estimated that approximately one third of these complaints related to welfare issues including maltreatment, physical and sexual abuse and inhumane working conditions. Obviously, these are not conditions widely shared by voluntary sojourning groups such as foreign students, international business people and volunteer aid workers. On the basis of the trends reported by Gonzalez (1995) and our own research findings, it is strongly recommended that further investigations of psychological and sociocultural adjustment of Filipina domestic helpers in Singapore be undertaken. This could prove beneficial for the development of more sophisticated acculturation theory as well as the formulation of significant social policy and effective therapeutic interventions.

References

Armes, K., & Ward, C. (1989). Cross-cultural transition and sojourner adjustment in Singapore. *Journal of Social Psychology, 12,* 273-275.

Asian Pacific Development Center. (1992, August). *The Philippines country report on the trading of maids in the Asia Pacific region.* Paper presented at the Asian Regional Dialogue on Foreign Women Domestic Workers: International Migration, Employment and National Policies, Colombo, Sri Lanka.

Aycan, Z., & Berry, J. W. (1994, July). *The influences of economic adjustment of immigrants on their psychological well-being and adaptation.* Paper presented at the XII International Congress of the International Association for Cross-Cultural Psychology, Pamplona, Spain.

Berry, J. W. (1997). Immigration, acculturation and adaptation. *Applied Psychology: An International Review, 46,* 5-34.

Berry, J. W., & Blondell, T. (1982). Psychological adaptation of Vietnamese refugees in Canada. *Canadian Journal of Community Mental Health, 1,* 81-88.

Berry, J. W. & Kim, U. (1988). Acculturation and mental health. In P. Dasen, J. W. Berry, & N. Sartorius (Eds.), *Health and cross-cultural psychology* (pp. 207-236). Newbury Park, CA: Sage.

Berry, J. W., Kim, U., Minde, T., & Mok, D. (1987). Comparative studies of acculturative stress. *International Migration Review, 21,* 490-511.

Brislin, R. (1981). *Cross-cultural encounters.* Elmsford, NY: Pergamon.

Celano, M. P., & Tyler, F. B. (1991). Behavioral acculturation among Vietnamese refugees in the United States. *Journal of Social Psychology, 131,* 373-385.

Chen, G.-M. (1992). Communication adaptability and interaction involvement as predictors of cross-cultural adjustment. *Communication Research Reports,* June, 33-41.

Church, A. T. (1982). Sojourner adjustment. *Psychological Bulletin, 91,* 540-572.

Dyal, J. A., Rybensky, L., & Somers, M. (1988). Marital and acculturative strain among Indo-Canadian and Euro-Canadian women. In J. W. Berry & R. Annis (Eds.), *Ethnic psychology: Research and practice with immigrants, refugees, native peoples, ethnic groups and sojourners* (pp. 80-95). Lisse: Swets & Zeitlinger.

Furnham, A., & Bochner, S. (1982). Social difficulty in a foreign culture: An empirical analysis of culture shock. In S. Bochner (Ed.), *Cultures in contact* (pp. 161-198). Oxford: Pergamon Press.

Furnham, A., & Bochner, S. (1986). *Culture shock: Psychological reactions to unfamiliar environments.* New York: Methuen.

Gonzalez, J. L. (1995). *The Philippine labor diaspora: Patterns and trends.* Paper presented at the ASEAN Inter-University Seminars on Social Development, Cebu, Philippines.

Gullahorn, J. E., & Gullahorn, J. T. (1966). American students abroad: Professional versus personal development. *Annals, 368,* 43-59.

Haley, W. D. (1985). Social skills deficits and self-evaluation among depressed and non-depressed psychiatric inpatients. *Journal of Clinical Psychology, 41,* 162-168.

Heyzer, N., & Wee, V. (1992, August). *Domestic workers in transient overseas employment: Who benefits, who profits?* Paper presented at the Asian Regional Dialogue on Foreign Women Domestic Workers: International Migration, Employment and National Policies, Colombo, Sri Lanka.

Hung, Y. Y. (1974). Sociocultural environment and locus of control. *Psychologia Taiwanica, 16,* 187-198.

Kealey, D. (1989). A study of cross-cultural effectiveness: Theoretical issues and practical applications. *International Journal of Intercultural Relations, 13,* 387-428.

Keon, T. L., & McDonald, B. (1982). Job satisfaction and life satisfaction: An empirical evaluation of their interrelationship. *Human Relations, 35,* 167-180.

Kuo, W. H., Gray, R., & Lin, N. (1976). Locus of control and symptoms of distress among Chinese Americans. *International Journal of Social Psychiatry, 22,* 176-187.

Lance, C. E., & Richardson, D. (1988). Correlates of work and non-work stress and satisfaction among American insulated sojourners. *Human Relations, 41,* 725-738.

Lazarus, R. S., & Folkman, S. (1984). *Stress, coping and appraisal.* New York: McGraw-Hill.

Lefcourt, H. M., Von Baeyer, C. L., Ware, E. E., & Cox, D. J. (1979). The Multidimensional-Multiattributional Causality Scale: The development of a goal specific locus of control scale. *Canadian Journal of Behavioral Science, 11,* 286-304.

Lester, D., Castromayor, I., & Icli, T. (1991). Locus of control, depression and suicidal ideation among American, Philippine and Turkish students. *Journal of Social Psychology, 131,* 447-449.

MacPhillamy, D. J., & Lewinsohn, P. M. (1974). Depression as a function of levels of desired and obtained pleasure. *Journal of Abnormal Psychology, 83,* 651-657.

Pilcher, K. (1994). *The work and non-work adjustment and adaptation of New Zealand business people while overseas on assignment.* Unpublished Masters' thesis, University of Canterbury, Christchurch, New Zealand.

Rotter, J. B. (1966). Generalized expectancies for internal and external control of reinforcement. *Psychological Monographs, 80* (1, Whole No. 609).

Sano, H. (1990). Research on social difficulties in cross-cultural adjustment: Social situational analysis. *Japanese Journal of Behavioral Therapy, 16,* 37-44.

Schmitt, N., & Bedeian, A. G. (1982). A comparison of LISREL and two-stage least squares analysis of a hypothesized life-job satisfaction reciprocal relationship. *Journal of Applied Psychology, 67,* 806-817.

Searle, W., & Ward, C. (1990). The prediction of psychological and sociocultural adjustment during cross-cultural transition. *International Journal of Intercultural Relations, 14,* 449-464.

Sykes, I. J., & Eden, D. (1987). Transitional stress, social support, and psychological strain. *Journal of Occupational Behavior, 6,* 293-298.

Torbiorn, I. (1982). *Living abroad: Personal adjustment and personnel policy in the overseas setting.* Chichester, UK: Wiley.

Ward, C. (1996). Acculturation. In D. Landis & R. Bhagat (Eds.), *Handbook of intercultural training* (2nd ed., pp. 124-147). Thousand Oaks, CA: Sage.

Ward, C., & Kennedy, A. (1992). Locus of control, mood disturbance and social difficulty during cross-cultural transitions. *International Journal of Intercultural Relations, 16,* 175-194.

Ward, C., & Kennedy, A. (1993a). Where's the "culture" in cross-cultural transition? Comparative studies of sojourner adjustment. *Journal of Cross-cultural Psychology, 24,* 221-249.

Ward, C., & Kennedy, A. (1993b). Psychological and sociocultural adjustment during cross-cultural transitions: A comparison of secondary students overseas and at home. *International Journal of Psychology, 28,* 129-147.

Ward, C., & Kennedy, A. (1994). Acculturation strategies, psychological adjustment, and sociocultural competence during cross-cultural transitions. *International Journal of Intercultural Research, 18,* 329-343.

Ward, C., & Kennedy, A. (1996a). Crossing cultures: The relationship between psychological and sociocultural dimensions of cross-cultural transitions. In J. Pandey, D. Sinha, & D. P. S. Bhawuk (Eds.), *Asian contributions to cross-cultural psychology* (pp. 289-306). New Delhi: Sage.

Ward, C., & Kennedy, A. (1996b). Before and after cross-cultural transition: A study of New Zealand volunteers on field assignments. In H. Grad, A. Blanco, & J. Georgas (Eds.), *Key issues in cross-cultural psychology* (pp. 138-154). Lisse: Swets & Zeitlinger.

Ward, C., Okura, Y., Kennedy, A., & Kojima, T. (in press). The U curve on trial: A longitudinal study of psychological and sociocultural adjustment during cross-cultural transition. *International Journal of Intercultural Relations.*

Ward, C., & Searle, W. (1991). The impact of value discrepancies and cultural identity on psychological and sociocultural adjustment of sojourners. *International Journal of Intercultural Relations, 15,* 209-225.

Wong, D. (1995, October). *Foreign domestic workers in Singapore.* Paper presented at the Asian Women in Migration Conference, Manila, Philippines.

Ying, Y.-W. & Liese, L. H. (1991). Emotional well-being of Taiwan students in the U.S.: An examination of pre- to post-arrival differential. *International Journal of Intercultural Relations, 15,* 345-366.

Zung, W. W. K. (1965). A self-rating depression scale. *Archives of General Psychiatry,* 12, 63-70.

Zung, W. W. K. (1969). A cross-cultural survey of symptoms in depression. *American Journal of Psychiatry, 126,* 116-121.

Author Notes

The research was supported by a grant (RP 92-0007) from the National University of Singapore. The authors would like to acknowledge the assistance of Gina Tuason for translation of the research instrument. The authors would also like to thank Norma Alegria, Liwliwa Baided, Maribeth Gapuz, and Florence Terro for their assistance with data collection, Agnes Malto for Tagalog data coding, and Catherine Eaw and Antony Kennedy for data preparation and analysis.

Requests for copies should be sent to Colleen A. Ward, Department of Social Work & Psychology, National University of Singapore, Kent Ridge, Singapore 119260.

Ethnic Identity and Enculturation/Acculturation

Peter Weinreich
University of Ulster, Northern Ireland, UK

ABSTRACT

Ethnic identity as a concept tends to be reified, whereas in reality individuals of an ethnicity express their ethnic identity in a variety of ways in accordance with differing patterns of identifications. In multicultural contexts, individuals of an ethnicity may identify with features of alternative cultures. The paper maintains that the nature of partial identification with other ethnic groups depends on biographical experiences within the socio-historical contexts of relationships between ethnic groups. Empirical studies demonstrate *enculturation* to be a partial and varying process, which should not be assumed to be *acculturation* towards the dominant culture. Hong Kong Chinese students reveal systematic relationships between partial identification with alternative ethnic groups and inter-generational continuity of identification, self-esteem and identity diffusion. Black youth in South Africa, partially identifying with another ethnic group, situated within specific oppressive ethnic context manifest vulnerable identities. Distinctive alternative orientations to their own ethnicity are strongly apparent in Muslim youth in Britain.

Ethnic identity is much in the news nowadays. In Britain, there are recognised to be a number of ethnic minority groups, such as Afro-Caribbean, Hindu, Sikh, Muslim and Greek Cypriot. From Bosnia-Herzegovina, we have acclimatised ourselves to a constant barrage of news of ethnic cleansing, in furtherance of territorial areas of a homogenous ethnic identity. As a result of stereotyping the ethnic groups in question, *ethnic identity* as a concept is all too often reified as an essentialist quality. Indeed, the act of social categorisation by others of people being of an ethnic group contributes to this reification. A study of ethnic identity and stereotyping of ethnic groups in the multi-cultural context of Hong Kong demonstrates that, as a social process, different ethnic groups —Japanese, British, Vietnamese— are each characteristically stereotyped by the Hong Kong Chinese students participating in the study (Weinreich, Luk, & Bond, 1996).

However, from the perspective of the individual member of an ethnicity, identity formation consists of socio-psychological and developmental *processes* situated within a particular socio-historical context in accordance with the person's biographical experiences. Socio-historical contexts differ greatly in terms of the particular distribution of multiple ethnic groups in a country and the nature of the relationships between the ethnic groups. The historical contexts of economic migrations, of conquest, apartheid ideologies and ethnic cleansing, and of genocide and refugee status will have profound impact on the statuses of the ethnic groups in question.

The aim of the current survey of three studies of ethnic groups located in contrasting socio-historical contexts is to demonstrate that psychological processes of ethnic identity development differ greatly according to such contexts. Important features of the contexts in question include the ambience of different cultural value and belief systems, and the variations on such cultural systems within an ethnicity. *Enculturation* of cultural elements of other salient ethnic groups into one's identity frequently occurs in people's elaboration of their own ethnic identity. By and large, for those from a recognisably distinctive ethnic group, individuals tend not to *acculturate* towards the dominant group. Instead, whilst enculturating features of a salient, often a dominant, group, they maintain their ethnic distinctiveness albeit in modified form.

Each instance of inter-ethnic relationships requires understanding in its own terms, that is, in terms of the history of the interaction between the ethnic groups in question, taking into consideration the variations in the cultural expression of ethnic identity within the ethnicities concerned. The development of a sense of ethnic identity varies according to the identifications that the child initially makes with ethnically salient individuals, which identifications form the underpinnings of subsequent ones, within and across ethnic boundaries, all within specific socio-historical contexts. The specific enculturation of elements of alternative ethnicities, often with modification, varies considerably according to the socio-historical context within which benign, hostile, or ambivalent relationships between ethnic groups evolve. In each case the individual's biographical experiences will be unique, but emerge within the pervasive social context of the era. The illustrative studies presented here refer to the Hong Kong Chinese in Hong Kong prior the transition to the People's Republic (Weinreich, Luk, & Bond, 1996), South African black youth prior to the ending of apartheid (Weinreich, Kelly, & Maja, 1988), and Muslim youth in Britain (Kelly, 1989).

Whatever the particular context, the young child will identify for good or ill with a plethora of role models that are perceived to be powerful and influential. In the first instance, predominant role models will generally be of one's own ethnicity, such as parents and salient others within one's community. Subsequently, others are likely to be significant people of alternative ethnicities, such as teachers, media and political figures, etc. Any one identification made by the child tends not to be an all or none process, but partial: the child identifies only to a degree with others in the community.

Ethnic identity is defined within the Identity Structure Analysis (ISA) conceptual framework. This definition emphasises the continuity between current expressions of ethnicity, in relation to past conceptions of one's ancestry and future aspirations for one's progeny, that is, ethnic identity is situated within changing socio-historical contexts (Weinreich, 1986a). Formally:

One's *ethnic identity* is defined as that part of the totality of one's self-construal made up of those dimensions that express the continuity between one's construal of past ancestry and one's future aspirations in relation to ethnicity.

As a conceptual framework, ISA operationalises concepts pertaining to identity so as to integrate the *qualitative* aspects of identity, such as the discourses associated with specific cultural value and belief systems, with the *quantitative* aspects, such as the degree of empathetic identification with one's family members or people of a different ethnicity (Weinreich, 1980, 1986a,b, 1989a,b). In ISA, *etic* (culturally universal) concepts incorporate *emic* (culturally specific) values and beliefs. Incorporating emic features of ethnic identity constitutes a fundamental prerequisite for research on identity in cross-cultural and multi-cultural settings. In fieldwork, which uses the language and vernacular of the participants to a study, the Identity Exploration (IDEX) computer software (Weinreich, Asquith, Liu and Northover, 1989) facilitates ISA. *Qualitative* aspects of identity, such as the person's discourses on self and others, are integrated within the *quantitative* parameters of identity.

Method

Identity Instruments: Preliminary Ethnographic Work

ISA requires preliminary ethnographic pilot work to be undertaken in order to generate appropriate identity instruments that incorporate beliefs and values expressed in the vernacular of the participants. The theoretical concepts underlying the ISA parameters of identity and the standardisation procedures that provide for etic assessments of these parameters, irrespective of the emic content of the discourses incorporated, are outlined in detail elsewhere (Weinreich, 1980; Weinreich, Luk, & Bond, 1996).

In practice, ethnographic work within the cultural milieu of the study informs the specific content of each instrument. The customised instruments include the individuals, groups and institutions (collectively 'entities') thereby delineated as being salient participants and influential agents impacting on day to day affairs. The ethnographic work also provides the everyday discourses, expressed in the vernacular, used by local people to characterise and appraise the aforementioned salient contributors to community practices. Each instrument incorporates a judicious selection of such discourses, thereby engaging participants to the study with particular immediacy deriving from the instant familiarity with content and context.

Identity Instruments: Mandatory Features
However, each such instrument also incorporates mandatory features, informed by the ISA definition of identity. These represent self as located in a current context (current self), a view of self as being that towards which the person aspires (ideal self), and a memory of self as experienced in a personal biographical past (past self). Other mandatory features consist of two standard anchor individuals, 'an admired person' and 'a disliked person'.

The discourses to be used by the participants are evoked, one at a time, as bipolar constructs heading a page or screen of the identity instrument. A centre-zero scale between the two contrasting construct-poles of discourse enables participants, during their appraisal of self and others, either to deem the contrasting discourses as irrelevant (centre-zero), or to indicate the manner and extent to which the discourses apply. The social world so construed and appraised is represented by the entities that feature down the side of the instrument page or screen, against each of which the participant indicates an appraisal in terms of the discourses.

Analyses: Etic Parameters of Identity and Emic Perspectives
ISA procedures systematically analyse each person's appraisals of self and others, where these appraisals are obtained as described above by means of customised identity instruments. The resultant assessment of the individual's parameters of identity accord with the ISA definitions of psychological concepts pertaining to identity, and incorporate the individual's value and belief system, directly ascertained by reference to the person's aspirational (ideal) self. In this manner, the etic parameters of identity, subject to the standardisation of metrics taking into account individual response-biases, integrate the emic perspective of each participant. The emic characteristics remain manifest. The IDEX computer software conveniently assists the customised construction of identity instruments, obtains individuals appraisals of their social worlds and analyses these appraisals in terms of etic metric parameters, while

explicitly making manifest the emic, largely qualitative, perspectives held by individual participants[1].

The specific instruments used in the three studies from which results are excerpted here are given in the respective publications. Each instrument differs substantially in terms of the salient social worlds represented. The Hong Kong instrument, written in Chinese characters, included ten different ethnic groups. The South African instrument incorporated such relevant institutions as the then South African Government, Homeland Leaders and Town Councillors. Within the British Muslim instrument, the local Mosque and the Asian Society at College featured. In like fashion, the discourses represented in each instrument based on prior ethnographic work differed substantially according to the locality and emic perspectives.

Participants

The participants in the Hong Kong study were 156 ethnically Hong Kong Chinese students, aged from 17 to 22 years, with equal numbers of males and females. The South African study involved 160 Black youth in the Sovenga region, aged 15 to 16, equal numbers being urban or rural. The study of British Muslims was carried out with 40 young people, aged between 16 and 21, from a tertiary education college in Birmingham, and included for comparative purposes comparable Greek Cypriot and indigenous English samples. In all three studies, males and females participated in equal numbers.

Results

Excerpts of results from the three studies deal with contrasting socio-historical relationships between ethnic groups intertwined with cultural variations within the ethnicities. In the case of Hong Kong Chinese University students, Hong Kong as a British colony provides the historical context, one, which proved relatively benign to the development of a

---

1 The principal parameter of identity cited in these studies is empathetic identification, defined as the degree of similarity between the qualities one attributes to the other, whether 'good' or 'bad' and those of one's current self-image. Boolean algebra provides the underlying algebraic basis for computing empathetic identification, thereby retaining the discrete emic characteristics of individual perspectives, while deriving etic metrics. Identity diffusion is assessed as the magnitude and dispersion of identification conflicts with others.

Hong Kong Chinese ethnicity. Hong Kong Chinese cultural values predominate, but with partial degrees of identification with salient alternative ethnicities, thereby demonstrating variations in the expression of Hong Kong Chinese ethnicity. Partial identifications with various other ethnicities reflect differing kinds and degrees of enculturation of characteristics that are more typical of other ethnic groups within people's identities. These variations are related to students' identifications across generations and have ramifications for the students' self-evaluation and identity diffusion.

However, whether or not the students appraised themselves in different social contexts, interacting with their own kind or with Britons, was not examined in this study. The entities *me when I am with Hong Kong Chinese people* and *me when I am with British people* were not included in the Hong Kong identity instrument. Only the general socio-historical context of the then colony featured.

In the cases of the other two studies of South African black youth and the Muslim youth in Britain, the situated contexts were specifically included in the respective identity instruments. For the South African black youth, the entities *Me as I am with Afrikaners* and *Me as I am with the English* were included in the South African instrument. The British Muslim instrument included entities designating self with own group and self with the English. In other respects, the identity instruments used in these studies each conformed to the essential properties of ISA instrument construction (the characteristics of which are conveniently implemented by way of the IDEX computer software).

Enculturation in Hong Kong Students: Self-Esteem and Identity Diffusion

Using ISA, the earlier mentioned study of Hong Kong Chinese students in the multi-cultural context of Hong Kong demonstrates variations in the expression of Hong Kong Chinese ethnicity. ISA assesses degrees of empathetic identification with various people, in this case of one's own and alternative ethnicities. The findings are instructive since, while all of the students in the study recognise themselves as Hong Kong Chinese in ethnicity and ethnic identity, they express this ethnicity in rather different ways. The students identify with the various ethnic groupings that impinge on their daily lives in Hong Kong to a greater or lesser extent. The study investigates the relationship between their degrees of identification with one or other ethnic grouping[2] and their identification with

---

2 Preliminary cluster analyses of the students' stereotypical perceptions of the multiple ethnic groups impinging upon Hong Kong indicated that the following clusters were differentiated one from another: HK: Hong Kong

Table 1. *Correlation Coefficients between the Hong Kong Students'*
Empathetic Identification with Alternative Ethnic Groupings, and Their:
Parental and Peer Identifcation; Self-Esteem; and Identity Diffusion (N =
156) (excerpted from: Weinreich, Luk, & Bond (1996)

	Empathetic identification with				Self-esteem	Identity diffusion
	Father	Mother	Best friend	College student		
Empathetic identification with[a]						
HK	0.25*	0.32*	0.35*	0.50*	0.30*	0.11
WEST	0.18	0.14	0.47	0.61*	0.51*	-0.12
TC	0.20	0.28*	0.04	0.08	-0.11	0.26*
OR	0.36*	0.36*	0.26*	0.31*	0.08	0.26*
DE	0.02	0.06	-0.26	-0.15	-0.38*	0.63*

*$p < 0.01$.
[a] Where relevant for an ethnic grouping, the values entered into the analyses for the 156 respondents are based on the avarage of each individual's identification with the ethnic targets within an ethnic grouping.
HK   Hong Kong Chinese
WEST   Western grouping of British, American, and American-born Chinese
TC   traditional Chinese
OR   oriental grouping of Taiwanese and Japanese
DE   developing grouping of Guangzhou citizens, Filipinos and Vietnamese boatpeople

peers and parents (Table 1).

The closer the students identify with the mainstream Hong Kong people, the more they identify with both peers (best friend and college student) and parents, but with a greater emphasis on peers. There is inter-

Chinese; WEST: western grouping of British, American, and American-born Chinese; TC: traditional Chinese; OR: oriental grouping of Taiwanese and Japanese; DE: developing grouping of Guangzhou citizens (Republic of China), Filipinos and Vietnamese boatpeople

generational continuity, but peer identification dominates to some extent. The more they identify with the modern Orientals (Taiwanese and Japanese), again the closer they identify with both peers and parents, but with the emphasis on parents. Inter-generational identification is evident, but in this case, their identification with parents dominates somewhat.

Albeit with differing emphases, continuity of identification across generations features for students' closer empathetic identification with both mainstream Hong Kong people and modern Orientals. However, inter-generational discontinuities represent yet other patterns of identification with alternative ethnicities. Thus, students' greater identification with the western grouping of British, American and American-born Chinese, correlates only with closer identification with peers and *not* with parents. By contrast, their closer identification with the traditional Chinese correlates with parental, that is, maternal, identification only. Finally, but not least, closer identification with the developing grouping that includes the mainland Chinese along with Filipinos and Vietnamese boatpeople is accompanied by tendencies toward an alienated state of identity indicated in part by a negative correlation with identification with best friend.

In each instance, the findings of partial identification with other salient ethnic groupings demonstrate that differing features of the alternative ethnicities are to an extent enculturated by the students, who all maintain their Hong Kong Chinese distinctiveness. The variety of generational continuities and discontinuities in terms of just what features of alternative ethnicities are incorporated points to the complexity of relationships between generations in conjunction with the "influences" of other proximate ethnic groups. Much ongoing debate between Hong Kongers over what constitutes Hong Kong ethnicity will be apparent.

The differing patterns of partial identification with alternative ethnicities in Hong Kong have ramifications for individuals' *self-esteem* and *identity diffusion*, the latter corresponding to the degree to which the person's identifications with others are conflicted. Closer empathetic identification with both the western grouping and with the Hong Kong Chinese is associated with higher self-esteem. Closer identification with both the Oriental grouping and the traditional Chinese is correlated with identity diffusion. In respect of the developing grouping associated with the Mainland Chinese, students' greater identification with them is accompanied by lower self-esteem and greater identity diffusion, that is, increasingly towards identity crisis.

The Hong Kong study demonstrates variations in the expression of Hong Kong ethnic identity and how these are related to inter-generational continuities or discontinuities. Greater out-group identification does not necessarily diminish self-evaluation, if the out-group is an esteemed one (the westernised grouping of British, Americans, and westernised Chinese). Identity diffusion is demonstrated to be a different parameter of identity, largely unrelated to that of self-esteem, and in this context associated with conflicted identifications with aspects of oriental and traditional Chinese cultures.

Enculturation in South African Black Youth: Situated Contexts and Vulnerable Identities

The next study focuses more on the variation in expression of identity, when the person is situated with one ethnic group or another. Patterns of in- and out-group identification become modulated according to the immediate social context, but within the larger specific socio-historical context.

While the socio-historical context of Hong Kong at this time was relatively benign for the student sample, though with ominous implications when Hong Kong would return to the Republic of China, that of South Africa with the legacy of apartheid was psychologically deeply fraught. A study of Black youth in South Africa indicated somewhat differing patterns of identification in urban and rural youth. More importantly, however, was a major modulation in these identification patterns depending on the alternative social contexts of free-standing self, being with the English, and being with Afrikaners (Weinreich, Kelly, & Maja, 1988). The black youth manifested very different *situated* identity states.

In the presence of Afrikaners they identify with Afrikanerdom to a greater extent than when they are in the other contexts, but their identifications with Afrikaners are highly conflicted (op. cit.). When together with the English-speaking South Africans they identify more with them. However, free-standing, they empathetically identify closely with their own group, their families and friends, but their identifications in this context also cross ethnic boundaries, particularly with the English.

In this study, the socio-historical context is one of violent subjugation, such that the black youth's enculturation of despised elements of Afrikanerdom and English-speaking white South Africa, obtrude in a disturbing manner when activated in the respective social contexts. Thus, in general terms, they are without major identity vulnerability when with their own kind (Table 2). However, when cued into the Afrikaner context their identity state tends to become very vulnerable, with generally very low self-evaluation and high identity diffusion. Their greater vulnerability is also evident when cued into the English-speaking context, though to a much less pronounced effect.

By contrast with the case of the Hong Kong students who more closely identified with the highly regarded western grouping (of British,

Table 2. *Situated Identities of South African Black Youth (N = 160);*
Vulnerability According to Social Contact (excerpted from: Weinreich, Kelly, &
Maja, 1988)

Identity state	Social context		
	"Natural"; me as I am now	English: me as I am with the English	Afrikaner: me as I am with the Afrikaners
"Well adjusted"	50.6%	34.6%	15.5%
"Very vulnerable"	7.5%	35.9%	71.0%

American and westernised Chinese), black youth's greater identification
with the despised Afrikaner context, greatly diminishes their self-
evaluation and increases their identity diffusion. When situated within the
less despised English-speaking context, black youth's greater identification with the more favoured English-speaking South Africans is accompanied by a moderate diminution of self-evaluation and increase in
identity diffusion.

**Enculturation in Muslim Youth in Britain: Distinctive Cultural
Orientations within Islam**
In a relatively benign historical context, the Hong Kong study concen-
trated on variations in the expressions of ethnic identity in relation to
different degrees of identification with various salient alternative ethnic
groupings, ranging from oriental to western. In a historically violent and
fraught context, the South African study focussed more on the contrasting
social contexts for the expression of identity and the modulation of
patterns of identification with salient others according to context, being
free-standing, situated with Afrikanerdom, or situated with English-
speaking South Africa.

The next study referred to here, which is of British Muslim youth in a
historical context of some ambivalence, attends to two distinctive cultural
orientations within Islam expressed by these youth. The official avowed
ideology of the British State promotes multi-culturalism, regard for
cultural difference, equality of opportunity, and full civil rights. Racial
discrimination against ethnic groups is legally an offence. However,
relationships between the Muslims in Britain and Anglo-Saxons vary
considerably according to locality and during periods of high profile
events, such as the declaration of the fatwa on Salman Rushdie. The

study focuses on expressions of Muslim identity in youth according to their distinctively different cultural orientations in a historical context of some ambivalence.

With Pakistani Muslim youth in Britain, located in Birmingham, two major expressions of ethnic identity are delineated: *'progressive'* and *'orthodox'* in terms of the strictness of their orientation towards the opposite sex (Kelly, 1989). There are strong gender variations in the expression of both the 'progressive' and 'orthodox' orientations. Progressive young Muslim women show the greatest adaptability in their identifications when with the English or with their own group (op. cit.). Progressive young Muslim men also show adaptability, whereas orthodox young Muslim women demonstrate an unchanging state of identity, whether with the English or their own group. Orthodox young Muslim men are more vulnerable with the English compared with being with their own kind.

Depending on orientation, so do the young Muslim men and women identify with the other (Anglo-Saxon) ethnicity to a greater or less extent (Table 3). In this study the 'progressive' Muslim young women empathetically identify the closest with Anglo-Saxons (0.71 same sex; 0.65 opposite sex), while their 'orthodox' counterparts do so the least (0.31 same sex; 0.28 opposite sex). The disparity between the women of the two orientations is further emphasised by their empathetic identification with their own group ('progressive' 0.53 same sex, 0.58 opposite sex; 'orthodox' 0.89 same sex, 0.96 opposite sex). Both 'progressive' and 'orthodox' Muslim young men empathetically identify moderately with Anglo-Saxons ('progressive' 0.53 same sex, 0.59 opposite sex; 'orthodox' 0.63 same sex, 0.53 opposite sex). Though the 'orthodox' men empathetically identify with their own group more than do their 'progressive' counterparts, they do not do so to the great extent that the 'orthodox' young women do ('progressive' 0.56 same sex, 0.53 opposite sex; 'orthodox' 0.72 same sex, 0.70 opposite sex). Radically differing patterns of in-group and out-group identification, and modulations of them across ethnic contexts (op. cit.), distinguish the two cultural orientations, but in an asymmetrical manner according to gender.

These findings show that the particular elements of Anglo-Saxon culture enculturated in modified form by the Muslim males and females, differ according to both cultural orientation ('progressive' versus 'orthodox') and gender. The ambivalence of British/Islamic relationships in the current socio-historical era has a counterpart in two features emerging from the study. The first is the adaptability of those of 'progressive' orientation in terms of being situated with Anglo-Saxons or their own group, especially in females. The other is the high self-regard

Table 3. Muslim Youth's Current Empathetic Identification (excerpted from: Kelly, 1989)

	Muslim male		Muslim female	
	"Progress" $(N = 12)$	"Orthod" $(N = 8)$	"Progress" $(N = 12)$	"Orthod" $(N = 6)$
Own group, same sex	0.53	0.89	0.56	0.72
Own group, opposite sex	0.58	0.96	0.53	0.70
Other group, same sex	0.71	0.31	0.53	0.63
Other group, opposite sex	0.65	0.28	0.59	0.53

Progress = Progressive; Orthod = Orthodox.

and focussed identification of those who manifest the 'orthodox' orientation on the other hand, again especially in females.

Conclusion

Collectively, these results demonstrate that ethnic identity is expressed very differently according to socio-historical context (Chinese students in Hong Kong, Black youth in South Africa, and Pakistani Muslim youth in Britain). In each case, individuals identify to varying degrees with *elements* of other cultures, without however loosing their own distinctive sense of ethnicity with their own characteristic ethnic dimensions of identity. *Enculturation*, identifying with or adopting elements of an alternative culture, is a partial and varying process. This process, by means of which one's ethnic identity is *redefined* for contemporary times through the adoption of certain elements of an alternative culture, is to be distinguished from the process of *acculturation*, or identity redefinition towards the dominant culture (see Berry, Kim, Minde, & Mok, 1987; Berry, Trimble, & Olmeda, 1986).

In enculturation, individuals maintain conceptions of their distinctive ethnic identity, which include aspects that are newly created and uniquely novel. Individuals generate these novel features consequent upon grappling with synthesising enculturated elements with existing values and beliefs, and giving them new meanings within their continually evolving sense of identity. Within an ethnic group variations in the expression of an ethnic identity, in part influenced by elements of identification with alternative cultures, will provide points of departure for internal debate within an ethnic community as well as debates over the position of subordinate groups in relation to the dominant ones.

The findings of these studies also demonstrate that the orthodox notions of in-group and out-group identification have rather limited application. Such notions do not take account of the social realities of varying degrees of cross-ethnic identification, the situated contexts of modulations in these identifications, the differences in cultural orientation within an ethnicity, and the general historical contexts within which children initially identify with significant others and later with different others. Features of identity such as self-evaluation and identity diffusion can only be understood in terms of analyses of the history of inter-ethnic relations, ethnographic considerations of cultural orientations, and the current contexts of being situated with one or another ethnic group.

References

Berry, J., Kim, U., Minde, T., & Mok, D. (1987). Comparative studies of acculturative stress. *International Migration Review, 21,* 491-511.

Berry, J., Trimble, J., & Olmeda, E. (1986) Assessment of acculturation. In W. Lonner & J. Berry (Eds.), *Field methods in cross-cultural research*. Newbury Park, CA: Sage.

Kelly, A. J. D. (1989). Ethnic identification, association and redefinition: Muslim Pakistanis and Greek Cypriots in Britain. In K. Liebkind (Ed.), *New identities in Europe: Immigrant ancestry and the ethnic identity of youth*. London: Gower.

Weinreich, P. (1980). *Manual for identity exploration using personal constructs* (Reprinted 1986 and 1988). Coventry: University of Warwick/Economic and Social Research Council. Centre for Research in Ethnic Relations.

Weinreich, P. (1986a). The operationalisation of identity theory in racial and ethnic relations. In J. Rex & D. Mason (Eds.), *Theories of race and ethnic relations*. Cambridge: Cambridge University Press.

Weinreich, P. (1986b). Identity development in migrant offspring: Theory and practice. In L. H. Ekstrand (Ed.), *Ethnic minorities and immigrants in a cross-cultural perspective*. Lisse, the Netherlands: Swets & Zeitlinger.

Weinreich, P. (1989a). Variations in ethnic identity: Identity Structure Analysis. In K. Liebkind (Ed.), *New identities in Europe: Immigrant ancestry and the ethnic identity of youth*. London: Gower.

Weinreich, P. (1989b). Conflicted identifications: A commentary on Identity Structure Analysis concepts. In K. Liebkind (Ed.), *New identities in Europe: Immigrant ancestry and the ethnic identity of youth*. London: Gower.

Weinreich, P., Asquith, L., Liu, W., & Northover, M. (1989). *IDEX-PC* (identity exploration-pc) computer software, (IBM-PC compatible) and *User-guide* (Weinreich, P., Northover, M., & McCready, F.) Jordanstown: University of Ulster.

Weinreich, P., Kelly, A. J. D., & Maja, C. (1988). Black youth in South Africa: Situated identities and patterns of ethnic identification. In D. Canter, C. Jesuino, L. Soczka, & G. Stephenson (Eds.), *Environmental social psychology*. Dordrecht: Kluwer Academic.

Weinreich, P., Luk, C. L., & Bond, M. H. (1996). Ethnic stereotyping and identification in a multicultural context: "Acculturation", self-esteem and identity diffusion in Hong Kong Chinese university students. *Psychology and Developing Societies, 8*, 107-169.

Personality and Social Behavior across Cultures

Exploring Indigenous Spanish Personality Constructs with a Combined Emic-Etic Approach

Verónica Benet-Martínez
University of Michigan, USA

ABSTRACT

The present study identified indigenous Spanish personality constructs using a combined emic-etic approach. Factor analyses of self-ratings on indigenous Spanish personality adjectives yielded a seven-factor solution that closely resembled the North American Big Seven factor model. Culture-specific elements of the seven indigenous Spanish personality dimensions were: (a) the organization of affect in terms of hedonic valence and intensity (rather than the Extroversion and Neuroticism dimensions usually found in English); and (b) the emphasis on worldliness and spirituality in the Conventionality dimension. Correspondence between the seven indigenous Spanish personality constructs and imported (i.e., Spanish-translated) Big Seven and Big Five personality structures was assessed via correlational, and joint exploratory and confirmatory factor analyses. These analyses revealed that, at a broad level of analysis, seven common latent personality factors representing the Big Seven structure best capture variance shared by the indigenous and imported personality scales. Findings from this study underscore both the cross-cultural applicability of the Big Seven factor model in Spanish at a broad level *and* the cultural specificity of its affective components at a narrower level.

Researchers from many countries have relied on the natural language when developing taxonomies of personality (see Katigbak, Church, & Akamine, 1996, for a review). Numerous English-language lexical studies (see McCrae & John, 1992, for a review) have replicated a five-factor structure, the so-called 'Big Five' model of personality (Goldberg, 1981), which is said to encompass most of the covariation among personality-descriptors used in personality ratings. Common labels for these five dimensions are: I. Extraversion, II. Agreeableness, III. Conscientiousness, IV. Neuroticism or Emotional Stability, and V. Openness to Experience or Intellect. The replicability and ubiquity of the Big Five, also known as the Five Factor Model (McCrae & Costa, 1987), have led many personality psychologists to adopt this model as the basic paradigm for the description and assessment of personality (McCrae & John, 1992).

One of the various theoretical and methodological limitations attributed to the Big Five (see Block, 1995, for a review) concerns the adequacy of the model to fully represent the personality domain (Benet & Waller, 1995; Block, 1995; Tellegen, 1993; Waller, in press). That is, the Big Five was originally developed from a pool of personality-relevant terms that *excluded evaluative terms and many state-mood descriptors* (Allport & Odbert, 1936; Cattell, 1943; Norman, 1967) on the grounds that these terms do not refer to personality at all. This exclusion —based on traditional definitions of personality that overemphasized the enduring, "trait-like" elements of personality and shied away from "moral judgments" (Pervin, 1990)— is at odds with contemporary views of personality, many of which now recognize state-mood dispositions and evaluation as important components of personality (Borkenau, 1990; Hogan, 1982; Tellegen, 1985).

Avoiding such *a priori* exclusion criteria, Tellegen and Waller (1987) conducted an independent exploration of the English personality lexicon that did not exclude mood-related and evaluative terms and identified seven higher-order dimensions. Of these 'Big Seven' orthogonal factors, two were highly evaluative: Positive Valence and Negative Valence. Examples of the kinds of terms that load on these dimensions are: *excellent, special, impressive, skilled* (Positive Valence), and *wicked, awful, disgusting, immoral* (Negative Valence). The other five dimensions (Positive Emotionality, Negative Emotionality, Conscientiousness, Agreeableness, and Conventionality) clearly resemble the Big Five's dimensions of Extroversion, Neuroticism, Conscientiousness, Agreeableness, and Openness, respectively[1].

Just as importantly, Tellegen and Waller's (1987) non-restrictive selection criteria allowed emotion-laden descriptors (e.g., *peppy, spirited, jumpy, jittery*) to emerge in the Big Seven factor structure. This inclusion provided the Positive and Negative Emotionality dimensions with affective components that are not well represented in the Big Five's dimensions of Extroversion and Neuroticism. The use of a non-restrictive criterion in the selection of descriptors broadened the resulting lexical dimensions of personality in one more way. It allowed evaluative terms —such as *peculiar, odd,* and *unusual*— to emerge in the negative pole of the Big Seven's Conventionality dimension, next to other terms denoting progressive political-social attitudes and intellectual curiosity (i.e., Openness).

---

1 For labels and examples of marker items for each of the Big Seven dimensions see Table 1 in Benet & Waller (1995).

The Positive and Negative Valence dimensions apply to components of self-evaluation that are not represented in previous lexical models. As such, Positive and Negative Valence might prove to be useful for understanding Axis II personality disorders (American Psychiatric Association, 1994) such as narcissism (which involves a grandiose sense of self-importance), borderline personality (which involves alternation of extreme overidealization and devaluation of the self), or avoidant personality (which involves social discomfort and fear of negative evaluation by others). The psychological significance of Positive and Negative Valence is also supported by recent multidimensional models of self-esteem and self-concept (O'Brien & Epstein, 1988; Roid & Fitts, 1988), which include two dimensions representing 'personal power' and 'moral self-approval,' constructs that can be conceptually linked to Positive and Negative Valence, respectively.

Replications of the Big Seven have been obtained across samples, targets, and languages (Almagor, Tellegen, & Waller, 1995; Benet & Waller, 1995; Waller, in press; Waller & Zavala, 1993) using the Inventory of Personal Characteristics (IPC7; Tellegen, Grove, & Waller, 1991), a provisional 161-item measure of the Big Seven. Furthermore, the Big Seven have shown optimal levels of convergent and discriminant validity across different instruments and observers (Benet & Waller, 1996).

To summarize, the Big Seven is a dimensional model of personality that, while related to the Big Five, differs from it and challenges its comprehensiveness. Essentially, the Big Seven incorporates within the personality domain two large evaluative dimensions which were prevented from appearing in previous lexical studies due to the use of an overly restrictive selection criteria. The two evaluative dimensions, Positive and Negative Valence, comprise central, organizing aspects of personality functioning related to self-perceptions of worth.

Cross-Cultural Generality of the Big Seven Factor Model

In trying to assess the cross-cultural generality of dimensional models of personality, researchers have traditionally relied on two different kinds of approaches: (a) 'imposed-etic' approaches, which rely on translated personality instruments and allow answering questions related to the cross-cultural *psychometric applicability* of a particular inventory; and (b) 'emic' approaches, which involve the use of 'indigenous' personality taxonomies and allow answering questions related to the cross-cultural *validity* of a particular personality model or theory.

With the goal of first exploring the psychometric applicability of Big Seven instruments in Spanish, and thus using an 'imposed-etic' approach, Benet and Waller (1995) administered Spanish versions of Big Seven

(IPC-7; Tellegen et al., 1991) and Big Five (BFI; John, Donahue, & Kentle, 1991) questionnaires to a large sample of native Spanish-speakers from Spain. The results from this study revealed remarkable similarities between the Big Seven factor structure obtained from the Spanish sample and the American Big Seven, across both self and observer data. Benet and Waller's (1995) findings also revealed, however, some psychologically meaningful item-level differences between the American and Spanish Big Seven solutions.

Benet and Waller's (1995) study supported the robustness of the Big Seven structure in an additional way. Specifically, factor structures recovered from joint factor analyses of the Big Seven and Big Five questionnaires depicted Positive and Negative Valence factors that were defined exclusively by Big Seven items. These latter results provided strong evidence for the cogency of Positive and Negative Valence as psychologically differentiated personality factors that cannot be captured by the Five Factor Model.

Benet and Waller's use of translated forms of the Big Seven and Big Five questionnaires optimally served to address the main goal of their study: assessing the robustness of the American Big Seven in the Spanish language. However, because Benet and Waller's study used an imposed-etic approach, it is not clear whether the results obtained in their study prove that the Big Seven dimensions best represent the actual structure of the Spanish personality lexicon or merely that American Big Seven markers can be translated into Spanish and still retain their structure. Such issue can only be addressed by taking an 'emic' approach, that is, by identifying the basic dimensions of personality in Spanish from a pool of 'indigenous' personality descriptors. With that goal in mind, the present study applied a combined emic-etic approach (Hui & Triandis, 1985), with the goal of not only exploring the intrinsic structure of personality description in Spanish, but also comparing this structure to the American Big Seven factor model.

The use of a combined emic-etic approach in the present study entailed: (a) uncovering the emic (indigenous) dimensions that organize the Spanish personality lexicon from a representative pool of Spanish personality descriptors; (b) uncovering the imposed-etic (imported) dimensions underlying translated versions of Big Seven and Big Five inventories, and (c) assessing the amount of content overlap/specificity between the uncovered imported and indigenous dimensions.

Method

Subjects and Procedure

A sample of 894 native residents of Spain, 185 men and 709 women, participated in this study. The mean age of the sample was 21.24 years (*SD* = 3.91). Participants were psychology, economics, law, or education undergraduate students attending day or evening courses at the Universitat Autònoma de Barcelona (a large public university in Spain). Questionnaires were administered to subjects in group during class. Participation was voluntary and anonymous.

Instruments

All subjects provided self-reports on: (a) a personality-descriptor list extracted from an unabridged Spanish dictionary, (b) a Spanish-translated version of the Inventory of Personality Characteristics (IPC-7; Tellegen et al., 1991), and (c) a Spanish-translated version of the Big Five Inventory (BFI; John et al., 1991).

The Spanish personality descriptor list. This list included 299 personality adjectives selected from the widely used, unabridged Spanish dictionary Diccionario Manual e Ilustrado de la Real Academia de la Lengua Española (Real Academia Española, 1989). Descriptors for this list were culled in the following way: Every fourth page of the 1,666-page Spanish dictionary was carefully inspected to identify the presence of personality-descriptive adjectives. The first descriptor found on each fourth page was included in the list. When no personality descriptors were found on the selected page, the next fourth page was examined. A team of two expert judges (a Ph.D. in Spanish and the author, a native Spanish speaker) carried out the descriptor selection. Following Tellegen and Waller's (1987) method, we considered as personality-relevant those adjectives that could be: (a) used to distinguish the behavior, thoughts, or feelings of one human being from those of another, and (b) meaningfully inserted into one or both of the following sentences: Tends to be X, or, Is often X. No exclusion-criteria were applied to evaluative or state descriptors. We did, however, avoid non-distinctive terms that could apply to all individuals, such as terms referring to geographic origin, nationality, profession, social role, relationships, or physical qualities (see Angleitner, Ostendorf, & John, 1990, for similar criterion).

A total of 299 indigenous personality adjectives representative of the entire Spanish natural language of personality were identified. These 299 terms were assembled in random order in a research questionnaire. A 5-point scale response format was applied. To enhance the definitional clarity of the descriptors, each term was followed by a synonym or short definition. The complete list of 299 Spanish personality-descriptors is available from the author.

The Inventory of Personality Characteristics (IPC-7; Tellegen et al., 1991): This inventory is a 161-item measure of the Big Seven factor model of personality that was developed from previous lexical work with American-English personality descriptors (Tellegen & Waller, 1987). In order to simplify the analyses, the 10 best markers of each factor from a previous analysis of the IPC-7 (Waller, in press) were selected for the present study. Thus a 70-item (rather than a 161-item) Big Seven questionnaire was administered.

The Big Five Inventory (BFI; John et al., 1991): This inventory is a 44-item measure of the Big Five factor model that was developed from the Adjective Check List (ACL; Gough & Heilbrun, 1983). The 44 ACL adjectives that form the core of each of the BFI items have been shown in previous studies (John, 1990) to be univocal, prototypical markers of the Big Five dimensions: Extraversion, Neuroticism, Agreeableness, Conscientiousness, and Openness.

Spanish translations of IPC-7 and BFI: The back-translation (Brislin, 1980) method was employed. A detailed description of the procedure is included in Benet and Waller (1995). The complete list of IPC-7 and BFI items, along with their Spanish translations, is available from the author.

Results

Factor Analyses
A principal axis factor analysis followed by Varimax rotation was used to examine the structure of ratings on the 299 indigenous personality descriptors. The goal of this first analysis was to uncover the basic indigenous dimensions that define the Spanish natural language of personality description, so that these dimensions could be later compared to the imported dimensions obtained from the Spanish-translated Big Seven and Big Five questionnaires.

The scree plot of the eigenvalues suggested that a solution of between six and eight factors could optimally account for the primary sources variance. The first ten eigenvalues from the 299 x 299 interitem Pearson correlation matrix were: 24.17, 16.18, 8.55, 5.90, 5.37, 4.99, 4.29, 3.51, 3.19, 2.95. These values show moderate breaks after the fifth and seventh latent roots, indicating that five- and seven-factor solutions are highly plausible. Accordingly, the psychological meaningfulness of

Varimax rotated five, six, seven, and eight-factor solutions was examined[2].

This inspection revealed that a seven-factor solution yields the most appropriate structure for these data and that this solution, with some variations, represents the Big Seven. The adequacy of the seven factor solution was also supported by a parallel analysis (see Horn, 1965), which compared the empirically obtained eigenvalues with eigenvalues generated from a Monte Carlo simulation of the data. Given the large size of the Spanish sample, three Monte Carlo runs proved to be highly consistent and showed that the first seven factors had eigenvalues exceeding that of the largest of the random factors. The primary markers of the seven-factor solution with factor loadings $\geq$ .30 are shown in Table 1, which shows abbreviated English-translations of the original Spanish terms[3].

A comparison of the seven-factor structure depicted in Table 1 with Tellegen and Waller's American-English Big Seven structure (see Table 1 Benet & Waller, 1995) reveals that, with the exception of Positive and Negative Emotionality, the major features of the Big Seven are clearly represented in the Spanish structure. Corroborating Tellegen and Waller's (1987) previous findings on the natural organization of the English personality lexicon, two large evaluative factor emerged in the present solution as independent dimensions representing positive and negative aspects of self-evaluation. Arguably, there is an almost complete conceptual overlap between these two indigenous Spanish evaluative dimensions and Tellegen and Waller's Positive and Negative Valence dimensions. The Spanish Positive Valence dimension, for instance, appears as a large bipolar dimension primarily defined by descriptors

---

2 Alternative five-, six-, and eight-factor solutions failed to show adequate levels of interpretability and theoretical interest. In the five-factor solution, for example, Factor I was a large factor combining Positive Valence and descriptors representing different levels of affect hedonic value and activation. Factor II represented Conscientiousness, and Factors III, IV, and V represented Agreeableness, Negative Valence, and Conventionality respectively. The six-factor solution differed from the previous solution only in that Positive Valence represented an independent dimension. The eight-factor solution depicted an additional dimension represented by descriptors denoting different levels of talkativeness/quietness (e.g., chattering, gossiping, private, asocial).

3 For the sake of space, the original Spanish personality terms and the factor cross-loadings (this factor analysis included 1477 loadings) are not included in Table 1. These terms and the complete factor analysis are available from the author upon request.

Table 1. Primary Factor Loadings for the Indigenous Spanish Personality Dimensions (Decimal Points Omitted)

Positive valence

Amazing, 62
Superior, 58
Formidable, 56
Resplendent, 56
Admirable, 55
Brilliant, 52
Delightful, 52
Exemplary, 50
Marvelous, 48
Super, 48
Appetizing, 47
Radiant, 45
Supernatural, 43
Striking, 40
Astounding, 39
Pleasurable, 39
Favorite, 39
Arrogant, 35
Powerful, 35
Ostentatious, 32
Sloppy, -30
Lumbering, -30
Faulty, -30
Ordinary, -30
Clumsy, -34
Not special, -35
Secondary, -37
Mediocre, -40

Negative valence

Sickening, 43
Worn out, 41
Terrifying, 41
Filthy, 41
Greasy, 39
Cruel, 39
Wicked, 38
Vandalic, 38
Horrible, 36
Idiotic, 36
Harmful, 35
Wearing, 33
Coarse, 30
Unimportant, 30

Pleasantness

Shrewd, 56
Cheerful, 54
Reveling, 53
Independent, 52
Active, 50
Comical, 48
Mischievous, 48
Charming, 47
Fond of parties, 46
Jocose, 46
Cunning, 45
Shameless, 44
Sidespitting, 42
Dynamic, 42
Prankish, 42
Great, 41
Spontaneous, 40
Noisy, 39
Rascally, 38
Moves constantly, 38
Alert, 38
Friendly, 38
Wily, 38
Funny, 37
Dialectical, 36
Direct, 36
Likes traveling, 36
Perspicacious, 34
Challenging, 33
Liberal, 32
Fearless, 31
Fast, 31
Fed up, -30
Inexperienced, -30
Feels used, -30
Impressionable, -31
Of few words, -31
Chaste, -31
Softy, -31
Dumb, -33
Feels guilty, -33
Retiring, -34
Worried, -35
Withdrawn, -43
Stereotyped, -43
Distressed, -44
Sluggish, -46
Somber, -47
Asocial, -48
Bashful, -49
Discouraged, -49
Blushing, -49
Isolated, -53
Languid, -53
Dull, -54
Gloomy, -56
Shy, -58

Table 1. Primary Factor Loadings for the Indigenous Spanish Personality Dimensions (continued)

Engagement
Ardent, 43
Impulsive, 37
Seething, 36
Intense, 35
Fervent, 34
Heated, 34
Anxious, 33
Passionate, 30
Idle, -30
Lazy, -36
Unemotional, 37

Conscientiousness
Stable, 64
Moderate, 54
Reasonable, 53
Tranquil, 52
Reflective, 50
Proper, 49
Orderly, 47
Sensible, 45
Relaxed, 45
Patient, 44

Versatile, 43
Traditional, 41
Uncomplicated, 40
Family-oriented, 40
Natural, 39
Home-body, 39
Trustworthy, 39
Honest, 38
Frank, 37
Able to concentrate, 37
Thrifty, 37
Objective, 37

Courteous, 37
Punctual, 35
Convential, 34
Gentle, 33
Early-rising, 32
Capable, 32
Doesn't panic, 31
Skillful, 31
Reputable, 30
Trouble-maker, -30
Embroiling, -31

Entangled, -31
Wasteful, -33
Exaggerated, -33
Undisciplined, -34
Unmoderate, -35
Fickle, -38
Lunatic, -39
Contradicting, -40
Nonsensical, -42
Hasty, -42
Reckless, -43
Crazy, -49

Agreeableness
Easy-going, 54
Good-natured, 49
Docile, 46
Affectionate, 44
Manageable, 43
Loving, 40
Agreeable, 39
Naïve, 38
Kind, 36
Warm, 36

Servile, 35
Flexible, 32
Honeyed, 30
Disagreeable, -30
Rude, -30
Proud, -32
Rejecting, -32
Obstinate, -33
Attacking, -34
Quarrelsome, -39
Antagonistic, -39
Pigheaded, -40
Glowering, -40
Irascible, -41
Tyrannical, -41
Headstrong, -42
Stubborn, -43
Inflexible, -43
Vindictive, -43
Drastic, -44
Stormy, -45
Unreconciling, -47
Unyielding, -48

Conventionality
Chattering, 38
Gossiping, 36
Disclosing, 34
Nosy, 30
Inventive, -32
Creative, -36
Bizarre, -36
Spiritual, -37
Bohemian, -38
Mystical, -40
Strange, -41
Quaint, -42

denoting perceptions of personal worth and uniqueness. Representative markers of this dimension include: *superior, admirable, formidable,* versus *not special, mediocre,* and *ordinary* — terms which also serve as markers of Positive Valence in the American Big Seven. The Spanish Negative Valence dimension is unipolar and primarily defined by terms denoting perceptions of depravity (e.g., *sickening, cruel, wicked, harmful*), which are also markers of Negative Valence in the American Big Seven.

Two independent affect dimensions including numerous state-emotion terms as primary markers are also recognizable in the current Spanish seven-factor structure. A closer look at these two factors reveals that, rather than representing Big Seven's Positive and Negative Emotionality dimensions, these factors delineate a different organization of affect. Specifically, they seem to represent the hedonic tone and intensity qualities of affective experience, and thus portray a structural model very similar to the Pleasure-Displeasure and Arousal-Sleepiness two-dimensional structure included in the circumplex model of emotion (Larsen & Diener, 1992; Russell, 1980). The emergence of these two dimensions (which I labeled as Pleasantness and Engagement) is quite unexpected given the large body of evidence from the questionnaire and lexical traditions supporting Positive and Negative Emotionality as the major affect-based personality dimensions (Tellegen & Waller, in press; Watson & Tellegen, 1985; see also Larsen & Diener, 1992, for a review).

The Pleasantness dimension appears as a large factor representing a wide range of pleasurable and unpleasurable affective states and traits; the positive pole of this dimension contains numerous terms related to the experience of pleasurable affects such as joy (e.g., *cheerful, charming, comical, great*), energy (e.g., *active, dynamic, flitting*), sociability (e.g., *reveling, fond of parties, friendly*), and self-assurance (e.g., *independent, shameless, challenging*). Noteworthy is the absence of terms denoting pleasant disengagement (e.g., relaxed, calm), which appear instead as markers of Conscientiousness (e.g., *stable, tranquil, relaxed*). Another psychologically meaningful peculiarity of the Pleasantness pole is the presence of various descriptors denoting social and intellectual craftiness (e.g., *prankish, rascally, wily, cunning, shrewd, perspicacious*). This association between pleasurable affect and social and intellectual craftiness might be due to differences (relative to the American culture) in the social value given to these attributes. Accordingly, one could speculate that for Spaniards these attributes are highly instrumental in that they foster culturally-valued interpersonal and achievement-related successes (e.g., persuasive charm, foreseeing of opportunity), which, in turn, enhance pleasurable affect. Opposite to the Pleasantness pole are numerous state-emotion terms denoting both unpleasant engagement (e.g., *distressed, confused, easily upset, worried*) and unpleasant disengagement (e.g., *shy, gloomy, somber, dull, sluggish*). Orthogonal to Pleasantness is the other affect dimension, Engagement, a rather small factor representing high levels of affective activation (e.g., *ardent, passionate, seething)* and disengagement (e.g., *lazy, idle, unemotional*).

The remaining dimensions from the indigenous Spanish seven-factor solution depicted in Table 1 can be easily recognized as Conscientiousness, Agreeableness, and Conventionality. Several aspects about the Conventionality dimension are worth mentioning. First, the negative pole of this dimension mirrors Tellegen and Waller's (1987) Conventionality dimension, containing several evaluative descriptors denoting extreme levels of openness (e.g., *strange, bizarre, quaint*). The positive pole of this dimension, however, differs quite significantly from its American counterpart, and is defined by descriptors such as *nosy, gossiping, or disclosing*. These terms describe a fault finding, intrusive attitude that is generally associated with narrow-mindedness and which, at least in the Spanish structure, represents the opposite of being unconventional. Interestingly, in the Spanish structure, terms such as *traditional, family-oriented*, and *conventional* (primary markers of Conventionality in the American Big Seven) load significantly on Conscientiousness instead.

Next, factor analyses of the Spanish-translated Big Seven and Big Five inventories were performed to identify the imported Big Seven and Big Five personality dimensions. These analyses yielded seven-factor and five-factor structures similar to these uncovered in Benet and Waller (1995) using identical sets of markers, and for the sake of space will not be described here.

Interrelations Among the Indigenous and Imported Dimensions
What is the overall degree of content overlap and specificity between the indigenous Spanish personality constructs and the imported Big Seven and Big Five dimensions? To address this question, correlations among the indigenous and imported factors were first computed. Scale scores were computed for each person's self-ratings on every imported and indigenous dimension, and these scores were then correlated across subjects to provide an index of the overlap between the structural models. These correlations are presented in Table 2.

The top portion of Table 2 reports correlations among the indigenous and imported Big Seven factors. Notice that for the common dimensions (Conscientiousness, Agreeableness, Conventionality, Positive Valence and Negative Valence) the validity correlations (i.e., the convergent correlations) are the highest values in all but one column. For the indigenous Conventionality dimension, the validity correlation is only slightly smaller than the indigenous Conventionality—imported Positive

Table 2. *Correlations Between Indigenous and Imported Spanish Personality Dimensions*

Imported Spanish Big Seven	Indigenous Spanish Big Seven						
	PVAL	NVAL	PLEA	ENGA	CONS	AGRE	CONV
Positive Valence	**79**	-14	46	22	-06	01	-15
Negative Valence	-15	**47**	-08	01	-28	-06	05
Positive Emotionality	*43*	-15	*75*	*45*	-06	19	25
Negative Emotionality	*-31*	-03	*-43*	06	*-33*	-11	06
Conscientiousness	13	-02	-07	-02	**60**	09	07
Agreeableness	01	06	-10	-05	*41*	**71**	-08
Conventionality	-12	06	-29	-19	*36*	15	**22**
Imported Spanish Big Five							
Extraversion	*46*	-15	*76*	*50*	-09	14	12
Neuroticism	-28	-02	*-36*	11	*-40*	-19	06
Conscientiousness	*30*	-06	15	19	**49**	03	-04
Agreeableness	04	-07	-03	00	*50*	**58**	-18
Openness	*32*	-14	*41*	21	-08	00	**-44**

Note. N = 894 Spaniards. PVAL = Positive valence; NVAL = Negative valence; PLEA = Pleasantness; ENGA = Engagement; CONS = Conscientiousness; AGRE = Agreebleness; CONV = Conventionality. |Correlations| > .30 are in italics. Correlations between corresponding dimensions that are common to indigenous and imported structures (val coefficients) are in boldface.

Emotionality correlation. Notice that although the indigenous Pleasantness and Engagement dimensions have no direct imported counterparts, their correlations with Positive Emotionality and Negative Emotionality are substantial. This correlational pattern suggests that the indigenous Pleasantness and Engagement dimensions may be rotated composites of the imported Positive and Negative Emotionality dimensions (Larsen & Diener, 1992).

The bottom portion of Table 2 reports correlations among the indigenous Big Seven and the imported Big Five factors. The results here are similar to those reported above. Because the Big Seven factors subsume the Big Five, these results are not entirely surprising. None of the imported Big Five factors correlate appreciably with the indigenous Negative Valence dimension, and that although several imported Big Five factors correlate with the indigenous Positive Valence dimension, none of these approach the magnitude of the Positive Valence validity correlation reported in the top half of the table[4].

In summary, the convergent-discriminant validity patterns derived from the correlational analyses revealed that, with the exception of the affect dimensions (Pleasantness and Engagement) and Conventionality, a notable overlap exits among the indigenous and imported Big Seven dimensions. Particularly significant were the convergences found between the indigenous and imported Positive and Negative Valence dimensions, a finding that testifies to the applicability of these personality constructs in Spain. The pattern of interrelations also supported the indigenous Positive and Negative Valence as psychologically differentiated constructs that cannot be subsumed by the Five Factor model.

To corroborate further the previous convergent and discriminant correlational patterns and explore the latent structure of the variance shared by the indigenous and imported Spanish personality scales, exploratory and confirmatory joint factor analyses of the indigenous Spanish Big Seven and the imported Big Seven and Big Five scales were also performed. To ensure replicability, a split-sample cross-validation procedure was used: The derivation sample included 500 participants randomly selected from the total Spanish sample of 894, and the

---

4 This finding can be quantified via multiple regression. A multiple regression of Negative Valence on the imported Big Five factors produced an R^2 of .02 (see Benet, 1995, p. 109, for a variance-overlap analysis of these batteries). Furthermore, although 32% of the variance in the indigenous Positive Valence can be predicted by the imported Big Five dimensions, the imported Big Seven dimensions predict 68% of the variance in Positive Valence. Clearly, a significant portion of Positive Valence variation is not captured by the imported Big Five constructs.

Table 3. Joint Factor Analysis of Indigenous and Imported Spanish Personality Scales

	Common Personality Dimensions						
Scale	PEM	NEM	AGRE	CONS	CONV	PVAL	NVAL
Imported Positive Emotionality (IPC-7)	**90**	-07	07	-04	13	14	-13
Imported Extraversion (BFI)	**89**	-11	06	-06	-03	16	-07
Indigenous Pleasantness	**80**	**-31**	-10	00	-13	28	-16
Indigenous Engagement	**70**	**34**	-04	20	-26	08	05
Imported Negative Emotionality (IPC-7)	-12	**92**	-06	-05	05	-09	02
Imported Neuroticism (BFI)	-05	**91**	-14	-11	02	-09	01
Indigenous Agreeableness	09	-03	**90**	02	05	00	-13
Imported Agreeableness (IPC-7)	-05	-07	**88**	03	03	-03	-07
Imported Agreeableness (BFI)	00	-09	**77**	18	-18	-04	-18
Imported Conscientiousness (IPC-7)	-04	-03	03	**89**	14	05	-07
Imported Conscientiousness (BFI)	17	-08	00	**87**	-13	11	-08
Indigenous Conscientiousness	-09	-19	**44**	**69**	06	00	**-31**
Indigenous Conventionality	17	-01	-10	00	**87**	-09	-05
Imported Conventionality (IPC-7)	-23	15	20	**44**	**49**	-05	-01
Imported Openness (BFI)	**30**	-05	02	-03	**-73**	21	-13
Imported Positive Valence (IPC-7)	18	-12	-05	03	-21	**91**	06
Indigenous Positive Valence	**37**	-08	-02	15	-10	**86**	-01
Indigenous Negative Valence	-16	02	-14	-17	06	-02	**87**
Imported Negative Valence (IPC-7)	-08	02	-23	-09	-02	06	**86**

Note. N = 500 Spaniards (derivation sample). See Table 2 for explanation of the symbols.

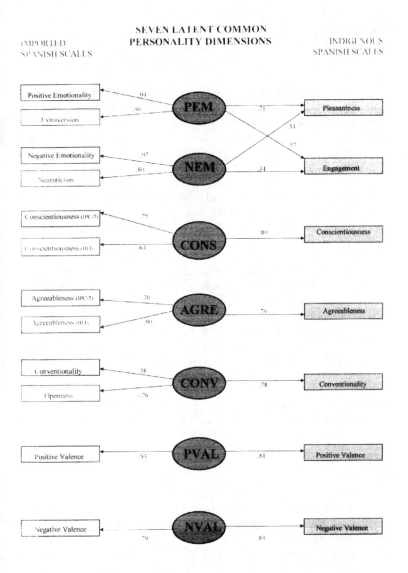

PVAL = Positive Valence; NVAL = Negative Valence; PEM = Positive Emotionality; NEM = Negative Emotionality; CONS = Conscientiousness; AGRE = Agreeableness; CONV = Conventionality

Figure 1. Common Latent Structure of the Indigenous and Imported Spanish Personality Scales

remaining 394 were used for the cross-validation sample. Using the derivation sample, an exploratory joint factor analysis of the indigenous and imported scale scores was first conducted. A clear seven-factor structure representing the familiar Big Seven factors emerged, which is depicted in Table 3.

The factor structure from Table 3 depicts seven common personality dimensions that, corroborating the patterns found in the correlational analyses, attest to the (a) content overlap between the corresponding indigenous and imported Agreeableness, Conscientiousness, and, to a lesser extent, Conventionality scales, (b) the cultural specificity of the indigenous Spanish dimensions of Pleasantness and Engagement, which represent rotations of the imported Positive Emotionality and Negative Emotionality dimensions, and (c) the correspondence between the indigenous and imported Positive and Negative Valence dimensions, which emerge as constructs independent from the other five personality dimensions.

The findings thus far provide robust evidence for the convergent and discriminant validity of the Spanish indigenous dimensions and suggest that the Big Seven optimally represents the major sources of variance in the indigenous and imported instruments. Using the 394 remaining subjects as a cross-validation sample, a more formal test of these structural findings was conducted via confirmatory joint factor analyses. Specifically, structural models representing seven and five personality factors were tested and statistically compared using the chi-square difference test ($\Delta\chi^2$). A model specifying seven common factors similar to these found in the exploratory joint factor analysis was first tested and is schematically depicted in Figure 1. This model yielded satisfactory practical fit indices (CFI = .945 and χ^2/df = 2.3). An examination of the latent-factor intercorrelations for this model revealed sizable correlations ($> .30$) between Positive Valence and Conventionality (-.45), Positive Valence and Positive Emotionality (.32), Negative Valence and Agreeableness (-.45), and Negative Valence and Conscientiousness (-.41), suggesting that perhaps a five-factor model where Positive and Negative Valence scales are subsumed by the Big Five would be more plausible. Accordingly, a second model specifying five factors representing the Big Five was tested. In this model, the indigenous and imported Positive and Negative Valence scales had primary loadings on Positive Emotionality and Conventionality, and Conscientiousness and Agreeableness, respectively. This model resulted in a significant decrease in overall fit, $\Delta\chi^2$ (11) = 735, and unacceptable fit indices (CFI = .787 and χ^2/df = 7.7). Overall, joint exploratory and confirmatory factor analyses corroborate that seven latent personality factors representing the

Big Seven structure capture the major sources of variance in both the indigenous and the imported Spanish personality scales.

Discussion

The objective of this psycholexical study was to identify indigenous Spanish personality constructs using a combined emic-etic approach. At a broad level, the findings from this study indicate that, with some variations in the affect domain, seven indigenous constructs clearly representative of the Big Seven factor model (Tellegen & Waller, 1987) underlie the Spanish natural language of personality.

Even so, at a narrower level of analysis, and as expected from the use of emic designs, the indigenous Spanish Big Seven dimensions also revealed several psychologically meaningful structural and item-level departures from the American Big Seven structure. These emic departures are particularly informative with regard to possible culture-specific aspects of Spanish personality organization. Especially notable is the organization of the affect domain in terms of hedonic quality and activation level (i.e., Pleasantness and Engagement), rather than in terms of Positive and Negative Emotionality. The implications of this finding for the study of personality structure in general, and more particularly, for the description and assessment of personality in Spain, are next discussed.

Pleasantness and Engagement as Indigenous Spanish Personality Constructs: Conceptual and Methodological Issues

A large body of research supports Pleasantness and Engagement (commonly known as Pleasure and Arousal), and Positive and Negative Affect as the two-dimensional reference axes defining the affect circumplex (see Larsen & Diener, 1992). Although in a true circumplex no set of dimensions can be any more 'primary' than any other set (because of the lack of simple structure), different kinds of evidence seem to support each set of dimensions. Pleasantness and Engagement usually emerge as the first *unrotated* factors in factor analyses of mood self-ratings and also as the first two dimensions underlying semantic categorizations of affect (see Russell, 1980, for a review). Positive and Negative Affect dimensions, on the other hand, are usually found after an orthogonal *Varimax rotation* of mood self-ratings (Watson & Tellegen, 1985). One consequence of these divergences has been the debate over which conceptual/rotational scheme should be considered 'primary,' a controversy further aggravated by recent methodological arguments suggesting that the emergence of one affect structure over the other is heavily influenced by response bias (Green, Goldman, & Salovey, 1993).

Positive and Negative Affect have been repeatedly related to individual differences in Extroversion and Neuroticism —or Positive and Negative Emotionality— (Meyer & Shack, 1989; Watson & Clark, 1992). Personality correlates of Pleasantness and Engagement have also been established, although to a less significant extent: Global measures of life satisfaction, subjective well-being, and happiness have been related to affects from the Pleasantness octant of the circumplex (Pavot & Diener, 1993), and individual differences in depression, for instance, are found to align with the Unpleasant octant (Watson, Clark, & Carey, 1988). Significant correspondences have also been found between Engagement and the personality dispositions of high affect intensity (Larsen & Diener, 1987) and high activity level (Buss & Plomin, 1984), and between affects from the Disengagement octant and the personality disposition of high emotional control (Watson & Greer, 1983).

In summary, different external personality correlates line up in a meaningful pattern all around the affect circumplex. This pattern seems to support a broader affect framework in which neither particular rotational/conceptual schemes are more basic in an absolute sense, although particular schemes relate more optimally than the others to certain basic cognitive, temperamental, or biopsychological variables (Diener & Larsen, 1992). Analogously, upon the notion that cultural differences may exist for the prevalence, categorization, and even social value of certain affects, one could speculate that particular affect dimensional structures will represent more optimally than others the modal affect organization of a particular cultural context (Scherer, Wallbot, & Summerfield, 1986). Cross-cultural research in the structure of mood (Shaver, Wu, & Schwartz, 1992; Watson, Clark, & Tellegen, 1984) shows that different cultures may combine basic affects in idiosyncratic ways to form culture-specific complex emotions, and that specific linguistic terms may emerge to represent the experience of these emotions. Findings in the current study suggest that, at least for Spaniards, a Pleasantness and Engagement conceptual scheme (rather than Positive and Negative Emotionality) best represents the affective core of the personality individual differences organized by the Spanish Big Seven structure. These findings also delineate Pleasantness and Engagement as the basic coordinates of the Spanish affect-descriptive natural language, supporting existing evidence for the emergence of these dimensions in affective categorizations of words and objects (Corraliza, 1987; Herrmann & Raybeck, 1981).

Spaniards' emphasis on the hedonic tone of affective experience suggests that the 'happy-sad' construal constitutes a *hypercognized* psychological experience in the Spanish culture. 'Hypercognized' being a term used in the emotion literature (Levy, 1984) to describe affects for which a society possesses an elaborate cognitive structure, and which are represented by a large number of lexical entries. The emergence of a small, but robust, dimension representing extreme levels of affective and behavioral engagement-disengagement (e.g., *impulsive, passionate*, or *idle, unemotional*) also speaks to the particular psychological and lexical significance this construct may have in the Spanish culture. In fact, in their observations of the Spanish character, novelists (Hemingway, 1926), news correspondents (McVeagh, 1990), and sociologists (Crow, 1985; Hooper, 1987; Shubert, 1990) have described Spaniards as *passionate* people with a strong commitment to the *pleasures* of life. Indeed, Spain is frequently advertised to the visitor as a land of intense and pleasurable experiences; a country that not only celebrates gastronomy, art, socializing, and risk-taking, but also performs them intensely (McVeagh, 1990).

Conventionality as Indigenous Spanish Personality Construct

The idiosyncrasies found in the indigenous Spanish Conventionality dimension, unlike Pleasantness and Engagement, are not so accessible to cultural interpretations. As shown in Table 2, this construct did not correspond to any of the imported Big Seven dimensions, although it related moderately to the imported Big Five dimension of Openness to Experience. This asymmetry is not so surprising considering the low correspondences for this dimension also reported in numerous other cross-cultural studies (Almagor et al., 1995; Bond, 1979; Hofstee, Kiers, De Raad, Goldberg, & Ostendorf, 1996; Yang & Bond, 1990).

How do the indigenous Spanish and American Conventionality dimensions differ from each other? The negative pole of the Spanish dimension is relatively similar to its American counterpart, in that it is primarily defined by evaluative terms denoting unconventionality (e.g., *strange, quaint, bizarre*) and openness to experience (e.g., *bohemian, inventive, creative*). However the negative pole of the Spanish Conventionality also includes terms alluding to spiritual and philosophical interests (e.g., *spiritual, mystical*) not represented in the American Conventionality dimension. Further differences can be seen in the positive pole of the indigenous Spanish dimension, which rather than denoting conservative and conforming attitudes (as in the American structure), represents attributes referring to indiscretion and garrulousness (e.g., *nosy, gossiping, disclosing*). Moreover, the terms *conventional* and *traditional* (markers of Conventionality in the American Big Seven) load most heavily on Conscientiousness, suggesting that for Spaniards these attributes are more associated with having a responsible disposition than they are with being conservative (i.e., for Spaniards, being *traditional* is not necessarily inconsistent with being *strange* or *bohemian*). Together, these patterns, suggest an interpretation of the indigenous Spanish Conventionality which is markedly different from the 'traditionalism-radicalism' interpretation offered by the American Big Seven's Conventionality dimension.

Conclusions

The present study indicates that seven natural language dimensions best represent indigenous Spanish constructs of personality. These seven dimensions, with some variations in the emotionality and openness domains, show significant overlap with the American Big Seven factor model of personality description (Tellegen & Waller, 1987). Because the indigenous dimensions were derived independently of any content or structural considerations, this correspondence provides support for the cross-cultural applicability of the Big Seven model in Spanish.

Ultimately, future research is necessary to support the construct validity of the indigenous Spanish Big Seven by relating these dimensions to non-lexical personality taxonomies. Meanwhile, this study adds to the available knowledge on the cross-cultural status of dimensional models of personality and introduces the *Siete Grandes* as primary indigenous constructs of personality description in Spanish.

References

Almagor, M., Tellegen, A., & Waller, N. G. (1995). The Big Seven Model: A cross-cultural replication and further explorations of the basic dimensions of natural language trait descriptors. *Journal of Personality and Social Psychology, 69*, 300-307.

Allport, G. W., & Odbert, H. S. (1936). Trait names: A psycho-lexical study. *Psychological Monographs, 47*, (n 211).

American Psychiatric Association. (1994). *Diagnostic and statistical manual of mental disorders: DSM-IV* (4th ed., DSM-IV). Washington, DC: Author.

Angleitner, A., Ostendorf, F., & John, O. P. (1990). Towards a taxonomy of personality descriptors in German: A psycho-lexical study. *European Journal of Personality, 4*, 89-118.

Benet, V. (1995). *Towards a Spanish taxonomy of personality descriptors: Generality of the 'Big Seven' model with indigenous and imported constructs.* Unpublished Doctoral Dissertation, Department of Psychology, University of California, Davis.

Benet, V., & Waller, N. G. (1995). The Big Seven factor model of personality description: Evidence for its cross-cultural generality in a Spanish sample. *Journal of Personality and Social Psychology, 69,* 701-718.

Benet, V., & Waller, N. G. (1996, August). *Positive and negative valence: Meaningful lexical dimensions of personality description outside the Big Five.* Poster presented at the annual convention of the American Psychological Society, San Francisco.

Benet-Martinez, V., & John, O. P. (in press). Los Cinco Grandes across cultures and ethnic groups: Multi-trait multi-method analyses of the Big Five in Spanish and English. *Journal of Personality and Social Psychology.*

Berry, J. W. (1980). Introduction to methodology. In H. Triandis & J. W. Berry (Eds.), *Handbook of cross-cultural psychology* (Vol. 2, pp. 1-28). Boston: Allyn & Bacon.

Block, J. (1995). A contrarian view of the five-factor approach to personality description. *Psychological Bulletin, 117,* 187-215.

Bond, M. H. (1979). Dimensions used in perceiving peers: Cross-cultural comparisons of Hong Kong, Japanese, American and Filipino university students. *International Journal of Psychology, 14,* 47-56.

Borkenau, P. (1990). Traits as ideal-based and goal-derived social categories. *Journal of Personality and Social Psychology, 58,* 381-396.

Brislin, R. W. (1980). Translation and content analysis of oral and written materials. In H. Triandis & J. W. Berry (Eds.), *Handbook of cross-cultural psychology* (vol. 2, pp. 389-444). Boston: Allyn & Bacon.

Buss, A. H., & Plomin, R. (1984). *Temperament: Early developing personality traits.* Hillsdale, NJ: Erlbaum.

Cattell, R. B. (1943). The description of personality: Basic traits resolved into clusters. *Journal of Abnormal and Social Psychology, 38,* 476-506.

Cliff, N. (1987). *Analyzing multivariate data.* Orlando, FL: Harcourt Brace Jovanovich.

Corraliza, J. A. (1987). *La Experiencia del Ambiente* [The experience of the environment]. Madrid, Spain: Tecnos.

Crow, J. A. (1985). *Spain: The root and the flower.* Berkeley, CA: University of California Press.

Goldberg, L. R. (1981). Language and individual differences: The search for universals in personality lexicons. In L. Wheeler (Ed.), *Review of personality and social psychology, 2,* 141-165.

Gorsuch, R. L. (1983). *Factor analysis.* Hillsdale, NJ: Erlbaum.

Gough, H. G., & Heilbrun, A. B., Jr. (1983). *The Adjective Check List manual* (revised). Palo Alto, CA: Consulting Psychologists Press.

Green, D. P., Goldman, S. L., & Salovey, P. (1993). Measurement error masks bipolarity in affect ratings. *Journal of Personality and Social Psychology, 64,* 1029-1041.

Hemingway, E. (1926). *The sun also rises.* New York: Grosset & Dunlap.

Herrmann, D. J., & Raybeck, D. (1981). Similarities and differences in meaning in six cultures. *Journal of Cross-Cultural Psychology, 12,* 194-206.

Hofstee, W. K., Kiers, H. A., De Raad, B., Goldberg, L. R., & Ostendorf, F. (1996). *Comparison of Big-Five structures of personality traits in Dutch, English, and German.* Unpublished manuscript, University of Groningen, The Netherlands.

Hogan, R. (1982). A socio-analytic theory of personality. In M. M. Page (Ed.), *Nebraska Symposium on Motivation, 1982: Personality — Current theory and research.* Lincoln, NE: University of Nebraska Press.

Hooper, J. (1987). *The Spaniards: A portrait of the new Spain.* London: Penguin Books.

Horn, J. L. (1965). A rationale and test for the number of factors in factor analysis. *Psychometrika, 30,* 179-185.

Hui, C. H., & Triandis, H. C. (1985). Measurement in cross-cultural psychology: A review and comparison of strategies. *Journal of Cross-Cultural Psychology, 16,* 131-152.

John, O. P. (1990). The "Big Five" factor taxonomy: Dimensions of personality in the natural language and in questionnaires. In L. A. Pervin (Ed.), *Handbook of personality: Theory and research* (pp. 66-100). New York: Guilford.

John, O. P., Donahue, E. M., & Kentle, R. L. (1991). *The "Big Five" Inventory — Versions 4a and 54.* Technical Report. IPAR. University of California at Berkeley.

Katigbak, M. S., Church, A. T., & Akamine, T. X. (1996). Cross-cultural generalizability of personality dimensions: Relating indigenous and imported dimensions in two cultures. *Journal of Personality and Social Psychology, 70,* 99-114.

Larsen, R. J., & Diener, E. (1987). Affect intensity as an individual difference characteristic: A review. *Journal of Research in Personality, 21,* 1-39.

Larsen, R. J., & Diener, E. (1992). Promises and problems with the circumplex model of emotion. In M. S. Clark (Ed.), *Review of personality and social psychology* (Vol. 13, pp. 25-59). Newbury Park, CA: Sage.

Levy, R. I. (1984). The emotions in comparative perspective. In K. R. Scherer & P. Ekman (Eds.), *Approaches to emotion* (pp. 397-412). Hillsdale, NJ: Erlbaum.

McCrae, R. R., & Costa, P. T. (1987). Validation of the five-factor model of personality across instruments and observers. *Journal of Personality and Social Psychology, 52*, 81-90.

McCrae, R. R., & John, O. P. (1992). Introduction to the five-factor model and its applications. *Journal of Personality, 60*, 175-215.

McVeagh, V. (1990). People. In K. Wheaton (Ed.). *Inside guides: Spain*. Singapore: APA Publications

Meyer, G. J., & Shack. J. R. (1989). Structural convergence of mood and personality: Evidence for old and new directions. *Journal of Personality and Social Psychology, 57*, 691-706.

Norman, W. T. (1963). Toward an adequate taxonomy of personality attributes. *Journal of Abnormal and Social Psychology, 66*, 574-583.

O'Brien, E. J., & Epstein, S. (1988). *MSEI: The Multidimensional Self-Esteem Inventory*. Odessa, FL: Psychological Assessment Resources.

Pavot, W., & Diener, E. (1993). The affective and cognitive context of self-reported measures of subjective well-being. *Social Indicators Research, 28*, 1-20.

Pervin, L. A. (1990). A brief history of modern personality theory. In L. A. Pervin (Ed.), *Handbook of personality: Theory and research*. New York: Guilford.

Real Academia Española (1989). *Diccionario manual e ilustrado de la Real Academia de la Lengua Espanola (Manual and illustrated dictionary of the Royal Spanish Academy of Language)*. Cuarta Edicion Revisada. Madrid: Espasa-Calpe.

Roid, G. H., & Fitts, W. H. (1988). *Tennessee Self-Concept Scale* (revised manual). Los Angeles: Western Psychological Services.

Russell, J. A. (1980). A circumplex model of affect. *Journal of Personality and Social Psychology, 39*, 1161-1178.

Scherer, K. R., Wallbot, H. G., & Summerfield, A. B. (1986). *Experiencing emotion: A cross-cultural study*. Cambridge: Cambridge University Press.

Shaver, P. R., Wu, S., & Schwartz, J. C. (1992). Cross-cultural similarities and differences in emotion and its representation: A prototype approach. In M. S. Clark (Ed.), *Review of Personality and Social Psychology Vol. 13. Emotion* (pp. 175-212). Thousand Oaks, CA: Sage.

Shubert, A. (1990). *A social history of modern Spain*. Boston, MA: Unwin Hyman.

Tellegen, A. (1985). Structures of mood and personality and their relevance to assessing anxiety, with an emphasis on self-report. In A.

H. Tuma & J. Maser (Eds.), *Anxiety and the anxiety disorders* (pp. 681-706). Hillsdale, NJ: Erlbaum.

Tellegen, A. (1993). Folk concepts and psychological concepts of personality and personality disorder. *Psychological Inquiry, 4,* 122-130.

Tellegen, A., Grove, W. M., & Waller, N. G. (1991). *Inventory of Personal Characteristics #7 (IPC).* Unpublished documents, University of Minnesota.

Tellegen, A., & Waller, N. G. (1987, August). *Reexamining basic dimensions of natural language trait descriptors.* Paper presented at the annual meeting of the American Psychological Association, Boston.

Tellegen, A., & Waller, N. G. (in press). Exploring personality through test construction: Development of the Multidimensional Personality Questionnaire. In S. R. Briggs & J. M. Cheek (Eds.), *Personality measures: Development and evaluation* (Vol. 1). Greenwich, CT: JAI Press.

Waller, N. G. (in press). Evaluating the structure of personality. In C. R. Cloninger (Ed.), *Personality and psychopathology.* Washington DC: American Psychiatric Press.

Waller, N. G., & Zavala, J. (1993). Evaluating the Big Five. *Psychological Inquiry, 4,* 131-134.

Watson, D., & Clark, L. A. (1992). On traits and temperament: General and specific factors of emotional experience and their relation to the Five-Factor model. *Journal of Personality, 60,* 441-476.

Watson, D., Clark, L. A., & Carey, G. (1988). Positive and negative affectivity and their relation to anxiety and depressive disorders. *Journal of Abnormal Psychology, 97,* 346-353.

Watson, D., Clark, L. A., & Tellegen, A. (1984). Cross-cultural convergence in the structure of mood: A Japanese replication and a comparison with the U.S. findings. *Journal of Personality and Social Psychology, 47,* 127-144.

Watson, D., & Greer, S. (1983). Development of a questionnaire measure of emotional control. *Journal of Psychosomatic Research, 27,* 299-305.

Watson, D., & Tellegen, A. (1985). Toward a consensual structure of mood. *Psychological Bulletin, 98,* 219-235.

Yang, K., & Bond, M. H. (1990). Exploring implicit personality theories with indigenous or imported constructs: The Chinese case. *Journal of Personality and Social Psychology, 58,* 1087-1095.

Author Note

I am deeply indebted to the psychology faculty at the Universitat Autonoma de Barcelona (especially to Jordi Bachs, Montse Goma, Maite Martínez and Merce Mitjavila) for allowing me access to their students. Furthermore, I thank Niels Waller, David Lopez Palenzuela, Virginia Kwong, and Catherine Clark for their valuable feed-back about the ideas and methods described in this paper.
Correspondence concerning this paper should be addressed to Verónica Benet-Martínez, Department of Psychology, University of Michigan, 525 East University, Ann Arbor, MI 48109-1109, USA.
E-mail:veronica@umich.edu

Attitudes, Beliefs, and Opinions about Suicide: A Cross-Cultural Comparison of Sweden, Japan, and Slovakia

Anna D. Eisler and Mia Wester
Stockholm University, Sweden

Mitsuo Yoshida
Osaka University, Japan

&

Gabriel Bianchi
Slovak Academy of Sciences, Bratislava, Slovakia

ABSTRACT

The cultural influence on attitudes, beliefs and opinions about suicide was investigated in Sweden, Japan, and Slovakia. Subjects from these three cultural groups (total $N = 193$) completed a suicide scale (Lester & Bean, 1992) consisting of five components: 1) beliefs in intrapsychic causes, 2) beliefs in interpersonal causes, 3) beliefs in societal causes, 4) personal attitudes, and 5) normative beliefs. A profile analysis showed significant main effects among the three cultural groups over the five components. Moreover, a mixed model analysis of variance revealed that Slovak participants were most inclined to attribute suicide to intrapsychic and interpersonal causes, and the Japanese, least to intrapsychic causes. The Japanese and Swedish groups did not differ in attribution to interpersonal causes. Slovak participants were most negative toward suicide in terms of their personal attitudes and normative beliefs; and the Swedish, least negative. Also, gender differences were obtained, between as well as within cultures, except that in the Swedish group, there was no difference between female and male subjects. In the Swedish group, the components of attitudes, beliefs, and opinions about suicide were also considered in relation to personality assessed with Eysenck's EPQ-I test. The only significant correlation was between personal attitudes (Component 4) and impulsiveness, indicating a more positive attitude towards suicide in impulsive individuals. The results are discussed with reference to theoretical approaches in social and cognitive psychology, focusing on cultural, cognitive, and social contexts.

From a historical perspective, attitudes and beliefs about suicide and suicidal behavior have differed greatly. This diversity existed among the ancient Greeks and Romans and is still evident today (Rosen, 1975). In general, suicide and suicidal behavior have been studied with different approaches, including philosophical, biological, medical, psychological, psychiatric, and sociological perspectives. The problem of suicide has also engaged many thinkers. For example, Camus discussed advantages and disadvantages of suicide and wrote that "suicide is prepared within the silence of the heart, as is a great work of art" (Alvarez, 1975; Camus, 1942). Schopenhauer (1851), on the other hand, claimed that moral freedom, the highest ethical ideal, is attainable only through denial of the will to live. However, according to Schopenhauer, suicide is not such a denial, for the essence of negation lies in shunning the joys of life, not its sorrows. The suicide is willing to live, but is dissatisfied with the conditions under which life is offered.

Reviewing the risk factors associated with suicide raises the problem that much of the research literature on suicidal behavior is conducted with suicide attempters, for the simple reason that suicide completers are unavailable for interviews. Risk factors for attempted and completed suicide may differ. Another problem in suicide research is that, for various reasons, suicide tends to be underreported. Such underreporting may reflect attitudes and beliefs about suicide and respect for the family in a particular country. In general, therefore, incidence estimates for suicide are considered to be too low (Garland & Zigler, 1993). It is important to note that underreporting varies between countries. Thus, comparisons based on statistical and epidemiological data are not very reliable.

Suicide occurs in a cultural context. In a recent study, for example, Piribauer and Etzersdorfer (1995) presented evidence that Hungary, Finland, and Austria had the highest global suicide mortality in Europe for the years of 1985-1989. On the basis of this finding, the authors claimed that suicide mortality in these countries involves cultural rather than socioeconomic factors. Yet, in spite of the importance of cultural factors, it seems that these are often disregarded in suicide research (Domino, Moore, Westlake, & Gibson, 1982).

Notwithstanding the plethora of definitions, there is general agreement that culture consists of shared elements that provide standards for perceiving, believing, evaluating, communicating, and acting among those who share a language, a historic period, and/or a geographic location. The shared elements are transmitted from generation to generation with modifications (Shweder & LeVine, 1984; Triandis, 1996).

Suicide and attempted suicide are the deepest expression of human suffering. Extensive knowledge about suicide is therefore needed and should include perceptions of suicide. Thus, knowledge of attitudes and beliefs about suicide, studied cross-culturally and with subjects not involved in any suicide attempt, can provide an empirical context and valuable predictions of vulnerability and risk factors useful in prevention programs. Furthermore, such an approach makes it possible to compare ways of looking at suicide in different cultural and temporal contexts; it elucidates the meaning of suicide for people with different cultural backgrounds (value systems, traditions, etc.). It reflects the present Zeitgeist, contemporary perspectives, and views on suicide.

For instance, Domino and Leenaars (1989) compared attitudes of college students in Canada and the U.S. toward suicide and found substantial attitudinal differences as well as similarities. Unlike their U.S. peers, Canadian subjects perceived suicide as a part of everyday life, an acceptable solution to incurable illness for the aged and infirm, not to be explained by recourse to religion, personality, or psychopathological constructs. In view of these findings, Leenaars and Lester (1992) conducted three studies on suicide in Canada and the U.S., for both genders between the years of 1960-1988. The results showed that the rates and patterns differed between the two countries, with Canada having the higher rate. Suggested possible explanations for these national differences are the reliability of suicide certification, the decriminalization of suicide in Canada in 1972, attitudes toward suicide, etc.

In another study of attitudes toward suicide using a "Suicide Opinion Questionnaire" (Domino & Takahashi, 1991), comparisons were made between female and male medical students in Japan and the U.S. Japanese students were more likely to believe in the right to commit suicide, with the view that suicide is normal behavior, while Americans were more likely to believe that suicide reflects aggression and anger. Males were more likely to believe that religious values are inversely related to suicide; and females, that suicide is basically an impulsive act. Noor and Mehilane (1991) likewise found that both psychological stressors and suicidality are culturally-bounded and correlated with political and national events.

In the present pilot study (the first step of a comprehensive project), both psychologists and social anthropologists participated as investigators. Thus, both psychological and social anthropological theories and methods are used. Programs aimed at promoting health and well-being must incorporate an understanding of culture, traditions, beliefs, values, etc. (Berry, Poortinga, Segall, & Dasen, 1992; Dasen, Berry, & Sartorius, 1988; Gantous, 1994; Pepitone, 1989). The study of suicide and suicidal behavior in different cultures may illuminate the following important questions: (1) Why do suicide rates differ among cultures (or sub-cultures)? (2) Is there any causal relation between cultural factors and suicide risk? (3) If so, which are the culturally specific patterns of beliefs and values that may contribute to suicidal behavior?

In this paper, we focus on attitudes, beliefs, and opinions about suicide in Swedish, Japanese, and Slovak cultures, because they differ widely in some respects but are similar in others. The Japanese people are concerned with their history and traditions (the samurai ethic with its loyalty to the master and the path of virtue to death). To commit suicide was never considered shameful, but rather a premeditated moral action, personally motivated and with a sense of responsibility. The commitment of the individual to the group is a dominant feature of Japanese society. Personal obligation and duty are regarded as more important than individual fulfillment. Japanese culture is collectivist and group-oriented, with the goal of maintaining group harmony (Hofstede, 1980; Hosaka & Tagawa, 1987; Iga & Tatai, 1975; Lewin, 1986; Triandis, 1994).

Persons in Swedish culture are regarded as individualistically-oriented. An individualistic culture like the Swedish tends to emphasize personal interests over group or collective interests. At the same time, self-reliance and individual competition contrasts with a humane attitude and the strong feeling of social justice and equality among people, which seems to be part and parcel of the Swedish cultural tradition. Social stratification is less pronounced in Sweden than other Western countries (Triandis, 1994).

In Slovakia (formerly a part of Czechoslovakia), during the forty or so years of its communist dictatorship, the society was closed to the outside world. Suicide was not officially recognized as a problem because it was regarded as nonexistent and, thus, taboo. The regime proclaimed that the government provides "adequately for its people, leaving them no cause for despair." The communist authorities used the rhetoric that all citizens in their country are "happy," so no one should have a reason to commit suicide. When it was mentioned by the authorities, suicide was portrayed explicitly as being a result of mental illness. The rationale behind this rhetoric was to stigmatize suicide. The communist regime dictated what people should think and feel; personal freedom was oppressed (see also Havel, 1989).

Slovakia is currently undergoing a political transition from an authoritarian to a democratic society. Unfortunately, although the isolation and the communist dictatorship have disappeared, much of the old pattern still holds in Slovakia or has been changing very slowly. Today, many Slovak people are encountering new problems. Living standards are declining for many individuals, people are losing their jobs and are thus afraid of the future. As in some other former socialist countries, the elements of a civil society are still weak. In contrast to the Swedish and Japanese cultures, the Slovak culture is both collectivistic or group-oriented as well as individualistic. However, the proportions of that combination are hard to assess. People used to live a double life in that country: the official life forced upon them by the communist regime, and the unofficial, private life apart from the communist society. Such life conditions give rise to double identities, thereby influencing behavior (see Havel, 1989).

A primary aim of this study was to compare the aforementioned three cultures regarding attitudes and beliefs toward suicide because they are culturally different but, in some respects, are also similar: (1) Japan is an open industrial society with a collectivistic culture, where suicide is not considered shameful, (2) Sweden is also an open industrial society, but with an individualistic culture, though with strong advocacy of social justice and equality among its people, and (3) Slovak culture is both individualistic and group-oriented, the latter being inherited from the totalitarian dictatorship that lasted for more than four decades.

Accordingly, we expected that (1) attitudes, beliefs, and opinions about suicide would differ among Swedish, Japanese, and Slovak participants, and (2) more specifically, that attitudes, beliefs, and opinions about suicide would be most positive in the Japanese sample and least positive in the Slovak sample, with the Swedish in between.

Method

Participants
Ninety-two Swedish participants (51 females and 41 males aged 19-70 years), 70 Japanese participants (39 females and 31 males aged 19-45 years), and 29 Slovak participants (16 females and 13 males aged 18-53 years) participated in this pilot study. Participants were not paid for their participation; and in all three countries, most were university students.

Procedure
The data were collected in 1994-1995 by Anna Eisler and Mia Wester at Stockholm University in Sweden, by Mitsuo Yoshida at Osaka University in Japan, and by Gabriel Bianchi at the Slovak Academy of Sciences in Bratislava, Slovakia. The subjects were asked to complete a questionnaire scale developed by Lester and Bean (1992) entitled "Attitudes, beliefs and opinions about suicide," which comprises five components and thirty-three items in a Likert response format. The components are: 1) belief in intrapsychic causes, 2) belief in interpersonal causes, 3) belief in societal causes, 4) personal attitudes, and 5) normative beliefs. The first three components are related to the causes to which people attribute suicide: intrapsychic problems ("People who commit suicide are usually mentally ill"), interpersonal conflicts ("Suicide is often triggered by arguments with a lover or spouse"), or societal pressures ("Those who are oppressed in a society are more likely to commit suicide"). In addition, the last two components were designed to measure the individual's personal approval ("I believe that suicide can be a rational act") or disapproval ("Only cowards kill themselves") of suicide, and the

Table 1. *Means of Transformed Scores and Standard Deviations for the Five Components**

Component	Japan			Sweden			Slovakia		
	Female	Male	All	Female	Male	All	Female	Male	All
1 M	0.43	0.44	0.44	0.49	0.51	0.50	0.60	0.58	0.59
SD	0.20	0.16	0.18	0.19	0.16	0.18	0.21	0.16	0.19
2 M	0.38	0.54	0.46	0.43	0.44	0.44	0.60	0.53	0.57
SD	0.17	0.21	0.20	0.18	0.19	0.18	0.17	0.22	0.20
3 M	0.47	0.48	0.48	0.47	0.46	0.46	0.56	0.44	0.51
SD	0.18	0.25	0.21	0.24	0.21	0.22	0.30	0.24	0.28
4 M	0.48	0.41	0.45	0.41	0.42	0.42	0.65	0.52	0.59
SD	0.21	0.21	0.21	0.21	0.25	0.23	0.17	0.26	0.22
5 M	0.78	0.70	0.75	0.66	0.66	0.66	0.82	0.75	0.79
SD	0.15	0.19	0.17	0.24	0.26	0.25	0.28	0.22	0.25

* 1 = Belief in intrapsychic causes; 2 = Belief in interpersonal causes; 3 = Belief in societal causes; 4 = Personal attitudes and 5 = Normative beliefs.

individual's perceptions of acceptance of suicide by peer and cultural groups ("Some of my friends think that suicide is an acceptable choice").

The aim of the present study was to investigate possible differences among the three countries, but it was also of interest to see whether there were gender differences. The Swedish participants, after completing the aforementioned questionnaire, were immediately administered the Eysenck Personality Questionnaire and Impulsiveness (EPQ-I) Test (Eysenck & Eysenck, 1975) to assess possible relationships between the five components of suicide attitudes and beliefs and personality. The EPQ-I test contains five personality scale dimensions: extraversion, psychoticism, neuroticism, lie, and impulsiveness.

Results

The raw data were transformed, using the procedure recommended by Lester and Bean (1992), and normalized to range between 0 and 1 because of varying numbers of questions per component. The means of the transformed scores and standard deviations are shown in Table 1.

Profile Analysis
Tabachnick and Fidell (1989) suggested three main questions that can be addressed by profile analysis: a) flatness, b) level, and c) parallelism. In the present study we examined whether the *pattern* of components differed between countries and gender, respectively, using MANOVA (SAS, GLM) and profile analysis over the five components [country(3) x gender(2)]. The hypothesis of parallelism could be rejected for countries but not for gender. The results showed significant main effects, $F(8, 364) = 2.41$, $p = .015$, between Japan, Sweden, and Slovakia. A profile analysis between countries in pairs showed only a significant difference between the Japanese and Swedish groups, $F(4, 182) = 3.71$, $p = .006$. The differences between the three profiles are illustrated in Figure 1.

However, the pattern is not simple. For *female subjects* alone, there is an overall significant effect, $F(8, 412) = 5.17$, $p < .0001$. A contrast between pairs of countries showed a significant effect between the Japanese and Swedish female groups, $F(4, 206) = 8.41$, $p < .0001$, between the Japanese and Slovak, $F(4, 206) = 3.64$, $p = .0068$, and between the Swedish and Slovak female groups, $F(4, 206) = 2.37$, $p < .05$, respectively.

For *male subjects,* the overall effect was also significant, $F(8, 328) = 3.59$, $p = .0005$. Significant differences were obtained in a contrast between the Japanese and Swedish male groups, $F(4, 164) = 5.71$, $p = .0003$, and between the Japanese and Slovak, $F(4, 164) = 3.82$, p

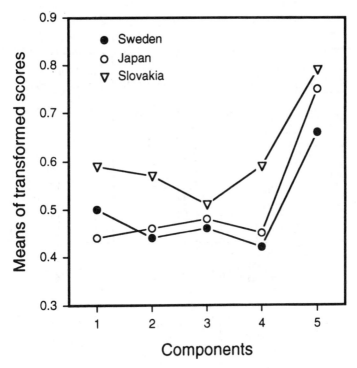

Figure 1. Profiles of Three Countries for the Five Components

= .0053. There was no significant difference between Swedish and Slovak male participants. It is also of interest that differences were less pronounced between the male than between the female cultural groups, as can be seen from the *F* values (see also the next section).

Finally, the profiles of the genders were studied for each country separately. The profiles showed significant differences only in the Japanese sample, $F(4, 135) = 8.41$, $p < .0001$. Gender differences for the three countries separately are illustrated in Figure 2. Note that the profiles in the Swedish sample are the same, as are the levels. In the next sections, the levels, overall as well as for each component separately, are compared.

Analysis of Variance using a Mixed Model (SAS, GLM)
Analysis of variance, using a mixed model [countries(3) x gender(2) x components(5)] with repeated measurements for components, yielded the following results: a significant overall effect for countries, $F(10, 362) =$

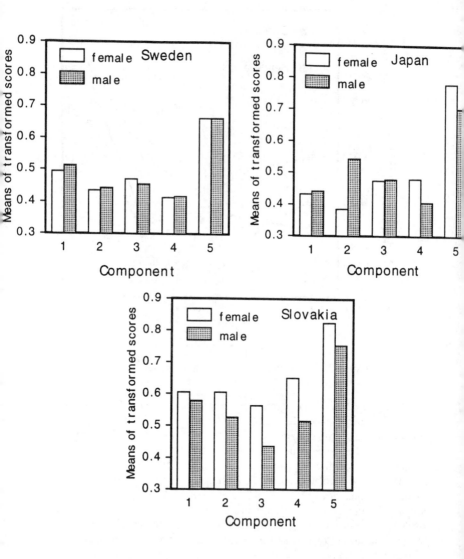

Figure 2. Means of Transformed Scores for the Five Components for Each Country and Gender

3.97, $p < .0001$, but not for gender, nor for the country x gender interaction. As to within-subjects factors, only one significant interaction emerged, between components and countries, $F(8, 740) = 2.08$, $p = .04$.

Finally, comparing the three countries on each of the five components separately yielded the following significant effects: 1) belief in intrapsychic causes, $F(5, 185) = 7.79$, $p = .0006$; 2) belief in interpersonal causes, $F(5, 185) = 5.46$, $p = .005$; in this component, gender effects approached significance [$F(1, 185) = 3.39$, $p = .067$] and the country x gender interaction was significant, [$F (2, 188) = 5.11$, $p = .007$]; 3) belief in societal causes, no significant difference; 4) personal attitudes, $F(5, 185) = 6.94$, $p = .001$; and 5) normative beliefs, $F(5, 185) = 4.82$, $p = .009$. [Note that the gender effect approached significance only in the belief in interpersonal causes (Component 2)].

Table 2 shows the outcome of comparing countries in pairs. The Slovak participants were most inclined to attribute suicide to intrapsychic and to interpersonal causes, the Japanese least to intrapsychic causes. The Japanese and the Swedish group did not differ in attribution to interpersonal causes. The Slovak participants were most negative toward suicide in their personal attitudes and normative beliefs, and the Swedish least.

Analysis of Variance for Gender using MANOVA (SAS, GLM)
The multivariate analysis of variance revealed overall significant gender differences between all three pairs of countries: (1) Japanese and Slovak, $F(5, 181) = 4.19$, $p = .001$, (2) Japanese and Swedish, $F(5, 181) = 3.11$, $p = .01$, (3) Swedish and Slovak, $F(5, 181) = 4.96$, $p = .0003$. Table 3 provides, for each component and each gender, the significance values for each of the three pairs of countries (see also Figure 2).

The patterns for two of the three countries showed gender differences; within the Japanese sample in belief in interpersonal causes, $F(1, 138) = 24.43$, $p < .0001$, in personal attitudes, $F(1, 138) = 4.29$, $p = .04$, and in normative beliefs, $F(1, 138) = 7.32$, $p = .007$. Within the Slovak sample, the gender difference in beliefs in societal causes approached significance, $F(1, 56) = 3.20$, $p = .079$, and was significant in personal attitudes, $F(1, 56) = 5.88$, $p = .02$. Unlike the Japanese and Slovak groups, the Swedish group did not show any gender differences (see Figure 2).

The results clearly showed that the Japanese men were more inclined to attribute suicide to interpersonal causes than the women, while the

Table 2. p-Values of Comparison of Mean Differences between Sweden, Japan, and SLovakia for the Five Components*

Component	Japan-Slovakia	Japan-Sweden	Sweden-Slovakia	Overall
1	.0002	.02	.03	.0006
2	.02	n.s.	.002	.005
3	n.s.	n.s.	n.s.	n.s.
4	.005	n.s.	.0005	.001
5	n.s.	.03	.01	.009

* Five Components (see Table 1). The direction of the differences can be seen in Figures 1 and 2.

Table 3. p-Values of Comparison of Mean Differences for Gender between Sweden, Japan and Slovakia for the Five Components*

Component	Gender	Japan-Slovakia	Japan-Sweden	Sweden-Slovakia	Overall
1	Female	.0001	.04	.006	.0002
	Male	.0003	.008	n.s.	.0007
2	Female	.0001	.056	.0001	.0001
	Male	n.s.	.004	n.s.	.01
3	Female	n.s.	n.s.	.05	n.s.
	Male	n.s.	n.s.	n.s.	n.s.
4	Female	.0001	.03	.0001	.0001
	Male	.05	n.s.	n.s.	n.s.
5	Female	n.s.	.0005	.0003	.0001
	Male	n.s.	n.s.	n.s.	n.s.

* Five Components (see Table 1). The direction of the differences in means can be seen in Figures 1 and 2.

Japanese women were more negative toward suicide in their personal attitudes and in normative beliefs than the Japanese men. The Slovak women were more negative toward suicide in their personal attitudes than the Slovak men.

Personality Correlates in the Swedish Sample

Extra-introversion in the Swedish sample was determined by the EPQ-I test, which contains five personality dimensions: extraversion (E), psychoticism (P), neuroticism (N), lie (L) and impulsiveness (I). Multiple stepwise regression, with the mean of each of the five components as dependent and test scores (EPQ-I test) as independent variables, showed only one significant, negative correlation: namely, between personal attitudes (Component 4) and impulsiveness, $r = -.20$, $p = .05$. Thus, impulsive individuals were most positive toward suicide in their personal attitudes (a low score in Component 4 denotes a positive attitude toward suicide). It may be that impulsive individuals are more emotional, impatient, and experience "time urgency" in a critical situation. Suicide may then be perceived as a possible immediate solution.

Discussion

In this study, we examined attitudes, beliefs, and opinions about suicide in a cross-cultural perspective among Sweden, Japan, and Slovakia. We found, as predicted, that the perception of suicide is influenced by the culture. Also, gender differences were found both between and within cultures, except in the Swedish group. It has been argued by Conwell (1993) that, considering the prevalence and nature of suicidal behavior, it seems self-evident that culture would exert a profound influence, both promoting risk and providing a protective factor. Our results do, in fact, suggest that the perception of suicide is in part a product of cultural influences.

An interesting finding concerns the item: "People who live under dictatorships are more likely to kill themselves." The Slovak participants generally answered "yes" to this question, as opposed to the Swedish and the Japanese participants, though in general, the Slovak participants were the most negative towards suicide. Another interesting finding concerns the item: "Suicide can be caused by work stress such as being fired from your job." The participants in all three countries generally answered "yes" to this question. It is perhaps hardly surprising that all the participants, independently of culture, perceive losing a job as having the same consequences: lowered self-esteem, fear, frustration, learned helplessness, etc., with the conclusion that it may have suicidal consequences.

Moreover, our results also unexpectedly showed no differences between Swedish female and male participants. A possible explanation is that this is a consequence of the dynamic process, currently underway in Sweden, of promoting equality between the genders. It is interesting to speculate about the gender differences in the Japanese and Slovak samples in contrast to the Swedish. Swedish culture reflects an individualistic view, while Japanese culture is collectivistic. Moreover, Japanese culture seems to have more systematic gender barriers. This polarization of gender may possibly explain why the attitudes and beliefs toward suicide in the Japanese sample express the common style of the relative roles in the female and the male group, respectively. Thus, gender differences in the perception of suicide could be partially determined by gender inequality.

The gender differences in the Slovak sample are not surprising; they seem to reflect the realistic scenario of a society in which oppression has been deeply rooted in everyday life. Under such conditions, women were at a disadvantage compared with men. Their need to take more personal responsibility for socially based problems could lie behind their more negative personal attitudes toward suicide. Of course, the Slovak sample is too small to arrive at firm conclusions. Future research with larger samples may clarify the issue of gender differences in Slovakia toward suicide.

Previous research has paid considerable attention to antecedents and motives of suicidal behavior (Bagley, 1991; Beskow, 1992; Domino & Takahashi, 1991; Eisler, 1986; Lester & Lynn, 1993). The large variation in suicide rates in different cultures (or subcultures) indicates that cultural and social contexts are critical variables, influencing suicidal behavior in some cultures more than in others. Why is this so? In certain cultural settings, people may find themselves in situations where attempting to behave in line with a certain reference value threatens to enlarge deviations from another reference value. Under such circumstances, a conflict between these two reference values can potentially interfere with other values and cognitive activities, thereby resulting in suicidal behavior. How people cope with such problems is often dependent on the cultural and social setting of traditions, learning, values, rules, and codes.

Research on suicidal behavior in a cross-cultural perspective has not made much progress. Perhaps because of methodological difficulties, researchers in psychology seem generally uninterested in finding new approaches to the study of suicide cross-culturally. Interest in this issue seems to have faded, perhaps because it entered a cul-de-sac. The present pilot study focused on the self-report questionnaire method and may support the view that attitudes and beliefs about suicide and suicidal behavior are variable, influenced by personal experience as well as by cultural learning, cultural patterns, and culturally dependent coping repertoires and coping strategies. This study, besides highlighting the contrasts among the three cultures and between the two genders, makes a valuable contribution to identifying aspects of vulnerability and predicting risk factors for suicide. Hopefully, the present findings can also contribute to the implementation of suicide prevention programs and services. In summary, our results confirm the importance of cultural differences in explaining and understanding the variation in suicide rates in different cultures.

References

Alvarez, A. (1975). Literature in the nineteenth and twentieth centuries. In S. Perlin (Ed.), *A handbook for the study of suicide* (pp. 31-60). New York: Oxford University Press.

Bagley, C. (1991). Poverty and suicide among native Canadians: A replication. *Psychological Reports, 69*, 149-150.

Berry, J. W., Poortinga, Y. H., Segall, M. H., & Dasen, P. R. (1992). *Cross-cultural psychology: Research and applications.* Cambridge, England: Cambridge University Press.

Beskow, J. (1992). *Självmord som existentiellt problem* [Suicide as an existential problem]. Stockholm: FRN.

Camus, A. (1942). *Le mythe de Sisyphe.* Paris: Gallimard.

Conwell, Y. (1993). Suicide in the elderly: Cross-cultural issues in late-life suicide. *Crisis, 14*, 152-153.

Dasen, P. R., Berry, J. W., & Sartorius, N. (1988). *Cross-cultural research and methodology.* Newbury Park, CA: Sage.

Domino, G., & Leenaars, A. A. (1989). Attitude toward suicide: A comparison of Canadian and U.S. college students. *Suicide and Life Threatening Behavior, 19*, 160-172.

Domino, G., Moore, D., Westlake, L., & Gibson, L. (1982). Attitudes toward suicide: A factor analytic approach. *Journal of Clinical Psychology, 38*, 257-262.

Domino, G., & Takahashi, Y. (1991). Attitudes toward suicide in Japanese and American medical students. *Suicide and Life Threatening Behavior, 21*, 345-359.

Eisler, A. D. (1986). *Kultur och beteende: är självdestruktivitet kulturellt betingad?* [Culture and behavior: Is self-destructiveness culturally determined?] Stockholm: Stockholm University, Department of Social Anthropology.

Eysenck, H. J., & Eysenck, S. B. G. (1975). *Manual of the Eysenck Personality Questionnaire.* London: Hodder & Stoughton.

Gantous, P. (1994). Stress drives high suicide rate among native Canadian Innu. *Psychology International, 4*, 3.

Garland, A. F., & Zigler, E. (1993). Adolescent suicide prevention. *American Psychologist, 48*, 169-182.

Havel, V. (1989). *En dåre i Prag* [A madman in Prague]. Stockholm: Symposion.

Hofstede, G. (1980). *Culture's consequences: International differences in work-related values.* Beverly Hills, CA: Sage.

Hosaka, T., & Tagawa, R. (1987). The Japanese characteristic of Type A behavior pattern. *Journal of Experimental Clinical Medicine, 12,* 287-303.

Iga, M., & Tatai, K. (1975). Characteristics of suicides and attitudes toward suicide in Japan. In N. L. Farberow (Ed.), *Suicide in different cultures* (pp. 255-280). Baltimore: University Park Press.

Leenaars, A. A., & Lester, D. (1992). Comparison of rates and patterns of suicide in Canada and the United States, 1960-1988. *Death Studies, 16,* 417-430.

Lester, D., & Bean, J. (1992). Attribution of causes to suicide. *Journal of Social Psychology, 132,* 679-680.

Lester, D., & Lynn, R. (1993). National character, suicide and homicide. *Personality and Individual Differences, 14,* 853-855.

Lewin, P. (1986). The Japanese life-plan and some of its discontents. *Hiroshima Forum for Psychology, 11,* 39-56.

Noor, H., & Mehilane, L. (1991). Sociopsychological situation and parasuicide incidence in Estonia. *Psychiatria Danubia, 3,* 345-348.

Pepitone, A. (1989). Toward a cultural social psychology. *Psychology and Developing Societies, 1,* 5-19.

Piribauer, F., & Etzersdorfer, E. (1995). Recent reversal of trends in suicide mortality in Austria and Hungary but not in Finland. *Crisis, 16,* 181-183.

Rosen, G. (1975). History. In S. Perlin (Ed.), *A handbook for the study of suicide* (pp. 3-30). New York: Oxford University Press.

Schopenhauer, A. (1851). Vom Unterschiede der Lebensalter [On the difference of periods of life]. In: *Parerga und Paralipomena: Kleine philosophische Schriften* (Aphorismen zur Lebensweishet), Vol. 1. Berlin: Hayn.

Shweder, R., & LeVine, R. A. (1984). *Culture theory: Essay on mind, self, and emotion.* Cambridge, England: Cambridge University Press.

Tabachnick, B. G., & Fidell, L. S. (1989). *Using multivariate statistics.* New York: Harper & Row.

Triandis, H. (1994). *Culture and social behavior.* New York: McGraw-Hill.

Triandis, H. (1996). The psychological measurement of cultural syndromes. *American Psychologist, 51,* 407-415.

Author Note

Anna D. Eisler and Mia Wester, Department of Psychology; Mitsuo Yoshida, Faculty of Human Sciences; Gabriel Bianchi, Department of Social and Biological Communication.

This investigation was supported by the Henrik Granholm Foundation, the Swedish Institute, the Osaka University and the Slovak Academy of Sciences.

Requests for reprints should be addressed to Anna D. Eisler, Department of Psychology, Stockholm University, 106 91 Stockholm, Sweden. E-mail can be addressed to: aaer@psychology.su.se.

Intergenerational Communication across the Pacific Rim: The Impact of Filial Piety

Cynthia Gallois, The University of Queensland, Australia
Howard Giles and Hiroshi Ota, University of California
 at Santa Barbara, USA
Herbert D. Pierson, St John's University, USA
Sik Hung Ng, Victoria University of Wellington, New Zealand
Tae-Seop Lim, Kwangoon University, Korea
John Maher, International Christian University, Japan
Lilnabeth Somera, De La Salle University, The Philippines
Ellen B. Ryan, McMaster University, Canada
and Jake Harwood, University of Kansas, USA

ABSTRACT

Most research and theory in communication and ageing is derived from North America. This investigation is one of a series of comparative attempts to redress this imbalance by studying intergenerational communication patterns in Southeast and East Asian cultures as well as the West. In this study, we focused on filial piety, and administered our own initial measure of normative beliefs about it to over 1400 students in four Western (United States, Australia, Canada and New Zealand) and four East and Southeast Asian (Japan, Korea, Hong Kong and The Philippines) sites. Three-mode factor analyses indicated that overall, participants in the study distinguished between younger and older people and family members and people outside the family in their judgements of filial piety. In addition, subjects' responses fell into dimensions of practical support versus communication, and respect versus contact and support. Results also indicated differences between what young people should give to their elderly parents (practical support), what parents expect (continued contact with their children) and what older adults in general expect (respect). Students from Asian cultures showed a sharper distinction than did Western students between what they intended to provide (practical support) and what they perceived their parents and older adults to expect (continued contact and respect), although this difference was not great. Finally, MANOVAs indicated that Asian students felt more obliged to give practical support than did Westerners, while the latter put more emphasis on continued communication and contact with older adults. Interestingly, Asian participants reported that their intentions to care for and communicatively support older people were lower than that expected of them, whereas Western participants claimed that they personally would provide more support of all types than was expected of them.

In the past decade, research and theory in intergenerational communication has increased greatly (e.g., Coupland, Coupland & Giles, 1991; Nussbaum & Coupland, 1995; Nussbaum, Hummert, Williams, & Harwood, 1995). Nevertheless, the majority of the research and theory has emerged from individualistic cultures (Hofstede, 1991; Triandis, 1995) such as the United States, Canada, Britain and Australia (e.g., Edwards & Noller, 1993; Harwood, Giles, Ryan, Fox, & Williams, 1993; Hummert, Garstka, & Shaner, 1995; Ryan & Cole, 1990). This research is grounded in a Western perspective on intergenerational relationships, represented by liberalism and individualism (Kim & Yamaguchi, 1994), as well as in Western stereotypes about ageism. An alternative perspective, derived from Confucianism and collectivism in East and Southeast Asia, has been neglected (Kim & Yamaguchi, 1994; Yum, 1988). The present paper is one of a series of programmatic attempts to take a more culturally inclusive perspective on intergenerational communication.

This study had two main goals. The first was to develop the conceptualisation of *filial piety* by exploring the relationships among some of its facets. More specifically, we examined the associations among perceived norms about filial piety, the perceived expectations of older people, and perceptions about the behaviour of peers, as well as personal norms and intentions to be filially pious with older people. Filial piety, generally known as care and respect for the aged, is the most prominent intergenerational concept shared across Southeast and East Asian nations. Furthermore, it should have high communicative potential, given that it is expressed symbolically through communication in intergenerational interaction. Our second aim was to examine filial piety cross-culturally. It is generally believed that the elderly in Asian nations receive more care and respect than their counterparts in Western nations (Kiefer, 1992; Palmore, 1975), yet some empirical studies of inter-generational relations suggest that a positive conception of the elderly in the East may be a myth (e.g., Koyano, 1989; Levy & Tsuhako, 1994; Tien-Hyatt, 1987). It is certainly time to visit filial piety cross-culturally in the context of this debate, as well as to bring this construct into the heartland of ageing and communication research.

Macro-Cultural Issues
Before beginning our discussion of filial piety and intergenerational relationships, it is important to situate them in a larger cultural context, as macro-level forces can influence intergroup/interpersonal interaction (see Gallois, Giles, Jones, Cargile, & Ota, 1995; Kim & Yamaguchi, 1994). Several relevant cultural-level variables have been suggested in the past (see Gudykunst & Ting-Toomey, 1988). Probably the most

relevant one for present purposes would be the philosophical orientations of Confucianism versus Liberalism, because (1) these orientations constitute the fundamental ground from which most other cultural variation, such as individualism-collectivism, emerges (e.g., Ho, 1994; Kim, 1994), and (2) they allude to a core foundation of intergenerational relationships.

Western nations tend to hold liberalism as their guiding principle of life (Kim, 1994; Kim & Yamaguchi, 1994). The sanctity of the individual is a core unit, represented by an independent construal of self (Markus & Kitayama, 1991). Thus, individuals are perceived to act rationally and to interact with one another as autonomous, equal individuals who pursue their own rights. Chinese Confucianism, on the other hand, provides a radically different and important philosophical orientation of life in many Asian nations (e.g., Kiefer, 1992; Kim, 1994; Kim & Yamaguchi, 1994). Five codes of ethics of Confucianism: affection between parent and child, righteousness between parent and child, a power distinction between husband and wife, order between old and young, and sincerity between friends prescribe the nature of social relationships and types of communication patterns displayed there. These five codes in combination emphasise interdependence between people and highlight status and role differentiation between people within the family (especially across generations) and among community relationships. Hence, a conception of self as an interdependent construal emerges (Markus & Kitayama, 1991).

To look specifically at intergenerational issues, negative perceptions and stereotypes of the elderly, such as the elderly as stigmatised, naturally follow from the independence and activity orientation in the West (Dowd, 1986; Goffman, 1963; Russel, 1981; Russel & Oxley, 1990). Interaction with the stigmatised tends to occur in limited contexts (Gardner, 1991). This is less the case in family settings, where the elderly are usually treated as ingroup members (see Ryan & Cole, 1990). Arguably though, family settings have been a more common ground for intergenerational communication in East and Southeast Asian than in Western nations (Sung, 1995). In Confucianist contexts, a parent-child relationship, especially father-son, is deemed most important (Tu, 1985). Kim and Yamaguchi argue that parents demand love, reverence, obedience, and respect from their children, while children expect love, wisdom, and benevolence from their parents. Parent-child relationships involve more than the family, as parents represent one's ancestors and a position within the community, and children represent one's progeny (1994, p. 176).

In sum, Confucianism and liberalism provide backdrops where distinctive forms of conceptions of self, interpersonal relationships, and communication styles emerge. As Yum (1988) argues, the differences between Eastern and Western nations are a matter of degree. Features of East and West actually exist in both cultural settings, but one tends to be more predominant than the other. Thus, it makes sense that the concept of filial piety is present in most of the cultures in the world, although its form, salience and importance may differ (Hamilton, 1990; Ho, 1994). Given the prevalence of Confucianist thought, one would predict that filial piety is more salient in East and Southeast Asian cultures than in the West.

That said, intergenerational relations and communication seem to be changing in East and Southeast Asia. We have found that young Asian adults have less favourable dispositions towards older people than their counterparts in Western societies. More specifically, Western young adults' stereotypes about the elderly (Harwood et al., 1996), their views of this age group's vitality (Harwood et al., 1994), and their past experiences of communicating with the elderly (Williams et al., 1996) are more positive than are those of their age peers in Southeast and East Asia. Hence, a question arises about whether filial piety may now be eroding in certain regions of Asia (as a number of commentators have also suggested recently). Indeed, if one were to follow through with the pattern of findings mentioned above, one might even anticipate the possibility of more filially pious norms and values among Western than East and Southeast Asian young people.

Conceptualisation of Filial Piety

Despite its importance in intergenerational relationships, filial piety has not been conceptualised very clearly or operationalised very well for research purposes. One perspective suggests that an emotional orientation constitutes the core of Asian filial piety (e.g., care and respect are given for the elderly simply *because* they are elderly), while a cognitive and more "rational" orientation is central to implicit Western notions of filial piety (e.g., caregiving is necessary because the elderly are weak, poor, and incompetent). Clearly, this characterisation is too simplistic to be useful in cross-cultural research.

Two scholars have contributed considerably to a more subtle understanding of filial piety. Ho (1994), from a Chinese perspective, argues that filial piety is a behavioural prescription that tells how "children should behave toward their parents, living or dead, as well as toward ancestors" (p. 351). His approach to the concept of filial piety is holistic, and includes obeying and honouring one's parents, as well as providing for the "material and mental well-being of one's aged parents, performing ceremonial duties of ancestral worship, taking care to avoid harm to one's own body, ensuring the continuity of the family line, and in general to conduct oneself so as to bring honour and not disgrace to the family" (p. 350). Nevertheless, some of the wording in his scale seems to be highly culture-specific and may be problematic if used in other cultures. Sung (1990) argues that filial piety, from a Korean perspective, is a value and is "a shared cultural standard, by which the moral relevance of filial attitudes and behaviour is judged" (p. 616). Sung offered three dimensions for filial piety. *Value commitments* refer to ethical and normative aspects of filial motives and are represented by religious beliefs, community harmony, family continuity, and saving face. *Service commitments* represent responsibility and care for parents. Finally, *emotional commitments* represent sympathy, concern for family harmony, and the desire to repay parental debts. In her empirical work, Sung (1995) found a two-factor structure for filial piety: behavioural orientation (sacrifice, responsibility and repayment) and emotional orientation (harmony, love and affection, respect). Although these distinctions are useful (and we have made use of them here), one can see problems in the overlap between motives and filial piety itself, so that ultimately it is not clear whether filial piety is an affect, behaviour, or the value that governs affect and behaviour.

The functions of filial piety appear to be clearer than their structural dimensions in previous work (Ho, 1994; Sung, 1990, 1995). One function involves a sense of mutuality representing reciprocity and inter-dependency, tangibly and affectively, between the young, the elderly and the community as well. This function is perhaps most commonly referred to as caregiving and social support (e.g., Cicirelli, 1992; Cutrona & Russell, 1990; Williams, Giles, Coupland, Dalby, & Manasse, 1990). The second function is positive identity support, which includes recognition, respect and enhancement of healthy identity. Both these functions are included in our work.

An Intergroup Approach to Filial Piety
A theoretically clearer conceptualisation of filial piety is now necessary, and this paper is an initial foray into exploring its dynamics cross-culturally. We conceptualise filial piety broadly as a special type of intergroup attitude (Tajfel & Turner, 1979) and, in this initial research, we take on only the perspective of young people. Based on the literature on filial piety, intergenerational attitudes may be isolated into affective and cognitive aspects. The affective aspect would be represented by one's symbolic attitudes towards the elderly, while the cognitive aspect would be represented by normative attitudes associated with roles "as young" (Herek, 1986; Hogg, Terry, & White, 1996). At present, we limit our research program to the cognitive aspect.

Norms are important in intercultural and intergroup communication, because violations of them can lead to negative consequences in communication (Burgoon, 1993; Gallois & Callan, 1991; Hall, 1959). Norms represent expectations about behaviour in particular situations, or "socially shared ideas about appropriate and inappropriate behaviour" (Gallois & Callan, 1991, p. 249). Normative attitudes about filial piety refer to one's attitudes toward the behaviours expected of young people in intergenerational encounters. Young individuals come to have a sense of identity as "the young" in their encounters with the elderly. Societal norms for young people's behaviour toward the elderly are associated with this identity. The more affirmative one's normative attitudes are, the more one is likely to be motivated to act according to them, by communicating accommodatively with the elderly and by providing care and a sense of support to them. Such normative attitudes may fulfil the elderly's practical needs, support their identity, and perhaps help young people to maintain their own distinctiveness (Brewer, 1991).

Hence, for us, filial piety is composed of at least five components. The first three of these are (1) peer norms about filial behaviours with the elderly in general, (2) perceived expectations of the elderly about filial behaviour towards them, and (3) intentions to engage in filial behaviour with the elderly. Peer norms and the elderly's expectations should be related to intentions (cf. the theory of reasoned action, Fishbein & Ajzen, 1975). Although it is not a component of filial piety itself, we also decided to examine the role of the perceived filial behaviour of other young adults (behavioural norms). Two other factors pertinent to orientations to one's own parents were also explored: personal norm about behaving towards one's own parents and parents' perceived expectations. The filial behaviours we examined included both nurturance and solidarity (i.e., respecting, looking after, taking care of, pleasing, listening to, keeping contact with the elderly). This study involved an exploration of the structure of these components in the perceptions of young adults. We expected Asians and Westerners to share some but not all aspects of this structure.

As outlined above, some comparative studies (including our own) about young people's attitudes toward the elderly suggest that positive perceptions of the elderly may not be currently characteristic of Asian youth (e.g., Chow, 1983; Koyano, 1989; Levy & Tsuhako, 1994; O'Leary, 1993). Given that filial piety has been such a core element in Southeast and East Asian intergenerational relations, however, we felt that it was more prudent to explore cultural differences, rather than making specific predictions about them. Thus, the study also examined the extent to which young adults across Western and Southeast Asian nations of the Pacific Rim differ in terms of their endorsement of filial piety.

Method

Participants
Participants from eight nations were involved. Four nations represented East and Southeast Asian nations: Japan, Hong Kong, Korea, the Philippines. The other four nations were Western (mainly Anglo-Saxon): Australia, New Zealand, the U.S., and Canada. These eight nations provide us with two distinct cultural clusters. According to Hofstede (1991), the U.S. is highest on his individualism index (with an individualism score of 91), Australia ranks second (90), Canada comes fourth (80), and New Zealand is ranked sixth (79). In contrast to highly individualistic nations, Japan is ranked 22nd (46), The Philippines comes 31st (32), Hong Kong 37th (25), and South Korea is ranked 43rd (18).

Data were gathered from one city in each of the nations: Tokyo, Japan; Shatin, Hong Kong; Seoul, Korea; Manila, The Philippines; Brisbane, Australia; Wellington, New Zealand; Santa Barbara, California, USA and Hamilton, Ontario, Canada. Altogether, 1445 young adults participated in the study. The number of participants from each of the nations was Japan, 228 (95 male, 133 female); Hong Kong, 205 (100 male, 102 female, 3 non-identifiers); Korea, 223 (109 male, 114 female); The Philippines, 191 (93 male, 98 female); Australia, 168 (72 male, 96 female); New Zealand, 150 (69 male, 81 female); the United States, 136 (46 male, 87 female, 3 non-identifiers); and Canada, 147 (54 male, 93 female). Their ages ranged from 16.2 to 30 years ($M = 20.1$, $SD = 1.93$), and age was relatively homogeneous across cultures. Samples from each nation were composed primarily of the dominant ethnic group, although there were two exceptions (considered theoretically non-problematic for our purposes): Canadians were mainly Anglos and French-Canadians, but other Euro-Canadians were included, and the Filipino sample was 50% Tagalog with the remainder comprising several different ethnolinguistic groups.

Questionnaire and Procedure
The questionnaire consisted of six *target scales*: (1) *intention* to engage in filial behaviour with elderly people in general, (2) *peer norms* about how young people should treat elderly people in general, (3) *behavioural norms*, or perceptions of how age peers treat elderly people, (4) perceptions of the *expectations by elderly people* about how they will be treated by young adults, (5) *personal norm* about filial behaviour toward

one's own parents, and (6) perceptions of *parents' expectations* regarding filial behaviour towards them.

Each of these six targets was made up of six items or *actions*, selected on the basis of extensive pilot work in Japan and Australia eliciting characteristics of filial piety, as well as from the literature. Each item was answered on a seven-point Likert-type scale, ranging from 1 = "strongly disagree" to 7 = "strongly agree." For instance, the actions in intention scale read: "I do/will look after older adults in general"; "I do/will financially assist older adults in general"; "I do/will respect older adults in general because of their age"; "I will/do listen patiently to the older adults in general"; "I do/will please older adults in general and make them happy"; and "I do/will retain contact with older adults in general". Each of the scales included these actions with a different opening target (e.g., peer norms, "Young adults should look after older adults in general;" behavioural norms, "Young adults whom I know do look after older adults in general;" older adults' expectations, "Older adults in general expect to be looked after;" personal norm, "When my parent(s) are older adults, I should look after them;" parents' expectations, "When my parent(s) are older adults, they will expect to be looked after").

The questionnaires were created in English and translated into the main language of instruction at the respective data collection sites. Reliabilities of each of the six targets were quite high across cultures (.80 to .85). Participants completed the questionnaires in large groups, either in undergraduate classes or in special research sessions at their universities. They were assured of anonymity and confidentiality, and their questions were answered by the researchers.

Results

Structure of Filial Piety

To examine the dimensionality underlying subjects' use of the filial piety targets and actions, we conducted a multi-mode principal components analysis. In this analysis, components or dimensions are computed for the use of the six targets (mode 1), use of the six actions (mode 2), and subjects (mode 3), but we will report only the first two modes here. The analyses reported were conducted using the program TUCKALS3 (Kroonen-berg & Brouwer, 1985). The basic aim of this program is reduction of the data to a limited number of components or dimensions for each mode, the assumption being that these components can describe the systematic variability in each mode. As well as conducting an analysis on subjects from all eight cultures, we conducted separate analyses for Asian

(Japanese, Korean, Hong Kong, and Filipino) subjects and Western (U.S., Canadian, Australian, and New Zealand) subjects. While this method does not compare Eastern and Western cultures directly, it provides a good picture of each.

A series of analyses were conducted to determine the number of components that provided both an adequate fit and a clear interpretation of the data. A solution with two components each for targets and actions, and four components for subjects, was selected. For the full sample, in terms of an ordinary principal components analysis, mode 1 accounted for 59% of the variance and mode 2, 62%. No formal procedures to decide the most appropriate solution are available at present, but the two by two by four solution gave the best improvement in fit, as well as providing a clear interpretation. In addition, this solution also gave good fits for the separate Asian and Western samples. The model is solved by least squares methods, so that it provides a standard division of sums of squares into fitted and residual, and a multiple correlation between data and fitted data is calculated. The solution reported here for the overall sample had an R^2 of .39, that for Asian subjects, an R^2 of .38, and for Western subjects, R^2 of 42; these results are fairly typical (Kroonenberg, 1983; Law, Snyder, Hattie, & McDonald, 1984).

Dimensionality of the Target Scales
The components of each mode partition the overall multiple correlation into independent contributions, and as would be expected in a principal components analysis, component one for each mode explains the most variance. For the overall sample, the first component of mode 1 contained four of the targets and opposed young people ("I do," "young adults do,") to older people ("older adults expect," "when my parents are older, they will expect"). The second component contained three targets and opposed family ("when my parents are older, I should," "my parents will expect") to other adults ("young adults do"). These same components, with slight variations in the targets included, also appeared for the separate Asian and Western samples.

Dimensionality of the Actions
For the overall sample, the second mode contained five actions in its first component, which opposed practical support ("look after older adults," "provide financial support") to communication ("respect," "listen patiently," "retain contact with older adults"). The second component contained two actions, and opposed respect ("respect") to support ("retain contact"). Once again, essentially the same components appeared for the Asian and Western samples.

Interaction of Targets and Actions

Multi-mode principal components analysis allows the relationship between the modes (in this case, the targets and actions comprising the filial piety measure) to be examined by calculating inner products, which represent the cosine of the angle between two vectors, and reflect the closeness of the vectors. Two vectors are highly and positively related if they are close together; such vectors have high positive inner products, and the concepts that the vectors represent are important to one another. Conversely, when two vectors have a high negative inner product, they are inversely related, and the two concepts have little or no importance to one another. These relationships can be illustrated graphically by means of a joint plot; the joint plot for the overall sample is presented in Figure 1. The dimensions of component one for targets and actions appear on the horizontal axis, and those of component two appear on the vertical axis. For ease of interpretation, ellipses have been drawn around clusters of targets and actions with high positive inner products (i.e., those which are important to each other).

As can be seen in Figure 1, there is a cluster connecting "older adults expect," "respect," and "young adults do," indicating that subjects perceived older people to expect to be respected by younger people, and indeed to receive this respect. A second cluster connects "when my parents are older, they will expect" and "retain contact.," The third cluster in the joint plot connects "I do," "young adults should," "when my parents are older, I should," "look after," and "support financially," indicating that subjects perceived a normative obligation to provide for their elderly parents, and to intend to do so.

The joint plots between scales for the Asian and Western samples revealed mainly the same pattern as for the full sample, although there were some interesting differences. The Western sample was almost identical to the overall sample. For the Asian sample, however, the clusters were somewhat different.

The cluster for parents expecting to retain contact with their children was also linked to "listen patiently," indicating that the Asian young people in the sample thought that their parents would want to communicate freely with their children when they grew older. The cluster connecting "older adults expect" and "respect" was also linked to "listen patiently," which suggests that the perception that older adults want communicative support is more general than just the family. Finally, the cluster connecting the personal and peer normative targets and practical support in this case also included "young adults do," which suggests that, unlike Western young people, the behavioural norm for the Asians holds that young people generally are prepared to do at least this much for their elders. Overall, compared to the Western sample, the Asians

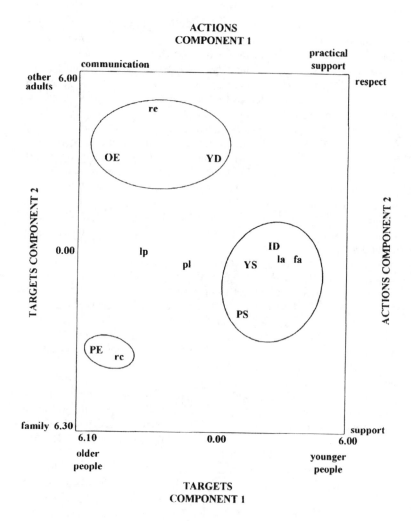

**ACTIONS
COMPONENT 1**

Figure 1. Joint Lot of Components 1 (Horizontal) and 2 (Vertical) for Targets (Mode 1) and Actions (Mode 2) for the Full Sample

Legend for targets: ID = I do; YS = Young adults should; YD = Young adults do; OE = Older adults expect; PS = When my parents are older, I should; PE = When my parents are older, they will expect;
Legend for actions: la = look after (older adults); fa = financially assist; re = respect; lp = listen patiently; pl = please; rc = retain contact.

appeared to have a more generalised idea of filial piety, as well as one which divides the expectations of older adults and the behaviour of young adults more sharply.

Cultural Differences in Perceptions of Filial Piety

In order to pursue some of the differences between Asian and Western young people further, and also to examine mean differences in perceptions of filial piety as a function of culture, a four-way multivariate analysis of variance was conducted (Bartlett's test of sphericity was significant, indicating that this was an appropriate course of action). Between-subjects variables were sex and culture (the eight original cultures), while target (six levels) was a repeated measure. The dependent variables were the filial piety actions. Because of the very large sample size, stringent significance criteria were used ($p < .001$ on both multivariate and univariate F-tests).

Results indicated a main effect on four targets for sex (Pillais = .042, $F(6, 1387) = 10.19$, $p < .001$), in which women showed higher means than did men. The other significant effects were all subsumed in a two-way interaction between culture and target (Pillais = .974, $F(210, 9583) = 7.37$, $p < .001$). Univariate tests for all six actions met the significance criterion. This interaction was followed up by complex comparisons between the four Asian cultures and the four Western ones, using confidence intervals to locate meaningful differences. Table 1 presents the means for each item for Asian and Western young adults. It also indicates the actions where means for the Asian and Western samples did not have overlapping confidence intervals.

It is easiest to interpret these results by action. For the actions "look after" and "financial support" (which were associated with the personal and peer norm targets in the three-mode principal component analysis), data for Asian subjects revealed higher mean scores than did those for Western subjects in all but two cases ("I do" and "young adults do" for the item "look after"). For the item "respect," Asian subjects had higher mean scores for the two targets dealing with parents and for the peer norm ("young adults should"), but had lower means on the behavioural norm ("young adults do") and on "older adults expect." The results for the fifth action, "please older adults" were very similar to those for "respect," as the table shows. Finally, for the fourth and sixth actions, "listen patiently" and "retain contact," means for Asian subjects were lower in most cases, the notable exceptions being "older adults expect" and "parents expect" for "listen patiently." Overall, Asian subjects appeared to endorse the actions relating to practical support more than did Western subjects, but to endorse those related to communication and contact less.

Table 1. Means for Filial Piety Actions by Asian and Western students

Target and Sample	Action					
	Look after	Fin.	Resp.	Listen	Please	Cont.
I *should*						
Asian stud.	5.04	4.83*	5.15	5.00	5.00	4.51*
Western stud.	4.89	4.53	5.11	5.63	5.12	5.53
Young adults *should*						
Asian stud.	5.41*	5.14*	5.25*	5.32*	5.12*	5.21*
Western stud.	4.67	4.33	4.90	5.58	4.79	5.71
Young adults *do*						
Asian stud.	3.92	3.57*	4.24*	4.00*	3.95*	3.66*
Western stud.	3.71	2.80	4.64	4.61	4.48	4.74
Older adults *expect*						
Asian stud.	4.83*	4.58*	5.46*	5.72*	5.03*	5.62
Western stud.	3.90	3.10	5.68	5.49	4.55	5.60
Parents, I *should*						
Asian stud.	6.16*	6.00*	5.70*	5.87	5.97*	6.21*
Western stud.	5.60	5.37	5.13	5.91	5.50	6.38
Parents *expect*						
Asian stud.	4.97*	4.52*	5.50*	5.84*	5.57*	6.14*
Western stud.	3.92	3.06	4.58	5.44	4.58	6.51

* This action and the one below it in the same column have a non-overlapping confidence interval ($p < .05$).
Fin. = Finance; Resp. = Respect; Cont. = Contact.

In terms of the targets, it is worth noting that the fewest cross-cultural differences appeared for the intention scale (three actions out of six were significantly different, as against five or six significant actions each for the other targets). The means show that subjects in both samples have positive intentions toward older people on all filial piety actions. The means also indicate that these young people, particularly the Asians, perceive that their family and non-family elders have high expectations of them. The lowest means appeared for the behavioural norm, "young adults do," indicating (not surprisingly) that these subjects believe that their own behaviour is better than that of their peers.

Discussion

The present study is a part of a large-scale program of research on ageing and communication across the Pacific Rim. In this study, the importance of understanding filial piety in intergenerational communication was emphasised, and an initial attempt at conceptualising its dynamics was undertaken. In addition, cross-cultural comparisons of filial piety were conducted to determine whether traditional endorsements of this value in East and Southeast Asian cultures still persist compared with the West.

In the first instance, these results show that filial piety has two distinct parts in the minds of these young people. The first centres around practical support and the financial maintenance of older people, particularly the parents. Both Asian and Western students perceived an obligation to look after and support older people, and they intend to meet it. On the other hand, they perceived the expectations of older people as different from their own; in their view, their parents and older people in general expect respect, communication, and contact. For all participants, but especially for Asians, this is a sharp distinction, and it may well be the source of future conflicts between these people and their elderly parents (and others). Such a tension is reflected in the polar opposition in the dimensions of the three-mode factor analysis between young and older people, which appeared for all three samples.

As well as the distinction between young and older people, these students also distinguished between obligations to their families and obligations to older people in general. In their perceptions, their parents deserve practical support, while older adults in general deserve respect. For these students, the specific demands of filial piety are largely restricted to the family. It should be noted that this was less true in the case of Asians, who perceived the expectations of older people in general to be linked more closely to those of their own parents. This finding may suggest that young Asian adults still maintain more traditional filial piety toward their own parents and the elderly in general. They feel they should engage in filial behaviours toward the elderly in general, and are also aware that they are expected to do so.

The results of the cross-cultural comparisons are also revealing. In general, these students intend to "do the right thing" by their parents and older adults. Nevertheless, Asian students endorsed the more practical aspects of filial piety more strongly than did Westerners, while the converse was true for the components of filial piety related to contact and communication. It may be that Western social policies of welfare and provisions for the elderly (pensions, superannuation) have taken the edge off the sense of personal obligation among their children, especially as the standard of living is perceived to have declined in the West in recent years. On the other hand, it seems that this loss of obligation to give practical help has been replaced by a stronger norm among Westerners of retaining contact with parents and the elderly in general.

Rather surprisingly, the results reveal that young Asian adults tend to think that they are not fulfilling social expectations and norms about filial behaviours. In this study, Asian students believed that the elderly have high expectations of filial behaviours from them which they believe to be acceptable, yet they are less likely to think they will engage in these behaviours themselves. On the other hand, Western students believed that they will engage in filial behaviours more than the elderly expect, and more than they think they should. It should be noted, of course, that should the expectations of the elderly become too high, there may be a backlash, an issue worthy of further study. In any case, these results indicate that young people in some Southeast and East Asian cultures may not willingly practice filial oehaviour toward the elderly in general, despite the fact that they are socially expected to and feel they should. Instead, these young adults may reluctantly accommodate to the elderly's expectations and social norms. On the other hand, young adults in Western cultures seem to feel that they go beyond social expectations and voluntarily accommodate.

These results are suggestive in at least two ways. First, young adults in East and Southeast Asian nations are not as positive about inter-generational communication as those in individualistic nations, even though they are very positive about their practical obligations. This interpretation coincides with findings from other parts of our research project. Harwood et al. (1996) found that young people in Japan, Hong Kong, Korea, and The Philippines have more negative stereotypes of the elderly than those in Australia, New Zealand, the U.S., and Canada, while Williams et al. (1996) found that young adults in the four Southeast and East Asian nations have more negative perceptions of the elderly during conversation than their Western counterparts. Taken together, these studies and others (e.g., Koyano, 1989, and Levy & Tsuhako, 1994), paint a picture of stress, and perhaps negative change, in Asian young people's communicative inclinations towards older people.

We might also draw a theoretical connection between these findings and young people's communicative orientations during intergenerational interaction. Young adults in East and Southeast Asian nations appear to be *under*accommodating to elderly people in general (see Gallois et al.,

1995; Williams et al., 1990). The data showed that they intend to act filially to a lesser extent than they are expected to and believe they should. Young people in individualistic nations, on the other hand, appear to be *over*accommodating, given that they intend to act filially more than they believe they should, and more than they are expected to. Such overaccommodation may result in the kind of "patronising speech" that has been documented as a common phenomenon in individualistic nations (e.g., Harwood et al., 1993; Ryan, Hummert, & Boich, 1995), but less so in Asian ones (e.g., Giles et al., in press). Obviously, future work needs to move us from intentions to the actual behaviour of these same informants in intergenerational communication.

In conclusion, this study provides an initial cross-cultural look at the structure of filial piety. For the future, it is important to improve the current instrument and to elaborate our construct of filial piety; notions such as reciprocity have yet to be incorporated. Moreover, the other side of filial piety —symbolic attitudes toward elderly people— must be studied in parallel; Sung (1995) suggests that filial piety is so called because of the presence of positive affect toward the elderly. Hence, future studies need to look at how filial piety is related to other constructs, such as stereotypes, vitality and intergenerational communicative beliefs, as well as how filial piety affects young adults' actual communication behaviours. Relatedly, it is important to investigate the reactions of the elderly to young adults' behaviour and communication. The role of filial piety, thus, should be investigated in ongoing intergenerational interaction. Non-student young and middle-aged adults need to be studied to see if the same patterns of filial piety emerge, and the extent to which the magnitude and nature of filial piety may be different. Last, but not least, it is important to expend more energy than we have in addressing filial piety as a gendered phenomenon interacting with culture.

References

Brewer, M. (1991). The social self: On being the same and different at the same time. *Personality and Social Psychology Bulletin, 17*, 475-482.

Burgoon, J. K. (1993). Interpersonal expectations, expectancy violations, and emotional communication. *Journal of Language and Social Psychology, 12*, 30-48.

Chow, N. W. (1983). The Chinese family and support of the elderly in Hong Kong. *The Gerontologist, 23*, 584-588.

Cicirelli, V. G. (1992). *Family caregiving*: Autonomous and paternalistic decision making. Newbury Park, CA: Sage.

Coupland, N., Coupland, J., & Giles, H. (1991). *Language, society, and the elderly: Discourse, identity and aging.* Oxford: Basil Blackwell.

Cutrona, C. E., & Russell, D. W. (1990). Type of social support and specific stress: Toward a theory of optimal matching. In B. R. Sarason, I. G. Sarason, & G. R. Pierce (Eds.), *Social support: An interactional view.* New York: John Wiley & Sons.

Dowd, J. J. (1986). The old person as stranger. In V. W. Marshall (Ed.), *Later life: The social psychology of aging* (pp. 147-189). Beverly Hills, CA: Sage.

Edwards, H., & Noller, P. (1993). Perceptions of overaccommodation used by nurses in communication with the elderly. *Journal of Language and Social Psychology, 12,* 207-223.

Fishbein, M., & Ajzen, I. (1975). *Belief, attitude, intention, and behaviour: An introduction to theory and research.* Reading, MA: Addison-Wesley.

Gallois, C., & Callan, V. J. (1991). Interethnic accommodation: The role of norms. In H. Giles, J. Coupland, & N. Coupland (Eds.), *Contexts of accommodation: Developments in applied sociolinguistics* (pp. 245-369). New York: Cambridge University Press.

Gallois, C., Giles, H., Jones, E., Cargile, A. C., & Ota, H. (1995). Accommodating intercultural encounters: Elaborations and extensions. In R. L. Wiseman (Ed.), *Theories of intercultural communication* (pp. 115-147). Thousand Oaks, CA: Sage.

Gardner, C. B. (1991). Stigma and the public self: Notes on communication, self, and others. *Journal of Contemporary Ethnography, 20,* 251-262.

Giles, H., Harwwod, J., Pierson, H. D., Clement, R., & Fox, S. (in press). Stereotypes of the elderly and evaluations of patronizing speech: A cross-cultural foray. In R. K. Agnihotri & A. L. Khanna (Eds.), *Research in applied linguistics IV: The social psychology of language.* New Delhi: Sage.

Goffman, E. (1963). *Stigma: Notes on the management of spoiled identity.* New York: Simon & Schuster.

Gudykunst, W. B., & Ting-Toomey, S. (1988). *Culture and interpersonal communication.* Newbury Park, CA: Sage.

Hall, E. T. (1959). *The silent language.* New York: Doubleday.

Hamilton, G. G. (1990). Patriarchy, patrimonialism and filial piety: A comparison of China and Western Europe. *British Journal of Sociology, 41,* 77-104.

Harwood, J., Giles, H., Ota, H., Pierson, H. Gallois, C. Lim, T-S., Ng, S., Ryan, E. B., Maher, J., & Somera, L. (1996, May). *Multiple stereotypes across cultures: Health issues.* Paper presented at the

Third International Conference on Communication, Health, and Aging, Kansas City.

Harwood, J., Giles, H., Pierson, H. D., Clement, R., & Fox, S. (1994). Vitality perceptions of age categories in California and Hong Kong. *Journal of Multilingual and Multicultural Development, 15*, 311-318.

Harwood, J., Giles, H., Ryan, E. B., Fox, S., & Williams, A. (1993). Patronizing young and elderly adults: Response strategies in a community setting. *Journal of Applied Communication Research, 21*, 211-226.

Herek, G. M. (1986). The instrumentality of attitudes: Toward a neo-functional theory. *Journal of Social Issues, 42*, 99-114.

Ho, D. Y-F. (1994). Filial piety, authoritarian moralism, and cognitive conservativism in Chinese societies. *Genetic, Social, and General Psychology Monographs, 120*, 349-365.

Hofstede, G. (1991). *Culture and organizations: Software of mind.* New York: McGraw Hill.

Hogg, M. A., Terry, D. J., & White, K. M. (1996). A tale of two theories: A critical comparison of identity theory with social identity theory. *Social Psychology Quarterly, 4*, 255-269.

Hsu, F. (1971). Filial piety in Japan and China: Borrowing, variation, and significance. *Journal of Comparative Family Studies, 22*, 67-74.

Hummert, M. L., Garstka, T. A., Shaner, J. L. (in press). Beliefs about language performance: Adults' perceptions about self and elderly targets. *Journal of Language and Social Psychology.*

Kiefer, C. W. (1992). Aging in Eastern cultures: A historical overview. In T. R. Cole, D. D. Van Tassel, & R. Kastenbaum (Eds.), *Handbook of the humanities and aging* (pp. 96-123). New York: Springer Publishing Company.

Kim, U., & Yamaguchi, S. (1994). Cross-cultural research methodology and approach: Implications for the advancement of Japanese social psychology. *Research in Social Psychology, 10*, 168-179.

Kim, U. (1994). Individualism and collectivism: Conceptual clarification and elaboration. In U. Kim, H. C. Triandis, C. Kagitcibasi, C. Choi, & G. Yoon (Eds.), *Individualism and collectivism: Theory, method, and applications.* (pp. 19-40). Thousand Oaks, CA: Sage.

Koyano, W. (1989). Japanese attitudes toward the elderly: A review of research findings. *Journal of Cross-Cultural Gerontology, 4*, 335-345.

Kroonenberg, P. M. (1983). *Three-mode principal components analysis: Theory and applications.* Leiden: DSWO Press.

Kroonenberg, P. M., & Brouwer, P. (1985). *User's guide to TUCKALS3.* Leiden: University of Leiden.

Law, H. G., Snyder, Jr., C. W., Hattie, J. A., & McDonald, P. M. (1984). *Research methods for multimode data analysis.* New York: Praeger.

Levy, B., & Tsuhako, S. (1994). *The status paradox of Japanese elderly.* A paper presented at Gerontology Society of America Annual Conference.

Markus, H., & Kitayama, S. (1991). Culture and self: Implications for cognition, emotion, and motivation. *Psychological Review, 98,* 224-253.

Nussbaum, J. F., & Coupland, J. (1995). *Handbook of communication and aging research.* Mahwah, NJ: Lawrence Erlbaum.

Nussbaum, J. F., Hummert, M. L., Williams, A., & Harwood, J. (1996). Communication and elder adults. In B. Burleson (Ed.), *Communication yearbook, 19* (pp. 1-47). Thousand Oaks, CA: Sage.

O'Leary, J. S. (1993). A new look at Japan's honorable elders. *Journal of Aging Studies, 7,* 1-24.

Palmore, E. (1975). *The honorable elders: A cross-cultural analysis of aging in Japan.* Durham, NC: Duke University Press.

Russel, C. (1981). *The aging experience.* Sydney: George Allen & Unwin.

Russel, C., & Oxley, H. (1990). Health and aging in Australia: Is there culture after sixty? *Journal of Cross-Cultural Gerontology, 5,* 35-50.

Ryan, E. B., & Cole, R. (1990). Evaluative perceptions of interpersonal communication with the elderly. In H. Giles, N. Coupland, & J. M. Wiemann (Eds.), *Communication, health, and the elderly* (pp. 172-190). Manchester, England: Manchester University Press.

Ryan, E. B., Hummert, M. L., & Boich, L. H. (1995). Communication predicaments of aging: Patronizing behaviour toward older adults. *Journal of Language and Social Psychology, 14,* 144-166.

Sung, K-T. (1990). A new look at filial piety: Ideas and practice of family-centered parent care in Korea. *The Gerontologist, 30,* 610-617.

Sung, K-T. (1995). Measures and dimensions of filial piety in Korea. *The Gerontologist, 35,* 240-247.

Tajfel, H., & Turner, J. C. (1979). An integrative theory of intergroup conflict. In W. G. Austin & S. Worchel (Eds.), *Social psychology of intergroup relations* (pp. 33-47). Monterey, CA: Brooks-Cole.

Tien-Hyatt, J. L. (1987). Self-perceptions of aging across cultures: Myth or reality. *International Journal of Aging and Human Development, 24,* 129-148.

Triandis, H. C. (1995). *Individualism & collectivism.* Boulder, CO: Westview.

Tu, W. M. (1985). *Confucian thought: Selfhood as creative transformation.* New York: SUNY press.

Williams, A., Giles, H., Coupland, N., Dalby, M., & Manasse, H. (1990). The communicative contexts of elderly social support and health: A theoretical model. *Health Communication, 2*, 123-143.

Williams, A., Ota, H., Giles, H., Pierson, H. D., Gallois, C., Ng, S-H., Lim, T-H., Ryan, E, B., Maher, J., & Harwood, J. (1996, May). *Young people's beliefs about intergenerational communication: An initial cross-cultural comparison.* Paper presented at the 46th Annual conference of the International Communication Association, Chicago.

Yum, J. O. (1988). The impact of Confucianism on interpersonal relationships and communication patterns in East Asia. *Communication Monographs, 55*, 374-387.

Kiasuism across Cultures: Singapore and Australia

Shee Wai Ho, Don Munro, and Stuart C. Carr
University of Newcastle, Australia

ABSTRACT

"Kiasu" is a term widely used in Singapore to describe a preoccupation with never allowing oneself to lose out on any opportunity to get more, to win, to be better than others. "Kiasuism" thus refers to the lengths to which people will go to make sure that they do not lose out. It has been suggested that Kiasuism is a uniquely Singaporean characteristic, but there has yet to be an academic or empirical study done on it. This paper takes the first step in that direction by developing a reliable scale to measure Kiasuism. It also attempts to shed light on the uniqueness of Kiasuism for Singaporeans by a cross-cultural comparison with Australians, using results from 136 Singaporean and 128 Australian university students. The resulting Kiasu scale shows high internal consistency reliability (coefficient alpha = .90 for the combined sample) and has acceptable face and content validity. Principal component analyses revealed two 6-component structural patterns for the two population samples, with five components in common (Greed, Value for Money, Being Number One, Preventing Others from Winning, and Rushing) and one unique component (Ensuring a Win for the Singaporeans, and Money Consciousness for the Australians). It is concluded that the phenomenon of Kiasuism is not unique to Singaporean culture; and assessment of other cultural groups is suggested.

"Kiasuism" is a term originally used by Singapore's National Servicemen to describe the behavior of recruits who tried extra hard to impress their sergeants at boot camp (Tripathi, 1993). It began trickling into civilian vocabulary about 1990 and was popularized by three enterprising Singaporeans —James Suresh, Johnny Lau, and Lim Yu Cheng— who created "Mr Kiasu," a comic character. To date, Mr Kiasu has been featured in five books, a quarterly magazine, and even a musical. The official Courtesy Campaign and the Traffic Police Road Safety Campaign have made use of the character and given him celebrity status in Singapore. Even the multinational corporation, MacDonald's, cashed in on Mr. Kiasu in 1993, by having the character promote the "Kiasu Burger" as "the extra Singaporean burger."

Kiasu is used in Singapore to describe a cultural phenomenon of a preoccupation with never allowing oneself to lose out on any opportunity to get more, to win, to be better than others, etc. It encompasses the elements of competitiveness, greed, and a concern with value for money. Truly Kiasu people are the first to board the bus and the first at the exit. When it is very crowded at a sale, they will get their family to queue at the paying line first while they do the rest of the shopping. At the supermarket, they are seen digging for the fruits at the bottom of the pile because they think they are fresher than those at the top, and Kiasu diners will stack their plates with food and eat too much just to get their money's worth.

Overall, it is an ambiguous concept (Tripathi, 1993). For some people it is defined in terms of not wanting to lose out; and for others, wanting to have more than other people (Lin, 1994). Many Singaporeans believe that Kiasuism reflects negatively on them: "The social phenomenon of Kiasuism is a fascinating example of affluent, technocratic Singapore gone haywire" (Lewis, 1991).

Literally translated from the Chinese dialect, Kiasu means "afraid to lose." The 1997 edition of the Australian Macquarie Dictionary defines Kiasuism as "an obsessive desire for value for money — hailed as a national fixation in Singapore." Neither are complete definitions. However, Kiasuism has been hailed as the one Singaporean national trait that most Singaporeans recognize and acknowledge:

"Singaporeans do have other values, but none, it seems, [is] as distinctive as Kiasuism. The great spirit of Kiasuism ... unites all Singaporeans, regardless of race, language, culture or creed. Just try to find another national value, ideology or sport in Singapore that is more widely embraced or more deeply entrenched than Kiasuism, and you would probably come up with a complete blank" (Lee, S.C., cited in Lewis, 1991).

Lin (1994) has argued that the Kiasuism phenomenon can be partly attributed to Singaporeans being brought up in an education system that encourages students to strive for academic excellence. Lim (1993) proposed viewing the trait of Kiasuism in the broader perspective of an ongoing process of national development and the growth of a national ideology that set the tone and direction for individual behaviors. In the early years, the dedication to technological advancement was perceived as the only means of survival for a little island with no natural resources of its own and therefore totally dependent on the development of its human resources. There thus arose a need to do things in a hurry, a fear of making mistakes, a need to be extremely cautious in decision making, a tendency to see things only in concrete, measurable and quantifiable terms, and a tendency to value things in purely monetary or utilitarian terms.

Some Possible Western Parallels to Kiasuism

There is no single concept in the mainstream psychological literature that is the replica of Kiasuism, though it can be thought of as having various aspects, some of which have Western parallels. These may include competitiveness, need for achievement, individualism, and uncertainty avoidance.

Competitiveness. Most writers define competitiveness in terms of the desire to win in interpersonal situations (Smither & Houston, 1992). Kiasuism is similar in that individuals are trying to be first, but different in that it involves striving in every situation and sometimes using devious means to get ahead of others. Kiasu individuals show two characteristic behaviors: Making sure that all means of keeping ahead have been covered (e.g., students read or write more than is required), and trying to prevent others from winning (e.g., by quitting while ahead so that others will not have a chance to catch up).

Need for achievement. The need for achievement was originally defined as "the desire to overcome obstacles, to experience power, to strive to do something difficult well and as quickly as possible" (McClelland, Atkinson, Clark, & Lowell, 1953), but more recently it has been suggested that there is more than one form of achievement behavior (Maehr, 1974; Maehr & Nicholls, 1980). Ability-oriented motivation is characterized by striving to maintain a favorable perception of one's ability by maximizing the subjective probability of attributing high ability to oneself. Task-oriented achievement behavior has the primary goal of producing an adequate product or solving a problem for its own sake rather than to demonstrate ability. Social-approval motivation is directed at maximizing the chances of attributing high effort and minimizing the chances of attributing low effort to the self. Every culture may demonstrate a unique mix of these aspects.

Although need for achievement appears similar to Kiasuism, the latter differs in that it is not only concerned with the result but with the process of achieving. Kiasu students need not be the first in class (although they try to be), but can be equally happy so long as they have done all the "Kiasu stuff" (such as being the first to sign up for tutorials, hogging notes, hiding library books, reading and writing more than required, etc.). It might even be argued that Kiasu individuals enjoy the process of achieving more than the result.

Individualism. The individualism-collectivism dichotomy (Hofstede, 1980) represents the relative emphasis that members of a culture place on personal versus collective goals and has become widely used to compare national groups. However, it is recognized as a simplistic classification, as there are few societies or organizations in which members are purely individualistic or collectivistic; and individuals within any society tend to have both individualistic and collectivistic tendencies (Kashima, 1990). According to Hui (1990), it also mistakenly assumes that collectivists treat most people alike. He argues that collectivism is target-specific in that individuals within a collectivistic culture favor certain ingroups such as family and close friends, or as Leung and Bond (1984) put it, collectivists are only collectivistic towards ingroup members.

In individualistic cultures, it is the individual who achieves; in collectivistic cultures, groups achieve (Triandis, Bontempo, & Villareal, 1988). Cooperation, interdependence, and even dependence within groups can and do exist comfortably with an achieving orientation towards the world in general. Similarly, Kiasu individuals are not wholly selfish. From their various behaviors (e.g., queuing overnight to buy tickets for friends and family), it can be said that they are very concerned about their ingroup. At other times, however, they seem to be trying to outdo everyone, including their own ingroup. This reflects the complex nature of Kiasuism.

Uncertainty avoidance. Uncertainty avoidance in a culture programs its members to feel uncomfortable in unstructured, novel, unknown, or surprising situations. Uncertainty-avoiding cultures try to minimize the possibility of such situations by adhering to strict laws and rules, safety and security measures, and a belief in absolute truth (Hofstede & Bond, 1988). Kiasu individuals, in wanting to avoid losing, might also be high on uncertainty avoidance. This is not supported by Hofstede's (1980) study, which found that Singaporeans had a very low score on the uncertainty avoidance scale, but the study was conducted in the period 1973-78, before the Kiasu phenomenon was identified, so its applicability to the fast-changing Singapore society twenty years later is questionable.

Aims of the Study

The main aims were the development of the first (reliable) Kiasu measure, the establishment of its relationship to other established constructs, and the investigation of the uniqueness of Kiasuism by way of cross-cultural comparison between a Singaporean sample and an Australian sample on the measure developed. It does not investigate the causes or effects of Kiasuism.

Development of the Kiasu Scale

An initial pool of more than 200 items for the draft versions of a Likert-scale questionnaire came from three main sources: (a) review of literature pertaining to Kiasuism [In particular, use was made of the examples provided by Suresh, Lau, Chong, and Cheng (1990), and Cheng, Lau, and Suresh (1991)], (b) the first author's personal experience and knowledge of the phenomenon, and (c) unstructured interviews with Singaporean students in Australia and personal acquaintances in Singapore. Convergent and divergent validity were explored in relation to four related constructs:

Social desirability. In the search for a valid social desirability measure in the cross-cultural context, it was found that the Lie Scale from the Eysenck Personality Questionnaire (Eysenck, 1974) had been cross-culturally validated. Specifically, Eysenck and Long (1986) reported high reliability (coefficient alphas of .81 and .80 for Singaporean males and females, respectively) and validity for the Lie Scale with a Singapore sample. The pilot questionnaire therefore included 19 items from the Eysenck Lie Scale to check for social desirability responding.

Competitiveness. To measure competitiveness, the 15-item Competitiveness Index developed by Smither and Houston (1992) was used. This appears to be the only psychometrically sound measure available that is independent of an achievement motivation scale and taps into settings other than sport.

Need for achievement. The more common projective measures of Need for Achievement were deemed unsuitable, as they do not conform to the Likert-type format of the Kiasu measure. A Need Achievement scale of 22 items was therefore compiled from the two achievement motivation scales from the Edwards Personal Preference Schedule (Edwards, 1953) and Jackson's (1974) Personality Research Form (PRF)-Form E.

Fear of success. Given that Fear of Success is proposed to be a construct in opposition to that of achievement motivation and competitiveness (Horner, 1972), a measure that taps into this construct is expected to diverge from the Kiasu measure. A literature review indicated that Ho and Zemaitis' (1981) Concern over the Negative Consequences of Success Scale was the only available scale that fits well with Horner's (1972) original conception of Fear of Success. It also had the advantage of being developed for the Australian population. However, two of the items were judged to be culturally inappropriate in Singapore, so only 25 of the original 27 items were used.

Pilot Study

A pilot study was undertaken with 20 Singaporean (10 of each gender) and 20 Australian (10 of each gender) students studying in various disciplines in Australia, with a mean age of 22.3 years. Satisfactory initial estimates of internal consistency reliability were obtained for the five scales: Kiasu Scale (116 items, $\alpha = 0.93$); Competitiveness Index (15 items, $\alpha = 0.75$); Need for Achievement Scale (22 items, $\alpha = 0.90$); Fear of Success Scale (25 items, $\alpha = 0.70$); and Eysenck Lie Scale (19 items, $\alpha = 0.68$).

Although the requirements were not met, an exploratory analysis was conducted to tentatively identify the underlying structures of the Kiasu construct. The data from the Kiasu Scale were submitted to a principal component analysis, and items loading on the first component (accounting for 17.2% of the variance) were used to form the revised Kiasu scale. Those items that correlated negatively with the scale and those that loaded less than 0.30 with the first component were eliminated. The remaining items were scrutinized with a view to including as wide a variety in content as possible while, at the same time, ensuring the component loadings and item-total correlations were high. This procedure resulted in forty nine Kiasu Scale items.

Method

Participants

The participants were Singaporeans and Australians who were students from the National University of Singapore and the University of Newcastle, New South Wales, Australia, respectively. Including those used for the initial pilot study, there were 136 Singaporeans (63 males and 73 females from 19 to 32 years old, with the mean age being 22.01 years) and 128 Australians (44 males and 84 females from 19 to 57 years old, with the mean age being 23.79 years).

A two-way, Gender by Nationality ANOVA performed on age revealed a significant difference between the nationalities, $F(1, 260) = 9.68$, $p < .01$, and a Gender X Nationality interaction effect, $F(1, 260) = 4.66$, $p < .05$. Post hoc comparisons indicated significant differences between the genders in the Australian sample, $F(1, 260) = 5.19$, $p < .05$, with the males ($M = 22.89$) being significantly younger than the females ($M = 24.27$), and also significant differences between the females of the two nationalities, $F(1, 260) = 14.39$, $p < .01$, with the Australian females ($M = 24.27$) being significantly older than the Singaporean females ($M = 21.48$).

Measures

Participants were administered the final version of the questionnaire, which consisted of 130 items in random order from the five scales described previously (the 49-item Kiasu Scale, the 19-item Lie Scale, the 15-item Competitiveness Index, the 22-item Need for Achievement Scale, and the 25-item Concern over Negative Consequences of Success Scale).

Table 1. Coefficients of Internal Consistency (alpha) for the Five Scales

Scale	No. Items	Singapore (N=136)	Austral (N=128)	Pooled (N=264)
Kiasu	49	0.91	0.87	0.90
Competitiveness	15	0.72	0.74	0.74
Need for achievement	22	0.89	0.87	0.89
Fear of success	25	0.85	0.80	0.85
Lie	19	0.60	0.63	0.61

Procedure
The Australian participants were recruited during one of the third year Psychology lectures. All the participants answered the questionnaire voluntarily and anonymously during the lecture and returned the questionnaire after the lecture. The return rate was 71.33%. The Singaporean participants were recruited by two tutors from the Psychology and Statistics departments. The participants answered the questionnaire voluntarily and anonymously in their own time and returned the questionnaire when they had finished. The return rate was 73.33%.

Results

Internal Consistency Reliability of the Scales
Table 1 presents the coefficients of internal consistency reliability as estimated by Cronbach's alpha for the five scales in the Singapore and Australia samples and the pooled data. As can be seen, most of the scales have a reasonably high reliability for both the pooled data and the separate samples, except for the Eysenck Lie Scale.

Intercorrelations Among the Instruments
As expected, the Kiasu Scale was moderately positively correlated across the combined national samples with the Competitiveness Index, $r = 0.26$, $p < .01$, and the Need for Achievement Scale, $r = 0.36$, $p < .01$, and the latter two scales were also significantly related, $r = 0.37$, $p < .01$. The Kiasu scale correlated negatively with the Lie Scale, $r = -0.31$, $p < .01$, showing that Kiasuism is generally interpreted as a socially undesirable trait.

Table 2. Corrrelations among the Five Scales for the Two National Samples

Scale	Kiasu	Comp.	Achiev.	Fear	Eys Lie
Kiasu	-	0.35**	0.39**	0.35**	-0.34**
Comp.	0.12	-	0.51**	-0.36**	-0.01
Achiev.	0.30**	0.19*	-	-0.07	0.16
Fear	0.37**	-0.38**	-0.10	-	-0.26**
Eys Lie	-0.29*	-0.13	0.20*	-0.24**	-

Note. Comp. = Competitiveness; Achiev. = Achievement; Fear = Fear of success; Eys Lie = Eysenck Lie Scale; $* p < .05$; $** p < .01$.

An unexpected finding was that the Fear of Success Scale was positively correlated to the Kiasu scale, $r = 0.32$, $p < .01$, in contradiction to the hypothesis that Kiasuism is related to a positive reaction to success. The Fear of Success Scale is significantly negatively correlated with Competitiveness, $r = -0.39$, $p < .01$, confirming that the two are somewhat antagonistic or that the Fear of Success Scale may measure fear of competition, and Fear of Success is negatively correlated with the Lie Scale, $r = -0.25$, $p < .01$, indicating its low social desirability. A principal components analysis conducted on the 25 items of the Fear of Success Scale yielded six components with eigenvalues greater than one, accounting for 56.1% of the total variance, suggesting that the scale is not unidimensional despite its acceptable alpha coefficients of above .80.

Correlational Analyses for the Two Samples Separately

To examine the differences, if any, between the two national samples, two separate correlational analyses were performed on the two samples. Table 2 presents the zero-order correlations among the five scales for the Singaporean and Australian samples. Comparison of the correlations between the Kiasu Scale and the Competitiveness Index for the Singaporean sample and the Australian sample, using Fisher's transformation to z, revealed that the pattern difference is significant, $z = 2.21$, $p < .01$. This is true also for the correlations between the Competitiveness Index and the Need for Achievement Scale for the two samples, $z = 3.04$, $p < .01$.

Regression Analysis

Given the fact that all the four scales are significantly correlated to the Kiasu scale, the four validation scales plus age, nationality, and gender

Table 3. Means and Standard Deviations by Nationality on the Five Scales

	Singaporean			
Scale	Males (*N* = 63)		Females (*N* = 73)	
	M	*SD*	*M*	*SD*
Kiasu	91.51	19.07	87.01	17.01
Competitiveness	37.86	5.72	35.71	6.02
Achievement	58.90	9.24	53.21	9.91
Fear of success	44.81	9.54	45.32	8.35
Lie	59.32	5.54	58.51	5.23
	Australian			
Scale	Males (*N* = 44)		Females (*N* = 84)	
	M	*SD*	*M*	*SD*
Kiasu	98.39	16.27	90.21	13.87
Competitiveness	40.93	5.80	37.82	6.06
Achievement	61.59	9.05	57.57	10.31
Fear of success	41.82	8.12	40.44	7.84
Lie	57.25	5.56	60.50	4.69

were regressed on the pooled Kiasu scale scores. Significant ($p < 0.01$) beta coefficients were obtained for Fear of Success (–0.42), Need for Achievement (0.33), the Competitiveness Index (0.25), the Eysenck Lie scale (–0.25), and (Australian) nationality (0.14). Beta coefficients for gender and age were close to zero.

Comparison of Scale Scores
Given high internal consistency reliability for the Kiasu Scale, results from the whole scale were first used to test whether there were nationality or gender differences. The design was a 2 X 2 (Nationality X Gender) between-subjects factorial ANOVA. The number of participants across the four cells ranged from 44 to 84. Univariate ANOVAs were conducted on the five scales. Table 3 presents means and standard deviations for the scales. Significant nationality effects were observed for all scales except Lie: $F(1, 260) = 5.20$, $p < .05$ for Kiasu, $F(1, 260) = 11.50$, $p < .01$ for Competitiveness, $F(1, 260) = 9.34$, $p < .05$ for Achievement, and $F(1, 260) = 14.45$, $p < .01$ for Fear of Success. For all the scales that showed a significant nationality effect, the Australians

scored higher than the Singaporeans, with the exception of Fear of Success. In the scales that showed a significant gender effect, males scored higher than females, the ratios being $F(1, 260) = 8.82, p < .01$ for Kiasu, $F(1, 260) = 11.96, p < .01$ for Competitiveness, and $F(1, 260) = 16.01, p < 01$ for Achievement. There was a significant nationality by gender interaction effect for the Lie Scale ($F(1, 260) = 9.50, p < .01$), with Australian females scoring significantly higher than males and Singaporean females lower than Australian females.

Principal Component Analysis of the Kiasu Scale

A principal components analysis was conducted on the Kiasu scale data using varimax rotation. The 49 Kiasu Scale items produced 15 initial components with eigenvalues greater than unity, accounting for 62.0% of the variance. Cattell's scree test was used as a guide but was not very clear, so a number of solutions extracting one to seven components were tried. The most interpretable result was found with the 6-component solution, accounting for 39.0% of the variance. Only those items with a loading of .50 or greater and relatively low loadings on other components were considered. This procedure resulted in 19 items being included (see Table 4). Value-neutral descriptive labels for each component are suggested.

Correlations between Kiasu Components and the Other Scales

A new Kiasu score was calculated for all the subjects by summing scores from items included in the six varimax rotated components. This had an almost identical correlation pattern as that which utilized the original full scale: i.e., significant positive correlations with the Competitiveness Index, Need for Achievement Scale, and Fear of Success Scale, and a significant negative correlation with the Lie Scale (see Table 5). This correlation pattern was also found in the Greed and Being Number One components. The Money Consciousness and Value for Money components were positively correlated with the Fear of Success Scale and Need for Achievement Scale, while the Rushing component was positively correlated with the Competitiveness Index and negatively correlated with the Lie Scale.

Separate Principal Component Analyses for the Two Samples

Two separate principal components analyses were conducted on the two sets of data using varimax rotation extracting six components. Again all of the 49 items had significant loadings of .30 or above on at least one of the components. When only those items with a loading of .50 and above were considered, it resulted in 23 items for the Singaporean sample (accounting for 43.7% of the variance) and 21 items for the Australian

Table 4 Varimax-Rotated Kiasu Scale Principal Components for Pooled Data (with loadings)

I. Greed (18.2% of total variance)
Eat your money's worth of food (0.73).
Pile up food in your plate every time you go for a helping (0.67).
Rush to be one of the first to get the food at a buffet (0.66).
Keep an eye out for any new dishes that the kitchen might bring out at a buffet (0.65).
Go for more than one helping at a buffet (0.63).
Take more than you can eat at a buffet (0.63).
Take the more expensive food at a buffet (0.60).
II. Money Consciousness (4.9% of total variance)
Go through a lot of trouble just to get something cheap (0.67).
Collect discount coupons to use (0.60).
Actively look for discounts (0.58).
Go out of your way to avoid wasting anything (0.58).
III. Being Number One (4.6% of total variance)
Try to be ahead of others in anything and everything (0.80).
Try to outdo everyone you know (0.76).
Try to find out everyone else's grade for test/examination (0.51).
IV. Preventing Others from Winning (4.2% of total variance)
Keep vital information/tips from your other classmates (0.56).
V. Rushing (even if there is no need to) (3.8% of total variance)
Speed up when driving if the traffic light turns orange (0.78).
Keep changing lanes when driving because the cars in front of you are too slow (0.74).
VI. Value for Money (3.3% of total variance)
Take as many photographs as possible when going on tour (0.67).
Go shopping on tour because things are so cheap (0.59).

Note: Loadings less than .50 not shown.

sample (41.0% of the variance). All items had high loadings on the main component and relatively low loadings on others.

Comparison between the two solutions indicated that the two samples had five common components: Greed (accounting for 21.7% of variance for Singaporeans and 16.4% for Australians), Preventing Others from Winning (5.6% and 3.8%), Value for Money (4.6% and 4.9%), Being Number One (4.5% and 4.7%), and Rushing (3.9% and 4.3%). However, the items that made up the components and the loadings for the two samples were slightly different, giving the components subtly different meanings. The unique components were Ensuring a Win for the Singa-

Table 5. Correlations between Six Kiasu Components and the Four Validity Scales (Pooled Data)

Component	Scales				
	Comp	Achiev	Fear	Eys Lie	Kiasu Total[1]
Greed	0.23***	0.23**	0.16**	-0.28***	0.86
Money	-0.01	0.19**	0.27**	-0.07	0.62
Be nr one	0.39**	0.42**	0.27**	-0.27**	0.57
Prev	0.04	0.16**	0.17**	-0.11	0.29
Winning					
Rushing	0.36**	0.11	-0.11	-0.25**	0.51
Value	0.04	0.14*	0.20**	-0.07	0.53

Comp = Competitiveness; Achiev = Achievement; Fear = Fear of Success; Eys Lie = Eysenck Lie scale.
Greed = Greed; Money = Money consciousness; be nr one = Being number one; Prev = Prevent others; Rushing = Rushing; Value = Value for money.
[1]Uncorrected; $*p < .05$; $**p < .01$.

poreans (accounting for 3.5% of variance) and Money Consciousness for the Australians (6.8%).

Finally, a new Kiasu score was computed by simple summation of the 23 items in the six components. For the Singaporean sample, the inter-correlations between the new Kiasu score and the six components with the original four marker scales showed similar patterns to that of the pooled results, though for the Australian sample only some of the components had significant positive correlations to one another. They were Greed and Money Consciousness, Value for Money and Money Consciousness, Greed and Being Number One, Being Number One and Value for Money, Being Number One and Rushing, and Greed and Preventing Others from Winning.

Discussion

The results of the study show that it is possible to construct a Kiasu measure that has high internal consistency reliability for both the pooled data and the two separate samples. Furthermore, the fact that Australians obtained scores which were higher than those of the Singaporeans, despite the fact that Kiasuism is taken to be a noteworthy feature of Singaporean culture, indicates that a similar measurable trait or attitude could be present in both cultures. However, it would be naïve to jump to the conclusion that this construct is equally important or of similar strength in both cultures because of their similar scores. In this study, no attempt has been made to equate the item or whole scale scores, an exercise which will require further data and analysis. Only then could any direct comparisons between cultures be contemplated (van de Vijver & Leung, 1997). All that was being sought was confirmation or disconfirmation that the construct could be detected in both cultures, and a first approximate indication of its meaning in terms of correlations with other reasonably well established scales, at least in Western countries.

The main problem with validation of such an instrument is that it depends on correlations with other measures that have themselves not been validated in both cultures. But by choosing a number of measures which can be expected to converge or diverge in relation to one another and the scale of interest, we may hope to provide some indication as to whether Kiasuism has common features in both cultures or not. In this case, the modest though significant correlations between the Competitiveness Index, the Need for Achievement Scale, and the Kiasu Scale, and the similarity of the pattern of correlations in both cultures, is some indication of convergence of meanings.

On the other hand, the significant correlation with Fear of Success in both cultures was unexpected. There was some indication that the Fear of Success scale has more than one dimension, possibly accounting for this effect, but it is more likely that one of the reasons for Kiasu behavior is a tendency to avoid conventional success. This may be suggested by its meaning in Chinese, "afraid to lose." In avoiding failure, the person may be attempting to gain a middle ground between failure and success rather than pursuing success wholeheartedly. From the correlation patterns, the Kiasu person is portrayed as being highly competitive but, at the same time, afraid of being successful. However, Australians, who scored higher on the Kiasu Scale than the Singaporeans, scored lower than Singaporeans did on the Fear of Success Scale. This is surprising given the correlation pattern and prevalence of the "Tall Poppy Syndrome" (a tendency to cut down high achievers) in Australia (Feather, 1994), and the emphasis on merit (or looking up to high achievers) in Singapore. Furthermore, the Fear of Success construct was originally proposed to be antagonistic to Need for Achievement (Horner, 1972), but these scales were unrelated in the present study. Instead, there was a significant negative correlation between the Fear of Success Scale and the

Competitiveness Index. The Fear of Success Scale may be measuring fear of competition rather than fear of success.

A negative correlation was also detected with the Lie scale, a measure of conventionality or social desirability. This means that only a person who is not too concerned about presenting the self in a socially desirable manner may admit to being Kiasu. Again, there is a problem with the validity of the Lie scale. Although it was in fact the most predictive for the Kiasu scores in the regression analysis, it showed unusually low reliability for these samples, thus preventing any clear conclusion to be reached as to the positive or negative implications of admitting to Kiasu behavior.

One small cross-cultural variation was observed, in that the Competitiveness Index was significantly correlated with the Kiasu Scale for the Singaporean sample but not for the Australian one. However, the difference between the correlations is itself not significant. The Competitiveness Index was also not significantly correlated with the Need for Achievement Scale for the Australians. Thus, there may be subtle differences between the Kiasu constructs in the populations that merit further study.

Principal component analyses conducted on both the pooled data and the two separate samples revealed six underlying components in the Kiasu measure, suggesting that Kiasuism is a multifaceted concept. Components derived from the pooled data were Greed, Money Consciousness, Being Number One, Preventing Others from Winning, Rushing, and Value for Money. The two separate six-component solutions and the correlation matrices revealed that while there are similar components for the two samples (Being Number One and Rushing), there are also components unique to each group (Ensuring a Win for the Singaporeans and Money Consciousness for the Australians). However, even the common components for the two samples may not have the same correlation patterns with the four other scales, again suggesting that the two samples may not have an identical concep-tualization of the Kiasuism construct.

From the components derived, Kiasuism can be said to incorporate elements of greed, a value-for-money mentality, competitiveness (by either trying to be number one or by preventing others from winning), and rushing even when there is no need to. This is very similar to the initial definition proposed. But the evidence is that Kiasuism is somewhat different in the two cultures: For Singaporeans but not Australians, Kiasuism involves utilizing all possible means to ensure a win; whereas for the Australians, the meaning of the (latent and not normally identified) construct incorporates thriftiness.

A project to be undertaken in the future is to investigate the generality of the construct in a variety of Asian and other cultures. Countries where Kiasuism may be prominent include the Asian economic "tigers" such as Hong Kong, Taiwan, and China, but the findings of the study suggest that Kiasuism as a motivator of behavior is not unique to Asia. In fact, it could be argued on the basis of these findings that Kiasuism is not a unique Singaporean phenomenon, merely a constellation of behaviors, values, and attitudes to which Singaporeans have uniquely drawn attention.

References

Cheng, Y., Lau, J., & Suresh, J. (1991). *Mr Kiasu: Everything also must grab*. Singapore: The Kuppies.

Edwards, A. L. (1953). *Edwards Personal Preference Schedule*. New York: The Psychological Corporation.

Eysenck, H. J. (1974). *Eysenck Personality Questionnaire Manual*. London, England: Pergamon.

Eysenck, S. B. G., & Long, F. Y. (1986). A cross-cultural comparison of personality in adults and children: Singapore and England. *Journal of Personality and Social Psychology, 50*, 124-130.

Feather, N. T. (1994). Attitudes towards high achievers and reactions to their fall: Theory and research concerning tall poppies. *Advances in Experimental Social Psychology, 26*, 1-73.

Ho, R., & Zemaitis, R. (1981). Concern over the negative consequences of success. *Australian Journal of Psychology, 33*, 19-28.

Hofstede, G. (1980). *Culture's consequences: International differences in work-related values*. Beverly Hills, CA: Sage.

Hofstede, G., & Bond, M. H. (1988). The Confucius connection: From cultural roots to economic growth. *Organizational Dynamics, 16*, 4-21.

Horner, M. S. (1972). Toward an understanding of achievement-related conflicts in women. *Journal of Social Issues, 26*, 59-66.

Hui, C. H. (1990). Work attitudes, leadership styles, and managerial behaviors in different cultures. In R. W. Brislin (Ed.), *Applied cross-cultural psychology* (pp. 186-208). Thousand Oaks, CA: Sage.

Jackson, D. N. (1974). *Manual for the PRF-Form E*. Port Huron, MI: Research Psychologists Press.

Kashima, Y. (1990). Cultural conceptions of the person and individualism-collectivism: A semiotic framework. In D. Keats, D. Munro, & L. Mann (Eds.), *Heterogeneity in cross-cultural psychology* (pp. 75-81). Lisse, The Netherlands: Swets & Zeitlinger.

Leung, K., & Bond, M. H. (1984). The impact of cultural collectivism on reward allocation. *Journal of Personality and Social Psychology, 47*, 793-804.

Lewis, M. (1991, October). Singapore: Kiasu capital of the world? *Asian Advertising & Marketing*, p.26.

Lim, C. (1993, October 30-31). Arise, the new Singaporean. *Straits Times*, p.11.

Lin, D. (1994). Kiasu Culture. In *Moving to Singapore - A Series by David Lin*. UseNet Newsgroup "Social-Cultural Singapore." http://www.mit.edu:8001/people/hot/move page.html.

Maehr, M. L. (1974). Culture and achievement motivation. *American Psychologist, 29*, 887-896.

Maehr, M. L., & Nicholls, J. G. (1980). Culture and achievement motivation: A second look. In N. Warren (Ed.), *Studies in cross-cultural psychology*. London, England: Academic.

McClelland, D. C., Atkinson, J. W., Clark, R. A., & Lowell, E. L. (1953). *The achievement motive*. New York: Appleton-Century-Crofts.

Smith, P. B., & Bond, M. H. (1993). *Social psychology across cultures: Analysis and perspectives*. New York: Harvester Wheatsheaf.

Smither, R. D., & Houston, J. M. (1992). The nature of competitiveness: The development and validation of the competitiveness index. *Educational and Psychological Measurement, 52*, 407-417.

Suresh, J., Lau, J., Chong, E., & Cheng, E. (1990). *Mr Kiasu: Everything also I want*. Singapore: The Kuppies.

Triandis, H. C., Bontempo, R., & Villareal, M. J. (1988). Individualism and collectivism: Cross-cultural perspectives on self-ingroup relationships. *Journal of Personality and Social Psychology, 54*, 323-338.

Tripathi, S. (1993, September). Capitalizing on Kiasu. *Asia, Inc.*, pp.16-18.

van de Vijver, F. J. R., & Leung, K. (1997). Methods and data analysis of comparative research. In J. W. Berry, Y. H. Poortinga, & J. Pandey (Eds.), *Handbook of cross-cultural psychology: Vol. 1. Theory and method* (2nd ed., pp. 257-300). Boston: Allyn & Bacon.

Author Note

Shee Wai Ho, Don Munro, and Stuart C. Carr, Department of Psychology; Stuart Carr is now at the School of Social Sciences, Northern Territory University, Darwin, NT 0909, Australia.

Correspondence concerning this article may be directed to the first two authors at the Department of Psychology, University of Newcastle, N.S.W. 2308, Australia, and the third author at the address above.

Collectivism in the Cultural Perspective: The Indian Scene

Jyoti Verma
Patna University, Patna, India

ABSTRACT

The paper presents the Indian scene as regards collectivism. It was observed that Indians describe themselves as allocentric and perceive the Indian system as more or less collectivistic. However, regional similarities and differences were also observed. The dominant themes of Indian collectivism appear to be relationship orientation, familialism, and belief in hierarchy. Some other themes were harmony and tolerance, inquisitiveness about others, support, concern for others' evaluation, and utilization of social contacts. Networking for mutual gain and Other-orientation were found to be important dimensions of allocentrism. Furthermore, it was contended that Indians look upon norms as accommodative rules for meeting the demands of the situation. The concept of a happy life for young students meant a good small family, nice social and physical environment, peace contentment, wealth and education. Their self-referents mirrored their immediate context and concerns but still could be placed under the category of social identity. Indian collectivism was positively related to psychological well-being but only in a socially supportive environment.

India has been termed collectivist in its cultural orientation (Bond, 1985; Hofstede, 1980; J.B.P. Sinha et al., 1994; J.B.P. Sinha & Verma, 1987; Triandis et al., 1986; Verma, 1989, 1992a). However, the majority of the above studies pointed out that Indians were located either somewhat towards the higher side of the collectivism end of the individualism-collectivism (I/C) spectrum or somewhere close to its midpoint. Recently, Hofstede (1994, p.xii) pointed out that, though India scored midway on the I/C index scale in his 1970 data, according to the average poverty level it could have been expected to score as even more collectivist.

Indians have been assigned to the category of "vertical collectivists" (Triandis, 1995) where the characteristics of embeddedness and power distance appear prominently in their personal and social dispositions. Indian psychologists (Mishra, 1994; D. Sinha & Tripathi, 1994) describe India as a "co-existence of dichotomies," while some recent empirical studies (J.B.P. Sinha et al., 1994) have not been able to present an articulated or clear pattern of Indian collectivism. Moreover, in our attempt to examine individual level variation in I/C (that is, idio-centrism/allocentrism) (Triandis, Leung, Villareal, & Clack, 1985), we have found Indian students scoring as idiocentric (J.B.P. Sinha & Verma, 1994). On the other hand, we also found a high positive correlation between the self-rating measures of allocentrism and idiocentrism in another group of Indian college students (J.B.P. Sinha et al., 1994).

It seems that Indians appraise themselves as collectivist, in general. However, there is a definite streak of individualistic tendencies in their apparent life style (Mishra, 1994; Tripathi, 1988). The harsh social reality of India, the upsurge of consumerist values, a combination of higher education and urban background, and the deeply ingrained spiritual values of duty, right action and self-growth, create a very complex context for the "context sensitive" Indians to decide what to do and whom to be.

Indian Collectivism: Unraveling the Construct

Some Indian psychologists tried to examine empirically the structure of Indian collectivism on an adult sample. Their aim was to develop measures of collectivism and allocentrism and check their validity by relating them to variables of (a) relative salience of the various in-groups, (b) the extent of individuals' embeddedness in the group, © the perception of collectivism in the Indian people, and (d) the nature of relationship orientation of three kinds (J.B.P. Sinha & Verma, 1987). The study provided some useful information regarding the validity of the measures. I shall come back to the findings of this study while discussing relation-ship orientation and family as the most important in-group for Indians.

In another empirical study, Verma (1992a) looked into the factor structure of the Collectivism Scale (J.B.P. Sinha & Verma, 1987). The seventeen scale items contained description of normative behavior of Indian people in general. The criterion used for deciding the number of factors yielded six factors named Inquisitiveness about others, Support, Concern for others' evaluation, Utilization of social contacts, Emotional affinity, and Tolerance. The Scree test (Cattell, 1966) suggested a four factor solution (see Table 1). Accordingly, the last two factors were not taken into account. The range of common factor variance explained by each of the four factors was between 17.3% to 7.1%, and the constituent factors were highly correlated with the total collectivism score. The scale's odd-even reliability was .76, but the factors did not seem to explain enough of the common factor variance.

We also attempted to look into the factor structure of the Allocentrism Scale. For this purpose, 16 items were added to the above Collectivism Scale. The idea was to examine whether the subjects who agreed to certain normative behaviors for collectivist people would also endorse

Table 1. Cultural Collectivism Scale, Its Factors and Item Loadings

Items Factor Name	Factor No.	Loadings
Inquisitiveness about others	1	
People take interest in the personal lives of other people		.71
People like to chat all the time		.69
Support	2	
Close relatives provide monetary help in case of serious illness		.78
People leave their work to visit sick friends and relatives		.66
There is no end to the hopes and expectations of close relatives		.45
People go to friends and relatives for help		.38
Concern for Others' Evaluation	3	
Nobody wants to speak unpleasant truth on face		.71
People are concerned about what others think of them		.61
People even tolerate guests they do not like		.53
Utilization of Social Contacts	4	
People visiting another city stay with their close relatives and friends		.83
When going to a new place people take recommendations of close relatives and friends		.60
People consult each other before taking any important decision		.42

such behaviors for themselves too. However, it was decided to use only the first two factors —namely, Networking for mutual gain and Other-orientation— out of the resulting 11 "weak" factors. With seven high loading items, Networking for mutual gain featured sociability, help, and interdependence in social relationships. On the other hand, Other-orientation, defined by five items, represented themes of helping others at one's own cost and concern for closeness with friends.

This exercise of looking into the dimensions of collectivism and allocentrism made us more or less accept the following conclusion: viz., the importance Indians give to other people could be due to the personal gratification it gives them, and the fact that it helps them get things done in a system where institutional and infra structural facilities are either weak or dysfunctional. Furthermore, people are sought for social comparison.

Our latest empirical work is based on a large sample of 759 students from different parts of India, where we made an attempt to understand the nature of Indian collectivism by examining the students' perception of what people in general believe, practice, and prefer (i.e., operative values) and the extent to which they attach importance to others' opinions, desires and interests over their own (J.B.P. Sinha et al., 1994).

The findings are striking because the subsamples showed significant mean differences among themselves and led us to identify three clusters of cities: namely, the North, the South, and the Central. Furthermore, the North and the South presented a contrast with one another. Northerners manifested strong orientations to meet unjustifiable and inconvenient social obligations and preferred to cultivate personalized relationships. On the other hand, they showed disregard for idealized values of tolerance and harmony. The Central cluster (consisting of one city each from West, East and North regions) showed pride in family heritage but not unduly high respect for age or seniority. There was much within cluster variation in this cluster too. Nevertheless, there were some items on which the subsamples did not differ, and such items formed a general factor of collectivism consisting of themes of familialism, relationship orientation, and hierarchy.

Familialism and Embeddedness

That family is the most important in-group in India finds support in empirical studies (Katju, 1986; Mishra & Tiwari, 1980; Roy & Srivastava, 1986; S.K. Singh, 1986). Parents and spouse are considered to be the most influential persons in an individual's life followed by friends. Coworkers and close relatives have average to below average degree of influence, while neighbors and acquaintances do not have much influence at all (J.B.P. Sinha & Verma, 1987). Indians' strong embeddedness with their family may be termed 'familialism.' People holding this value consider the family as the basic social unit. The major goal underlying familialism is maintaining the well-being and continuity of the family.

However, there is also evidence to show that "unlike the older generation who regard 'near' and 'other' relations also as part of the family, among the young there is a distinct trend towards nuclearization, that is, greater individualist orientation" (D. Sinha & Tripathi, 1994, p. 131). And though the individual is increasingly oriented toward the nuclear family, he/she does not want to lose the benefits of the extended family (D. Sinha, 1988). Verma (1992a) did not find a positive relationship between collectivism and home satisfaction, which could be some indication of the attitudinal change taking place regarding the family.

Often the individual's embeddedness within his/her collectivity becomes the individual's identity, and some prefer to use the terms 'embeddedness' and 'collectivism' almost interchangeably (J.B.P. Sinha & D. Sinha, 1990). J.B.P. Sinha (1990) notes the following important features of embeddedness for Indians. First, intimacy within an in-group is contrasted with indifference towards out-group members. Second, important in-groups are ascribed in nature. Third, the salience of an in-group varies with situations and conflicts of interest. Fourth, embeddedness in-groups may create problems of coordination and cooperation in contexts where persons from different in-groups have to interact with each other.

Relationship Orientation in Indians
It is typical of Indians to prefer a personalized relationship. Roland (1984) observed that their relationships have the character of "affective reciprocity" where exchanges are viewed in a long term perspective, and the evaluation processes do not involve calculations of instant gain and loss. In our studies (J.B.P. Sinha & Verma, 1987; Verma, 1992b), we have observed that both allocentrism and collectivism were associated with complementary relationships. That is, those who perceived themselves as allocentrics and the culture as collectivistic reported enjoying social interactions without thinking of any exchange or reciprocity. The other preferred orientation for the respondents was the obligatory relationship. In the obligatory relationship, accounting of immediate gain or loss is ignored in social transactions, and one feels a sense of obligation towards those with whom one is engaged in relationship of mutual interdependence. Finally, the least preferred relationship orientation for the respondents who scored as allocentrics was the contractual type, which refers to contract like, nonemotional association between people for accomplishing some task. We found an overlap between obligatory and contractual relationships, which could mean that the obligatory relationship is probably in a transitional phase, in which those starting to become disenchanted with cultural collectivism still conform to the norms in order to avoid social cost. The Indians' strong preference for complementary relationships could have been made with the close in-group members in mind. Otherwise, for outsiders, the principle of exchange may often be applied.

The relationship orientation of Indians along with their tendency to distinguish between 'own' and 'other' creates hurdles for the smooth functioning of the social system. In work organizations, caste-based informal groups may be formed due to emotional closeness felt towards one's in-group members (J.B.P. Sinha, 1990; S.K. Singh, 1986). On the other hand, out-group members may be distrusted. Favoritism and nepotism are practices where the code of morality is ignored for benefiting one's friends and relatives.

Hierarchy and Vertical Collectivism
Kothari (1970) observed that the Indian system is steeply hierarchical. According to Kakar (1978), Indians acquire early in childhood a tendency to locate their relative social positions as superior to some and subordinate to others. Triandis (1995) suggests that the Indian self may be categorized as "interdependent different from others" due to the following combination. First, being born in a caste-based society, a person is ascribed a caste status which makes him/her "stand out" from the other caste groups. Second, as an Indian, one feels obliged to fulfill one's family duties and live interdependently with relevant others all through life. Triandis (1995) notes further that in the case of India and especially so in Indian villages, the expected political system is "communalism" due to (a) values of Low equality-Low freedom (Rokeach, 1973), (b) Communal sharing-Authority ranking (Fiske, 1990; 1992), and (c) Interdependent self-Independent self (Markus & Kitayama, 1991).

The "Context Sensitivity" of Indians: Coexistence of I/C Orientations
Some leading Indian psychologists suggest that it is erroneous to label the Indian cultural system as collectivist (D. Sinha & Tripathi, 1994). They argue that both individualist and collectivist orientations may coexist within individuals and cultures and contend that exigencies of the situation almost always prevail over other concerns (such as values). The typical way in which an Indian might respond and react is contextual (also see Ramanujan 1990; Roland, 1984; J.B.P. Sinha, 1990). Similarly, Tripathi (1988) points out that the apparently contradictory values and attitudes are integrated in one scheme on the basis of some higher moral principle where "... I/C act like figure and ground. Depending on the situation, one rises to form the figure while the other recedes into the background" (p.324).

D. Sinha and Tripathi (1994) studied the coexistence model empirically and showed that university students chose the "mixed orientation" options more than the options representing either individualist or collectivist orientations. In fact, the only item on which a collectivist

orientation appeared to be prominent referred to a purely personal
relationship issue. Triandis (1995) contends that morality among
collectivists is more contextual. D. Sinha and Tripathi (1994) observed
that: "Rightness and wrongness appear to be determined by the context in
which the behavior takes place" (p.129). In sum, correct behavior is
expected in specific contexts of variety of roles and relationships rather
than any unchanging norms for all situations (Roland, 1984, p. 114).

Culture and Self: Self and Indian Collectivism

Dhawan, Roseman, Naidu, Thapa, and Rettek (1995) observe that
research has now begun to focus on the self as a cultural product. There
is evidence in the literature to suggest that members of collectivist
societies tend to define the self primarily by referring to aspects of their
social roles and membership and to their relatedness to others. This
relatedness of the individual to others is made possible by keeping the
internal, private or independent aspect of the self subordinate to the
collectivist or interdependent component of the self (Cross & Markus,
1993; Markus & Kitayama, 1991).

Roland (1991) has emphasized the familial and communal character of
the Indian self. Recently, Dhawan et al. (1995) studied self-concepts of
individuals across India and the U.S. with the Twenty Statements Test
(Kuhn & McPartland, 1954). They categorized respondents' self-statements into five categories of social identity, ideological beliefs, interests,
ambitions, and self-evaluation (along with their subcategories) and
arrived at the following results. First, the largest cultural difference was
observed in the greater prevalence of "social based" self-statements for
the Indian sample in comparison to the more clearly "self-evaluation
based" self-concept structure of the American sample. Second, in the
subcategories of social identity, Indian students described themselves
more in terms of role, group, caste, class, and gender role identity in
contrast to Americans, who chose to describe themselves in the
self-identity category. The authors contend that the above findings can be
interpreted within the individualist-collectivist value distinction identified
by Hofstede (1980) and Triandis (1989) and may be seen as supporting
the interdependent conception of the self in which self is defined in terms
of its relationship to others.

Verma and J.B.P. Sinha (1993) studied "self-referents and the concept
of a happy life" using the same Twenty Statements Test. However, the
categories for self-referents were derived after content analyzing the
statements of 110 students who were told that they could use persons,
themes, or objectives as referents to describe the self. The data yielded
18 categories for the self-referents. The most frequently mentioned
self-referents for students were psychological well-being; college, subject

of study (discipline), and class; independence and job. On the other hand, the students did not mention spouse, relative and a good family in defining the self very often. In another study (J.B.P. Sinha & Verma, 1994), we observed that students made frequent reference to their immediate context and concerns in response to the "Who Am I Test." Accordingly, some of the frequently mentioned self-referents were discipline (i.e., subject of study), job, and independence. The students' concerns were more "private" and mirrored in their self-referents. Nevertheless, the intercorrelations between self-referents suggested sampling of the collective self (or social identity) to some extent. For example, psychological well-being formed a cluster with in-group-related referents such as home and friends.

A decade ago, Verma (1985) observed that women referred to their identity as bound by their social roles. Moreover, children, husband, and family always remained the top priority for all generations of women. Younger women, however, considered education as very important too. Recently, reporting three case histories of three generations of women belonging to the same family, Verma (1995) found that the first-generation woman never questioned her existence beyond her housemaker's role in a close-knit, joint family but could also affectively extend herself to the larger collective of the village folks and chose spiritualism as the ultimate goal for herself. The second-generation woman too, saw herself basically as a daughter-in-law, wife and mother. Nevertheless, she felt that being a perfect social role player is not necessarily what a woman looks for. The third-generation, well educated, urban woman of modern India believed in being a good housemaker, but at the same time her self-referents had definite elements of the individualist self.

Values and Concept of a Happy Life

Support for Indians preferring both individualist and collectivist values is available in the literature. The source of values for Indians, and more so for the urban elite, has been their traditional moorings, on the one hand, and sources relating to personal growth, efficiency and collaborative work such as education, professional training, and modern technology, on the other (Parikh, 1979). Data from students, managers and professionals suggest that individualist values such as independence, freedom, autonomy in work, achievement of goals, willingness to take risk, challenge and creativity, power, competitiveness, and high economic motivation, etc. have been preferred or endorsed. At the same time, there is no dearth of studies substantiating the survival of traditional values. Again, data from students, people in different professions, and managers suggest that Indians subscribe to conservatism, fatalism, authoritarianism and "groupism," and values may be taken up as the basis for subcultural or religious identity (Solanke & Kadam, 1986).

Some traditional values preferred by Indians are (as already seen) relationship orientation, belief in hierarchy, and embeddedness. Furthermore, status consciousness, authority orientation, and belief in power distance are also endorsed and may be seen as correlates of belief in hierarchy. Harmony and tolerance are the other salient, traditional values recommended for maintaining peace in intergroup relations. Perhaps one way to articulate the value orientation of Indians would be to explain their value preferences in the light of their context sensitive way of functioning and take into account the determinants of their social behavior; that is, the norms they feel obliged to follow and the social obligations they decide to meet.

At the same time, one cannot ignore the contextual parameters of a society that can be very harsh (i.e., poverty, overpopulation, scarcity of resources, etc.) and take a toll on the finer values in life (J.B.P. Sinha, 1982). Indian collectivism represents a combination of a "prescriptive system" and "confining roles" that are under flux. For the urban elite, the core values are still deeply agrarian and traditional. Precisely for this reason, the value of "dynamism" seem to be preferred (Garg & Parikh, 1993).

Concept of a Happy Life

Verma and J.B.P. Sinha (1993) delineated twelve components of a happy life by content analyzing a few lines written by college students in response to the question as to 'what comprised a happy life for them?' The most frequently mentioned components were good small family, good spouse, good social and physical environment, wealth, peace and contentment, and education. The clustering of the components revealed a pattern. Peace and contentment together with spouse and companion formed the axis for the happy life. Related to this axis was health, on one hand, and wealth and affluence, on the other. The latter was related to honor and prestige, which was connected to peace and contentment.

Perhaps the concept of a happy life for Indians has conflicting components where materialistic and spiritual orientations can coexist (D. Sinha, 1969). Garg and Parikh (1993) aptly observe the dilemma faced by the educated urban elite (MBAs) who are at a crossroads mainly because of pressure from familial values, on the one hand, and Western values of an aggressive, achievement-oriented, self-enhancing life, on the other. Their problem appears to be wanting to build their own life and at the same time, retaining a sense of emotional continuity through ritual observations of role obligations.

Psychological Well-Being and Collectivism

J.B.P. Sinha and Verma (1994) observed that allocentrics experience a sense of psychological well-being only under the conditions of high social support. Verma (1992a) found that collectivism factors of Support and Emotional affinity were moderate, positive predictors of well-being of the self. Interestingly, ideas like a sense of detachment and self-control to define the variable of psychological well-being, were unrelated to allocentrism (J.B.P. Sinha & Verma, 1994). However, in general, Indian adults reported a moderate degree of psychological well-being for themselves (Verma, 1992a).

Some Observations: Beyond the Data

If one were to describe the striking features of the Indian scene, one would say the following: First, for Indian collectivists, "other people" are important. Others are needed for self-evaluation, social comparison, getting things done, and fulfillment of one's affiliative needs. Second, a debate seems to be going on in the minds of Indians between core values that are traditional and other-oriented, and those that are self-centric and promise economic success, name, fame, and power. In this debate, other-oriented values seem to have taken a back seat. Third, the much applauded value of familialism has had a setback. Furthermore, in the name of the values of freedom and equality, the younger generation is responding to messages that make them arrogant, disrespectful, and forgetful of their duties and obligations.

At times, a deep pessimism overpowers the common people. It appears that at the macro level, Indian collectivism has found a new and violent identity by being associated with caste, community, and opportunist political ideologies. Consequently, the finer values of collectivism that held hope for the flow of constructive social energy has changed places with negative collective forces. A country which once boasted of nonviolence and spiritualism is reeling under the forces of aggression, hedonism, and a self-centric, materialistic outlook leading to large-scale violence and corruption. Perhaps all this cannot be fully explained through the own-other distinction or the "co-existence of opposites." One wonders whether a decomposition of Indian psyche and character has begun, making us insensitive and unresponsive towards the chaos. The harsh social reality of deprivation and overpopulation could have a role in all this, but what has become of the masses who are the value watchers of the system?

Religion and spiritualism are still very much part of the Indian scene but they have become very much ritualistic and like a fad, especially in the urban setting, instead of a mind pacifying, self-transcending affair. Moreover, collectivism in remote villages of India, abode of poor and deprived Indians, is still unexplored by the social scientists in any substantial way. We cannot claim that our information is valid for 70 to 80 percent of our counterparts who live in the villages of India. There is some evidence that rural people tend to remain collectivistic despite higher education; whereas with higher education, the orientation of urban people tends to shift towards individualism (Mishra, 1994). Mishra (1994) found that salvation and enduring relationships (categorized as collectivist values) were given a prominent place by old, rural and less educated people. And perhaps Indian collectivism rests with them.

References

Bond, M. (1985). *Teasing etics out of emics: The case of Chinese values.* Available from the author, Department of Psychology, Chinese University of Hong Kong, Shatin, N.T., China.

Cattell, R. B. (1966). The scree test for the number of factors. *Multivariate Behavioural Research, 1,* 245-276.

Cross, S., & Markus, H. (1993, October). *Views of the self: Chinese and American perspectives.* Paper presented at the Annual Meeting of the Society of Experimental Social Psychology, Santa Barbara, CA.

Dhawan, N., Roseman, I. J., Naidu, R. K., Thapa, K., & Rettek, S. I. (1995). Self-concepts across two cultures: India and the United States. *Journal of Cross-Cultural Psychology, 26,* 606-621.

Fiske, A. P. (1990). *Structures of social life: The four elementary forms of human relations.* New York: Free Press.

Fiske, A. P. (1992). The four elementary forms of society: Framework for a unified theory of social relations. *Psychological Review, 99,* 689-723.

Garg, P., & Parikh, I. (1993). *Young managers at the cross-roads: The Trishanku complex.* New Delhi, India: Sage.

Hofstede, G. (1980). *Cultures' consequences.* Beverly Hills, CA: Sage.

Hofstede, G. (1994). Foreword. In U. Kim, H. C. Triandis, C. Kagitcibasi, S. C. Choi, & G. Yoon (Eds.), *Individualism and collectivism: Theory, method and application.* Newbury Park, CA: Sage.

Kakar, S. (1978). *The inner world: A psycho-analytic study of childhood and society in India.* New Delhi, India: Oxford University Press.

Katju, P. (1986). *Certain factors related to member integration in a multinational organization.* Doctoral Dissertation, University of Allahabad, India.

Kothari, R. (1970). *Politics in India.* New Delhi, India: Orient Longman.

Kuhn, M. H., & McPartland, R. (1954). An empirical investigation of self attitudes. *American Sociological Review, 19,* 68-76.

Markus, H. R., & Kitayama, S. (1991). Culture and self: Implications for cognition, emotion and motivation. *Psychological Review, 98,* 224-253.

Marsella, A. J., DeVos, G., & Hsu, F. L. K. (1985). *Culture and self: Asian and Western perspectives.* New York: Tavistock.

Mishra, R. C. (1994). Individualist and collectivist orientations across generations. In U. Kim, H. C. Triandis, C. Kagitcibasi, S. C. Choi, & G. Yoon (Eds.), *Individualism and collectivism: Theory, method and application* (pp. 225-238). Newbury Park, CA: Sage.

Mishra, R. C., & Tiwari, B. B. (1980). *Dialogues on development.* New Delhi, India: Sage.

Parikh, I. J. (1979). *Role orientation and role performance of Indian managers.* Ahmedabad: Indian Institute of Management.

Ramanujan, A. K. (1990). Is there an Indian way of thinking? An informal essay. In M. Marriot (Ed.), *Indian thought through Hindu categories* (pp. 41-58). New Delhi, India: Sage.

Rokeach, M. (1973). *The nature of human values.* New York: Free Press.

Roland, A. (1984). The self in India and America. In V. Kavolis (Ed.), *Designs of selfhood* (pp. 170-191). Rutherford, NJ: Associated University Presses.

Roland, A. (1988). *In search of self in India and Japan: Towards a cross cultural psychology.* Princeton, NJ: Princeton University Press.

Roland, A. (1991). *The psychological and psychosocial in Indian organizational relationships.* Mimeograph, American Institute for Indian Studies.

Roy, R., & Srivastava, R. K. (1986). *Dialogues in development.* New Delhi, India: Sage.

Singh, S. K. (1986). *Social groups within a work organization.* Doctoral Dissertation. Patna University, India.

Sinha, D. (1969). *Indian villages in transition: A motivational analysis.* New Delhi, India: Associated Press.

Sinha, D. (1988). Family scenario in a developing country and its implications for mental health: The case of India. In P. R. Dasen, J. W. Berry, & N. Sartorius (Eds.), *Health and cross cultural psychology: Towards applications.* Newbury Park, CA: Sage.

Sinha, D., & Tripathi, R.C. (1994). Individualism in a collectivist culture: A case of coexistence of opposites. In U. Kim, H. C. Triandis, C. Kagitcibasi, S. C. Choi, & G. Yoon (Eds.), *Individualism and collectivism: Theory, method and application* (pp. 123-136). Newbury Park, CA: Sage.

Sinha, J. B. P. (1982). The Hindu (Indian) identity. *Dynamic Psychiatry, 15,* 148-160.

Sinha, J. B. P. (1990). The salient Indian values and their socioecological roots. *Indian Journal of Social Sciences, 3,* 477-488.

Sinha, J. B. P., & Sinha, D. (1990). Role of social values in Indian organizations. *International Journal of Psychology, 25,* 705-714.

Sinha, J. B. P., & Verma, J. (1987). Structure of collectivism. In C. Kagitcibasi (Ed.), *Growth and progress in cross cultural psychology* (pp. 123-129). Amsterdam, The Netherlands: Swets & Zeitlinger.

Sinha, J. B. P., & Verma, J. (1994). Social support as a moderator of the relationship between allocentrism and psychological well-being. In U. Kim, H. C. Triandis, C. Kagitcibasi, S. C. Choi, & G. Yoon (Eds.), *Individualism and collectivism: Theory, method and application* (pp. 267-275). Newbury Park, CA: Sage.

Sinha, J. B. P., Daftuar, C. N., Gupta, R. K., Jayseetha, R., Jha, S. S., Mishra, R. C., Verma, J., & Vijayakumar, V. S. R. (1994). Regional similarities and differences in peoples' beliefs, practices and preferences. *Psychology and Developing Societies, 6,* 131-150.

Solanke, G. K., & Kadam, K. P. (1986). Value orientation and job preference of agriculture college students. *Journal of Psychological Researches, 30,* 88-92.

Triandis, H. C. (1972). *The analysis of subjective culture.* New York: Wiley.

Triandis, H. C. (1989). The self and social behavior in differing cultural contexts. *Psychological Review, 96,* 506-520.

Triandis, H. C. (1995). *Individualism and collectivism.* Boulder, CO: Westview Press.

Triandis, H. C., Leung, K., Villareal, M., & Clack, F. L. (1985). Allocentrism vs idiocentric tendencies: Convergent and discriminant validation. *Journal of Research in Personality, 19,* 395-415.

Triandis, H. C., Bontempo, R., Betancourt, H., Bond, M., Leung, K., Bernes, A., Georgas, J., Hui, H. C., Marin, G., Setiadi, B., Sinha, J. B. P., Verma, J., Spangenberg, J., Touzard, H., & deMontmollin, G. (1986). The measurement of the etic aspect of individualism and collectivism across cultures. *Australian Journal of Psychology, 38,* 257-267.

Tripathi, R. C. (1988). Aligning development to values in India. In D. Sinha & H. S. R. Kao (Eds.), *Social values and development: Asian perspectives* (pp. 315-333). New Delhi, India: Sage.

Verma, J. (1985). Life patterns and thinking of three generations of middle class Bihari women. *Social Change, 15,* 25-28.

Verma, J. (1989). Marriage opinion survey and collectivism. *Psychological studies, 34,* 141-150.

Verma, J. (1992a). *Collectivism as a correlate of endogenous development.* Indian Council of Social Sciences Research Report. New Delhi.

Verma, J. (1992b). Allocentrism and relationship orientation. In S. Iwawaki, Y. Kashima, & K. Leung (Eds.), *Innovations in cross-cultural psychology* (pp. 152-163). Amsterdam, The Netherlands: Swets & Zeitlinger.

Verma, J. (1995). Transformation of womens' social role in India. In J. Valsiner (Ed.), *Child development within culturally structured environments* (Vol. 3, pp. 138-163). Norwood, NJ: Ablex.

Verma, J., & Sinha, J. B. P. (1993). Self-referents and the concept of a happy life. *Psychological Studies, 38*, 45-54.

Author Note

Correspondence concerning this article should be directed to the author, Road No. 5, Rajendra Nagar, Patna 800 016, India.

Homesickness:
Do Personality and Culture Play a Part?

Louise Horstmanshof and Prasuna Reddy
Swinburne University of Technology, Australia

ABSTRACT

In this survey, 52 male and 50 female sojourners responded to a questionnaire designed to measure personality, homesickness, and personal satisfaction with the current situation. The sojourners were classified into 3
groups: English speaking, non-English speaking, and Asian. All respondents had lived in Australia longer than 6 months but less than 5 years.
The results showed satisfaction with the current situation to be the most
important factor influencing homesickness. Personality type and cultural
background influenced means of coping with the situation. The results
have implications for counseling.

We live in an increasingly multicultural world, partly as a result of both
temporary and permanent migration. This paper deals with homesickness
that can be experienced by both migrants and sojourners. The term
'sojourner' is applied to people who are temporary residents in a foreign
environment, who may be migrants, refugees, tourists, business people,
diplomats, foreign workers, voluntary workers, or students.

Homesickness has been variously defined in the literature as a
cognitive state characterized by profound and frequent attention to home-
related thoughts. These thoughts are not focused on problems connected
to home or resulting from leaving home, but are instead uncontrollable
ideations of home. The concept seems to exist in many languages.

Some theories have drawn a comparison between the experience of
homesickness and temporary bereavement. Bowlby's (1980) theory of
separation and loss describes the anxiety, panic, and searching behavior
of an infant when deprived of the visual contact with its mother. Bowlby
described four phases of bereavement: (1) the numbing stage, which can
last hours or weeks, (2) the yearning stage, which may be accompanied
by outbursts of panic or anger, (3) a stage of disorganization and despair,
and (4) a final phase of reorganization. Similarly, Parkes (1972) views
homesick behavior as being similar to the anxious searching and panic of
the recently bereaved. He described the elements of search behaviors as
being: (1) the pining stage, characterized by preoccupation with thoughts
of the deceased, (2) the attentional focus phase with attention on places
and objects associated with the lost person, (3) a misinterpretation of

cues and signs as representing the deceased, and (4) a calling out stage often accompanied by bouts of tears similar to an infant in distress. In their study of the relationship between attachment and homesickness, Brewin, Furnham, and Howes (1989) found support for their hypothesis that a measure of anxious attachment and greater reliance on others is a predictor of homesickness. Arredondo-Dowd (1981) has put forward the theory that the sadness and loss associated with the loss of one's homeland might never be completely resolved, and that events in that homeland, like the death of a distant loved one, could trigger deep feelings of homesickness years after immigration.

Other theories view homesickness as a stressful experience. Fisher (1989) suggested that homesickness might be a response to unpleasant aspects of the new environment, which result in a mismatch in favor of the home environment. It involves a strong commitment to the previous environment and can be seen as a form of post-traumatic stress syndrome that follows the transition from home. Stokols, Shumaker, and Martinez (1983) maintain that in general, both the spatial and the temporal context of the environmental experience have an impact on personal well-being. Horstmanshof and Reddy (1997) found that the nature of the current environment is influential in determining the experience of homesickness.

The research findings on the relationship between personality and stressful events may be useful in understanding individual differences in coping with homesickness. A four-year longitudinal study by Magnus, Diener, Fujita, and Pavot (1993) examining the causal pathways between personality and life events found that extraversion predisposed participants to view their experience of objective life events in a more positive light, while neuroticism predisposed participants to experience objective life events more negatively. Headey and Wearing (1989) reported that participants with higher extraversion scores reported more favorable life events, those with higher neuroticism scores reported more adverse life events, while high openness was related to the experience of both positive and adverse events.

Stokols et al. (1983) showed that low exploratory tendency was connected to adverse effects of moves. In other words, openness to new situations and a commitment to new sources of information may be important prerequisites of adjustment. Kuhl and Kazen-Saad (1988, cited in Fisher & Cooper, 1990) suggested that depressed persons are perfectionists who are overly committed to a task, which in the case of the homesick could manifest itself as an overcommitment to the previous environment. Burns's (1993) study on expatriate employees showed a negative relationship between the trait of neuroticism and life satisfaction, and a positive relationship among the traits of extraversion, agreeableness, and life satisfaction.

Carden and Feicht (1991) found that several aspects of homesickness in students, such as dependence on parental guidance and low social presence transcended cultural boundaries. They confirmed that introverts were especially susceptible to homesickness, and that low self-reliance was a major factor that influenced vulnerability to homesickness. On the other hand, they also identified factors influencing homesickness that seemed to be culture-specific. Homesick Turkish student participants had higher socialization and lower flexibility scores than the homesick American students in their sample. American students with high home-sickness scores tended to exhibit higher neuroticism scores than nonhomesick, American students, while homesick Turkish students tended to score higher on the psychoticism scale than their nonhomesick counterparts. In their study of the initial adjustment of Taiwanese students to the United States, Ying and Liese (1994) found that partici-pants with high externality scores on the California Personality Index were more likely to engage actively in their new environment and subsequently adjusted better. Ward and Kennedy (1993) believed that personality traits are susceptible to culture-specific influences and should be viewed in a sociocultural context. Their study found that extraversion facilitated psychological adjustment in the case of Malaysian and Singaporean students in New Zealand, while appearing to be associated with increased depression and ill health in English-speaking sojourners in Singapore. Markus and Kitayama (1991) suggested a cultural difference in coping. Those from Asian cultures that value connectedness to others adopt ways of coping that emphasize harmonious interdependence, while those from cultures that value independence rely more on their own inner attributes.

We investigated the self-reported perception of environment changes in the new situation (satisfaction) and homesickness among English speaking, non-English speaking, and Asian sojourners on relocation to Australia from overseas countries. The aim of this study was to test predictors of homesickness and establish whether the three groups differed in their experience of homesickness. The study further aimed to investigate the role of personality and cultural differences in coping with homesickness.

The first hypothesis was that participants who reported positive perceptions of the current situation would have lower homesickness scores than those who perceived their current situation to be a negative change from their previous home situation. Low levels of satisfaction with several aspects of the current environment were found to influence the experience of homesickness (Fisher, Murray, & Frazer, 1985; Horstmanshof & Reddy, 1997). The second hypothesis was that person-ality factors would predict homesickness. As suggested by Stokol et al.

(1983), openness to new situations and a commitment to new sources of information were predicted to be important prerequisites of adjustment. Extraversion, on the other hand, as Searle and Ward (1990) found, could be more problematic and would have to be viewed in the Australian sociocultural context. As the sojourner is likely to be without formal social support systems, the personality trait of agreeableness with its relationship to a social network could be a predictor of homesickness. If the homesick are perfectionists who are overcommitted to the previous environment, as Kuhl and Kazen-Saad (1988) suggest, conscientiousness could predict high levels of homesickness. Neuroticism has been shown to predispose participants to view life events more negatively. These two hypotheses were examined in different cultural groups to identify whether the same pattern of homesickness occurred in persons from cultures similar to or different from the host nation.

Method

Participants
The sample comprised 52 male and 50 female participants. Participants were classified into three groups: 16-24 years (25.5%), 25-34 years (37.3%), and 35 years or older (37.3%). They were further classified into three groups according to country of origin: Forty-eight participants were from English-speaking countries (24 males and 24 females), 19 from Non-English-speaking countries (6 males and 13 females), and 35 from Asian Countries (22 males and 13 females). The classifications were arrived at after merging the earlier data, as the sample size of many of the earlier groups was too small.

Instruments
In addition to demographic information, the questionnaire contained the following measures:
Perception of self compared to self prior to arrival. This measure assessed gains and losses the participant perceived as a result of the transition. These questions were designed to provide an overall perception of the level of satisfaction in the new environment, as individual assessments of the various areas described: physical, lifestyle, family, social, work, material belongings, community, and personal aspirations. Participants were asked to consider each area and indicate the extent to which they believed their situation to be better or worse than before. In addition, they ticked a box to indicate the nature of change or not: positive, no change, or negative. Items were scored so higher scores would indicate greater satisfaction with the current situation: i.e., greater

Table 1. *Classification of Respondents by Region of Origin*

Value label	Frequency	%	Classification
Australia	3	2.9	English Speaking
United Kingdom	19	18.6	English Speaking
North America	14	13.7	English Speaking
South America	5	4.9	English Speaking
Melanesia	1	1.0	Non English in Asia
New Zealand	7	6.9	English Speaking
Southern Europe	1	1.0	Non-English in Europe
Western Europe	6	5.9	Non-English in Europe
Northern Europe	1	1.0	Non-English in Europe
Eastern Europe	2	2.0	Non-English in Europe
Soviet Republics	9	8.8	Non-English in Europe
South East Asia	11	10.8	Non-English in Asia
North East Asia	19	18.6	Non-English in Asia
Southern Asia	2	2.0	Non-English in Asia
Africa (except N & S)	2	2.0	Non-English
Total	102	100	

positive evaluation. This measure was regarded as reflecting satisfaction with the current situation. The measure had an internal consistency reliability (i.e., coefficient alpha) of .78 for this study.

The NEO Five-Factor Personality Inventory (Costa & McCrae, 1991). This personality inventory measures five broad domains of personality: neuroticism, extraversion, openness, agreeableness, and conscientiousness. It consists of 60 statements to which participants responded by circling one of the following: SD (strongly disagree), D (disagree), N (feel neutral about the statement), A (Agree) or SA (strongly agree). The internal consistency for the NEO Five-Factor scales, using coefficient alpha, is .89, .79, .76, .74 and .84 for N, E, O, A, and C, respectively. In this study the internal consistency for the NEO Five-Factor scales, using coefficient alpha, was .84, .78, .67, .79 and .82 for N, E, O, A, and C, respectively.

The Dundee Relocation Inventory Questionnaire F (Fisher & Murray, 1985). This questionnaire was used to measure the degree of homesickness experienced. This questionnaire consists of 24 statements to which the participants responded by circling one of the following: never, sometimes or often. Statements such as "I forget people's names," "I miss having someone close to talk to," and "I feel optimistic about life here," were included. Homesickness is regarded as a specific response to a transition that involves leaving home. As such, the measure involves a state characteristic that is likely to change as the participants adjust to the new circumstances.

Procedure
Questionnaires were distributed through schools, universities, relocation companies, and international companies in Melbourne and Sydney. The participants had to be born outside of Australia, older than 16 years of age, and able to complete the questionnaire unaided. They had to have lived in Australia for more than 6 months, but fewer than 5 years. The questionnaires were completed individually and returned by post. Of the 350 questionnaires distributed, 102 (28.5%) were completed and returned. A 30% return for postal surveys is regarded as average (Shaughnessy & Zechmeister, 1985).

Results

No significant gender differences were found on any variables. No significant nation group differences on homesickness scores were found, $F(2, 99) = .057$, ns. However, analysis of variance revealed a significant difference among nation groups on levels of perceived satisfaction with the current situation, $F(2, 99) = 10.56, p < .01$. A post hoc Scheffé test indicated that the Asian group differed significantly from the other two groups in reporting lower levels of satisfaction with the current situation. Specifically, the Asian group was significantly less satisfied with their current material situation, their current work situation, and their current life style.

A Pearson correlation coefficient was computed between the measure of homesickness and the overall perception of changed environment (satisfaction). Homesickness correlated negatively with satisfaction, $r = -.39, p < .001$.

Analysis of variance showed a significant difference among nation groups on Personality traits. The Asian group differed significantly from the English-speaking group on agreeableness, $F(2, 99) = 3.656, p < 0.05$, and extraversion, $F(2, 99) = 4.87, p < 0.05$, with the Asian group showing significantly lower scores in each case. The Asian group also differed significantly from both groups on the measure of conscientiousness, $F(2, 99) = 4.64, p < 0.05$, again showing lower scores. Differences on the measures of openness and neuroticism were not significant.

Table 2. Mean Scores on Major Variables for Nation Groups

Dependent variable	English speaking	Non-English speaking	Asian group
Homesickness	17.02	12.89	19.20
Overall satisfaction	31.79	32.05	22.78
Material satisfaction	4.15	3.91	1.72
Work (job satisfaction)	3.75	3.92	2.01
Life style	0.77	4.87	3.11

A multiple regression analysis showed that, taken together, the five personality factors were significant predictors of variations in homesickness scores, $R = .55$, $F(5, 96) = 8.22$, $p < .001$. Specifically, high conscientiousness and high extraversion were associated with low homesickness scores, while high neuroticism was associated with high homesickness scores.

As the non-English-speaking group was small ($N = 19$), the remaining analyses were conducted separately for the Anglo group and the Asian group only. A stepwise multiple regression analysis was conducted by entering the personality factors in the following order: neuroticism, extraversion, conscientiousness, openness, and agreeableness. The results showed that the personality factors were significant predictors of variation in Homesickness scores for the Anglo group. Specifically, high neuroticism scores were associated with high homesickness scores, $R = .51$, $F(1, 46) = 16.26$, $p < .01$.

For the Asian group, on the other hand, the stepwise multiple regression analysis, with the predictors entered in the same order as for the Anglo group, showed that the Five Personality Factors were significant predictors of the variation in homesickness scores, with low extraversion scores associated with high homesickness scores, $R = .43$, $F(1, 33) = 7.60$, $p < .01$.

Discussion

The results of this study suggested a relationship between perceived satisfaction and homesickness. As shown in previous studies, low levels of satisfaction with several aspects of the current environment were found to influence the experience of homesickness (Fisher et al., 1985; Horstmanshof & Reddy, 1997). The results supported the hypothesis that

Table 3. Significant Predictors of Homesickness Scores for the Anglo Group

Variable	Beta	t	p
Neuroticism	0.51	4.03	.000
Extraversion	-0.05	-0.393	0.696
Counscientiousness	-0.13	-0.920	0.363
Openness	-0.02	-0.158	0.875
Agreeableness	0.12	0.957	0.343

Table 4. Significant Predictors of Homesickness Scores for the Asian Group

Variable	Beta	t	p
Neuroticism	0.30	2.031	0.051
Extraversion	-0.43	-2.757	0.009
Counscientiousness	-0.19	-1.122	0.270
Openness	-0.29	-1.95	0.060
Agreeableness	-0.02	-0.150	0.881

participants who reported positive perceptions of the current situation would have lower homesickness scores than those who perceived it to be a negative change.

The English- and non-English-speaking groups were significantly more satisfied with the current situation than the Asian group. It can be speculated that for many of the non-English-speaking participants, life in Australia is considerably easier than what they had experienced previously in their home nation (e.g., the former Soviet Republics). The fact that most of these participants were also migrants, as opposed to those from the other two nation groups who were mostly sojourners, may also have contributed to a different attitude and to greater acceptance of the new situation. The Asian group, predominantly comprised of students, experienced the greatest dissatisfaction with the current situation. It could be presumed that these participants missed the family and social settings of 'home'; however, this was not the case. Their dissatisfaction seemed to spring from a drop in living standards, fewer satisfying job opportunities, and a less satisfying life style. The Asian group perceived themselves worse off in terms of their current material situation, the current working environment, and their current lifestyles compared to their situation before moving to Australia. As the Asian group was predominantly composed of students, future studies might examine whether Asian students are more homesick than other same age student samples of different cultures.

This study supports previous findings that extraversion is related to lower homesickness scores and neuroticism, to higher homesickness scores. The results support the hypothesis that personality factors are correlated with high/low levels of homesickness, as measured on the Dundee Relocation Inventory (Fisher & Murray, 1985).

Specifically, in the Anglo group, high neuroticism scores related to high homesickness scores; and in the Asian group, low extraversion scores related to high homesickness scores. As found in the literature, high neuroticism scores predispose participants to view their experience of objective life events more negatively, whereas high extraversion scores predispose participants to view their experience of objective life events more positively. It should also be noted that extraversion is favorably regarded in the Australian sociocultural context.

As shown by Ward and Kennedy (1993), personality has to be viewed in its sociocultural context. It was interesting to note, therefore, that the Asian group scored lowest on the agreeableness, conscientiousness, and extraversion scales. Markus and Kitayama (1991) illustrated a difference between Asian and Western cultures as follows: "In America, 'the squeaky wheel gets greased'. In Japan, 'the nail that stands out gets pounded down'" (p. 224). Consequently, Asian participants would not be expected to score highly on extraversion scales. However, although the Asian group could be expected to value harmonious interdependence and are known for their 'work ethic,' the low scores in the agreeableness and conscientiousness scales did not reflect these attributes. Caution has to be exercised in any analysis of the Asian group with respect to the personality scales. The NEO Five-Factor Personality Inventory (Costa & McCrae, 1991) is a Western, English language measure. A new direction in cross-cultural research suggests that Western personality scales may not be appropriate to tap into the personality dimensions of Asian participants. Future studies may do well to utilize personality scales especially designed for Asian participants.

From a counseling perspective, this study has highlighted the fact that homesickness is a response to unpleasant aspects of the new environment, which results in a mismatch in favor of the home environment. With this information, counselors are in a position to isolate the areas of dissatisfaction and attempt to ameliorate the situation, or at very least, assist with some degree of acceptance of it. Further, it may be important for the student selection process, as well as for any pre-arrival briefing, to note the findings that, in the Australian sociocultural setting, higher extraversion scores relate to greater reported satisfaction.

Although this study accords well with findings from other studies in this area, the sample size was very small. The greatest limitation of this study was the exclusive use of English language, Western scales with a multicultural sample. Many potential participants had to be excluded, as their command of English was insufficient to answer the questionnaire unaided. This exclusion means that much valuable data on homesickness was missed. Future studies must examine ways to tap into this potential source of information in culturally appropriate ways. In closing, it would appear that personality and cultural differences do play a role in homesickness. Exactly what that role is needs further investigation.

References

Arrendondo-Dowd, P. M. (1981, February). Personal loss and grief as a result of immigration. *The Personnel and Guidance Journal,* 376-378.

Bowlby, J. (1980). *Attachment and loss. Vol. 3: Loss, sadness and depression.* New York: Basic Books.

Brewin, C., Furnham, A., & Howes, M. (1989). Demographic and psychological determinants of homesickness and confiding among students. *British Journal of Psychology, 80,* 467-477.

Burns, J. A. (1993). *Psychological adjustment of Australian expatriates.* Unpublished Honors Thesis, Swinburne University of Technology, Melbourne, Australia.

Carden, A. I., & Feicht, R., (1991). Homesickness among American and Turkish college students. *Journal of Cross-Cultural Psychology, 22,* 418-428.

Costa, P. T., & McCrae, R. R. (1991). *NEO five-factor inventory.* Odessa, FL: Psychological Assessment Resources.

DeJong-Gierveld, J., & van Tilburg, T. (1990). Rasch-type loneliness scale. In J. P. Robinson, P. R. Shaver, & L. S. Wrightsman (Eds.), *Measures of personality and social psychological attitudes* (Vol. 1). Orlando, FL: Academic.

Fisher, S. (1989). *Homesickness, cognition, and health.* London, England: Erlbaum.

Fisher, S. (1990). The psychological effects of leaving home: Homesickness, health and obsessional thoughts. In S. Fisher & C. L. Cooper (Eds.), *On the move: the psychology of change and transition.* Chichester, England: John Wiley & Sons.

Fisher, S., Elder, L., & Peacock, G. (1990). Contextual determinants and homesickness reporting. *Children's Environment Quarterly, 7,* 15-22.

Fisher, S., & Murray, K. (1985). The Dundee Relocation Inventory Questionnaire F. In S. Fisher, *Homesickness, cognition, and health.* London, England: Erlbaum.

Fisher, S., Murray, K., & Frazer, N. (1985). Homesickness and health in first year student. *Journal of Environmental Psychology, 5,* 181-195.

Headey, B. W., & Wearing, A. J. (1989). Personality life events and subjective well-being: Towards a dynamic equilibrium model. *Journal of Personality and Social Psychology, 57,* 731-739.

Horstmanshof, L., & Reddy, P. (1997). Homesickness among overseas sojourners in Australia. In K. Leung, U. Kim, S. Yamaguchi, & Y. Kashima (Eds.), *Progress in Asian social psychology* (Vol. 1, pp. 345-356). Singapore: John Wiley & Sons.

Kuhl, J., & Kazen-Saad, M. (1988). A motivational approach to volition: Activation and de-activation of memory representations related to uncompleted intentions. In V. Hamilton, G. H. K. Bower, & N. Frijda (Eds.), *Cognition, emotion and affect: A cognitive science view.* Dordrecht, The Netherlands: Martinus Nijhoff.

Markus, H. R., & Kitayama S. (1991). Culture and the self: Implications for cognition, emotion and motivation. *Psychological Review, 98,* 224-253.

Magnus, K., Diener, E., Fujita, F., & Pavot, W. (1993). Extraversion and neuroticism as predictors of objective life events: A longitudinal analysis. *Journal of Personality and Social Psychology, 65,* 1046-1053.

Parkes, C. M. (1972). *Bereavement.* New York: International University Press.

Searle, W., & Ward, C. (1990). The prediction of psychologocial and sociocultural adjustment during cross-cultural transitions. *International Journal of Intercultural Relations, 14,* 449-464.

Shaughnessy, J. J., & Zechmeister, E. B. (1985). *Research methods in psychology.* New York: Knopf.

Stokols, D., Shumaker, S. A., & Martinez, J. (1983). Residential mobility and personal wellbeing. *Journal of Environmental Psychology, 3,* 5-19.

Ward, C., & Kennedy, A., (1993). Where's the 'culture' in cross-cultural transition? Comparative studies of sojourner adjustment. *Journal of Cross-Cultural Psychology, 24,* 221-249.

Ying, Y., & Liese, L. H. (1994). Initial adjustment of Taiwanese students to the United States. *Journal of Cross-Cultural Psychology, 25,* 466-477.

Author Note

Correspondence concerning this article should be addressed to the authors at the School of Social Behavior Sciences, Swinburne Institute of Technology, PO Box 218, Hawthorn, Melbourne, Victoria 3122, Australia.

Organizational / Work Psychology

Leader Characteristics and Motivations in Lebanese- and Anglo-Australians

Tony El-Hayek and Daphne M. Keats
The University of Newcastle, Australia

ABSTRACT

Characteristics and motivations for leadership in Lebanese-Australians (LA) and Anglo-Australians (AA) were studied using a questionnaire approach. Items were drawn from a range of previous studies. Subjects were 130 adults from each cultural group with equal numbers of males and females associated with either the community or organizational setting. Significant differences were found on characteristics of leaders: LA leaders were male, religious, family oriented and social, while AA leaders were independent, charismatic and approachable. The LA leaders were motivated by situations associated with other people, while the AAs were motivated by individualism and independence. Significant differences were also found between the organizational and community contexts. The findings are discussed in terms of Hofstede's construct of individualism-collectivism and Misumi's PM theory of leadership.

Although there has been extensive work on leadership characteristics, leadership traits, and qualities considered important in leaders (Mullins, 1994; Petzall, Selvarajah & Willis, 1993; Ribeaux & Poppleton, 1992; Silin, 1976; Stogdill, 1974), there has been little work on the reasons why people might wish to lead. Moreover, most work on leadership characteristics has been in the context of organizations in the work environment. Little attention has been paid to leadership in community settings.

Evidence (Holt & Keats, 1992) suggests that cultural differences in work values and cultural goals may affect motivations to lead. In that study it was shown that the Lebanese-Australians (LA) differed greatly from Anglo-Australians (AA). Whereas the most important cultural goals of work for the AAs were financial independence and achieving a high income level, the most important for the LA were maintaining family status and maintaining family needs; the most important personal goals for the AAs were self-fulfillment followed by maintaining family needs, whereas the two most important personal goals for the LA were maintaining family needs and community respect. On work values, AAs ranked in order: a sense of achievement, job security and income level as the highest of twelve items ranked, while the LA ranked intellectual stimulation, followed by a sense of achievement and work offering variety. Job security and income level were ranked eighth and tenth in their list.

Perhaps the most significant research on leadership in organizational settings is by Misumi and his colleagues (Misumi, 1985; 1992; Misumi & Peterson, 1985). Misumi's PM theory has received much cross-cultural support in the organizational context. In this theory P stands schematically for a high emphasis on performance and M stands for a high emphasis on maintenance of good relations; low levels of emphasis on performance are represented by p and low levels of emphasis on maintenance by m. Thus a leader may be high on both (PM), low on both (pm), or high on one and low on the other (Pm or Mp). It has been found in many studies that the most favored type of leadership is that where both P (i.e., Performance) and M (i.e., Maintenance) are high. However, in cultural contexts where interpersonal relations are regarded as more important than output, it is likely that the M aspects of leadership may be more highly valued. One example is the nurturant task leader style, found by Sinha (1990) to be the favored style for Indian managers. The nurturant task leader pays attention to both task performance and to caring in a nurturant way for the well-being of the subordinate. In this there is some similarity to the Misumi PM style, however in the early stages of the relationship more attention is given to the interpersonal aspects. When the subordinate becomes more skilled, more attention is paid to the performance aspects.

The Lebanese in Australia
The LA make up one of the largest ethnic minorities in Australia. They have settled mainly in Melbourne and Sydney, and in the latter city are mainly found in the western suburbs. Psychologists have paid little attention to this group, although not only do their cultural traditions differ greatly from the AA majority but the religious differences between Muslim and Christian LA are just as great. In this study we will be referring only to subjects from the Christian group. Culturally, one of the most important influences is undoubtedly the family. Hassan, Healy and McKenna (1985) state that the Lebanese family is traditionally "patrilineal, endogamous and extended, with wide and complex kin relationships known to all members of the kinship group" (p. 180). They can be characterized as collectivist.

A study conducted in Lebanon by Waines and Jenness (1987) on the mutual understanding between Lebanese parents and their children on social and personal attitudes showed the Lebanese family to be the basic unit of social structure: its standing contributes to the prestige of its individual members, as the primary unit it demands loyalty and conformity from its members and in return provides them with security and support. Central to the idea of the family was the question of parental control, and conformity, respect and consideration of parental wishes on important matters were expected.

In his study of migrant family structure in Australia, McDonald (1991) argues that the LA have a "masculine" conception of the family and its tradition. In this view, the family is a formal political entity: "a tool in the struggle for power and prestige" (p. 104). McDonald believes that the LA family dominates over all other forms of social organization; the LA attain their identity and their place in society through the family.

In the LA community in Australia, great emphasis is placed upon maintaining the family's needs and structure. In a study of LA settlement in Sydney, Humphrey (1984) found that nearly all LA youth interviewed said that they would remain at home until they married. In 1981, only 2% of LA women aged between 15 and 29 were living in a non-family situation (McDonald, 1991).

The Anglo-Australians

The AAs of British background form the majority of Australians. English is the native language, and many have a background of several generations in Australia. Although the group includes those of Scottish and Irish descent, there is little difference among them and those of English descent. Their shared cultural traditions are Western. Undoubtedly Australians of this background are more individualistic in cultural orientation than the LA. The family is nuclear, there is much stress on independence as a goal of development. In Hofstede's (1980) study, AA respondents scored much above the mean on individualism, below the mean on power distance, below the mean on uncertainty avoidance, and slightly above the mean on masculinity. Taft and Day (1988) say that they are seen to have "a pragmatic, anti-intraceptive orientation with a concentration on materialism, consumerism and leisure" (p. 377).

Business versus Community Leadership

In an earlier study on community leadership, El-Hayek (1994) found major differences between LA and AAs in the attributes associated with effective community leadership. The LA associated family, religion, and male dominance with successful leadership, while the AAs associated independence, self-fulfillment, and personal characteristics such as charisma with successful community leadership. These findings differed from those based on research in business organizational settings. It would seem therefore that, given the cultural differences between these two groups, there would also be differences in their perception of desirable leadership characteristics and leadership motivations in the two contexts.

Aims and Hypotheses

The general aim of this study was to examine the role of cultural differences in leadership characteristics and leadership motivation in community and organizational contexts. On the basis of the cultural differences and previous research reported above, several predictions were made:

1. In the LA, leadership positions will be male-dominated.
2. The LA and AA cultural groups will differ on the characteristics leaders are perceived to exhibit.
3. The characteristics considered important for leadership by LA and AAs will differ.
4. The LA and AAs will differ on what motivates their leaders.
5. In both the LA and the AAs there will be differences between organizational and community contexts on both characteristics of leaders and motivations to lead.

Method

Participants

Participants were recruited individually through personal contact via members of the LA and AA communities in similar suburban environments. The participants in the study were 65 LA and 65 AA adults living in the same suburban area of Sydney. Among the LA, 32 males and 33 females with a mean age of 39.5 years. Among the AAs there were 34 males and 31 females with a mean age of 40.2 years.

Approximately half of the participants from both groups were drawn from community contexts and half from organizational contexts. Participants did not belong exclusively to any specific community or business organization.

Materials

A Leadership Motivation Questionnaire consisting of four main parts was designed for the study. The Questionnaire was modeled after a similar survey used by El-Hayek (1994) to investigate concepts of community leadership among the LA and AAs. The questionnaire was adapted to account for the inclusion of participants from the organizational context. Part 1 obtained background information on gender, occupation, age, marital status, number of children, cultural background and country of birth. Part 2 asked questions about the subjects' leadership position. The first question asked whether they were in a leadership position in their community or business organization. If the answer was yes, the next series of questions asked about the context in which they led, their position and what it involved, the level of that position, how they attained it, whom they led, and the advantages and disadvantages of being in their leadership position. If not now in a leadership position, the respondent was asked whether he or she would like to be in a leadership position, and why or why not. Part 3 contained four sections on leadership characteristics. A list of 48 leadership characteristics was derived from the literature, previous research by El-Hayek (1994) and several pilot studies. The characteristics were rated on a 4-point Likert scale. The order of the items was determined randomly. Respondents were invited to suggest other characteristics that did not appear in the previous list. They were then required to choose from the list the five most important and the five least important characteristics for leadership. A Pearson correlation coefficient (r) was calculated to determine the reliability of the scale of the 48 characteristics. The statistic showed a fairly high level of reliability ($r = 0.62$). Part 4 addressed the issue of leadership motivation. A list of eighteen motivator items was collected (see Table 1) from the same sources as the list of leadership characteristics and from Holt and Keats (1992). Respondents were asked to give a definition of each item to check that the meaning was understood. Next, each item was rated using a 4-point Likert type scale, and then the 18 items were ranked in order of importance. Kendall's W showed that participants within each group ranked items significantly similarly. The statistics are presented in the Results section below. All items in the Questionnaire were translated into Lebanese using the back-translation method (Brislin, 1970).

Procedure
The Questionnaire was administered to each respondent in an individual interview. Each respondent was given a copy of the Questionnaire in their preferred language. The introduction and directions for all four parts were given orally. The respondent was given the option of responding orally to the structured questions as well as writing down the answer in the Questionnaire booklet provided. All probe questions were responded to orally. The interviewer recorded all oral responses.

Results

Leadership Positions
Approximately 30% of the respondents in each cultural group, indicated that they were in a leadership position, with slightly more leaders in the organizational than in the community context. Leadership was virtually evenly divided by gender in the AA group, whereas among the LA only

3 of the 20 leaders were female. All three of these subjects were born in Australia and were in their twenties.

Perceptions by Leaders of Advantages and Drawbacks to Leadership
For the LA leaders, the most frequently cited advantages were recognition, status, and money to improve the family's status, whereas the most frequently cited drawbacks were time away from the family, the personal politics involved, and commitment when the preferred commitment was to the family. For the AA leaders, the most frequently cited advantages were financial independence, power, and the contacts to use for personal promotion and advancement, whereas the most frequently cited drawbacks were less time for personal endeavors, the power of superiors, and pressure.

Of the respondents who were not leaders, 64% of the LA and only 20% of the AA said that they would not like to be in a leadership position. Of the 28 female LA who were not leaders, only 6 expressed a desire to lead. Four of the these were born in Australia and were in their twenties. The most frequently cited reasons for wanting to lead by the LA were money to improve the lifestyle of one's family, to help others, and the pleasure of leading a team, whereas time away from the family, politics, and "It's a man's job to lead" (given by the female respondents), were the most frequently cited reasons for not wanting to lead. For the AAs the most frequently cited reasons for wanting to lead were power, independence, and financial independence, whereas too much pressure, too much responsibility, and too much time leads to loss of independence were the most frequently cited reasons for not wanting to lead.

Leadership Characteristics
The normal approximation to Wilcoxin-Mann-Whitney tests with Bonferroni-alpha adjustments to account for family- wise error were conducted on each of the 48 leadership characteristics. The LA and AAs differed significantly on 15 items. Those which stood out most were religious ($W = 6028.5, p < .0001$), family oriented ($W = 5628, p < .0001$), social ($W = 5258.5, p < .0001$) and nurturant ($W = 5081.5, p < .0001$), which were rated higher by the LA, and independent ($W = 3002, p < .0001$), well-off ($W = 3554, p < .0005$), approachable ($W = 3158, p < .0001$) and charismatic ($W = 3346, p < .0001$), which were rated higher by the AAs. No regular patterns were found on the variables of age, gender or context.

The leadership characteristics considered most important by the LAs in order of frequency, were: family oriented, social, responsible, wise, and religious, whereas the characteristics ranked least important by the

LAs were independent, taller and charismatic. Further analysis showed that all of the 10 LA who listed religious as not important were in their twenties, nine had been born in Australia and the other one had emigrated to Australia at an early age. The characteristics ranked most important by the AAs were, in order of frequency, self-confident, approachable, dependable, charismatic, assertive, and independent, whereas the characteristics ranked least important were, in order of frequency: religious, taller, good at sport, attractive, and family oriented.

Leadership Motivations
The ratings for the 18 motivators were analyzed using the normal approximation to Wilcoxin-Mann-Whitney tests with Bonferroni-alpha adjustments of the significance level from .05 to .0028 to account for familywise error. The data showed significant differences between the LA and the AAs on personal promotion and advancement ($W = 3327.5$, $p < .0001$), which was rated higher by the AAs, and team spirit ($W = 5022.5$, $p < .0002$), group support ($W = 5011.5$, $p < .0002$) and religious reasons ($W = 5844.5$, $p < .0001$), which were rated higher by the LA.

From the 18 motivator items differences between organizational and community contexts, collapsed across culture, were found on financial reasons ($W = 5985.5$, $p < .0001$), status ($W = 5405$, $p < .0001$), personal promotion and advancement ($W = 5148.5$, $p < .0023$), and fringe benefits ($W = 5467.5$, $p < .0001$), which were rated higher by respondents in the organizational context. To help others ($W = 3498$, $p < .0001$) and to advance the image of the community or business organization ($W = 3899.5$, $p < .0025$), were rated higher by the respondents in the community context.

When the two variables, context and culture, were considered in combination, significant differences were found between LA and AA subjects. In the organizational context the motivators personal promotion and advancement ($W = 967.5$, $p < .0002$), rated higher by the AAs, and team spirit ($W = 1514$, $p < .0012$), group support ($W = 1536.5$, $p < .0004$), and religious reasons ($W = 1739.5$, $p < .0001$), were rated higher by the LA. The only significant difference between the LA and AA subjects in the community context was on the motivator religious reasons ($W = 1269$, $p < .0001$), which was rated higher by the LA.

Rankings of the 18 motivators within each cultural and contextual group are presented in Table 1. Spearman rank order correlations applied to these data yielded correlations between the LAs and AAs ($r_s = .100$), and between organizational and community contexts ($r_s = 0.263$), that were non-significant at the .05 level. These correlations indicate that there was little similarity among the four rankings of the motivator items.

Table 1. Rank Hierarchies of the 18 Leadership Motivator Items across Culture and Context

Motivator	Australian		Lebanese	
	Org.	Com.	Org.	Com.
For financial reasons	1	15	3	18
For personal promotion and advancement	2	3	8	13
For the status	3	2	1	4
For the power	4	9	6	15
For the recognition	5	1	2	5
To use and develop their skills	6	4	13	10
For the fringe benefits	7	16	16	17
Because they consider themselves to be leaders	8	5	15	9
To realise their executive potential	9	11	11	16
For their intellectual challenge	10	14	17	12
To advance the image of community or business organisation	11	6	9	2
For the responsibility	12	8	4	7
For personal reassurance	13	12	18	14
To help others	14	7	5	3
For the social scene	15	13	10	11
For team spirit	16	10	7	6
For group support	17	17	12	8
For religious reasons	18	18	14	1

Org. = Organizational context; Com. = Community context.

When examined together, nonsignficant rank order correlations at the .05 level indicated that LA subjects in the organizational context ranked the 18 motivators differently from the AAs in the organizational context (r_s = 0.370), and LAs in the community context ranked the 18 motivators differently from the AAs in the community context (r_s =0.304). In the organizational context, the motivators that showed the largest differences were team spirit and to help others, ranked higher by the LA, and personal promotion and advancement, and fringe benefits, ranked higher by the AA. In the community context, the motivators that showed the largest differences were religious reasons and group support, ranked higher by the LA, and power and personal promotion and advancement, ranked higher by the AA.

Discussion

The results show striking differences between the LA and the AA and between the views of leaders in organizational and community contexts. Compared with the balanced gender distribution among AA leaders, the LA had few leaders who were female, and seemed to associate the leadership role primarily with the male. The younger LA females, however, were more like the AA in their willingness to be leaders.

The two cultural groups differed on their perceptions of leader characteristics. Of 48 characteristics, 15 differed significantly between LA and AA. The differences were epitomized by the following interview responses: By a LA: "One who is not family oriented and religious is not qualified and would not be accepted to lead our community"; contrasted with this view is the response of an AA: "In order for leaders to be successful, they must exhibit strong personal characteristics, such as charisma, be able to carry the load on their own, and most of all be approachable to those they are leading."

This contrast in the LA and AA responses illustrates the more collectivist nature of LA culture and the more individualist nature of the AA. According to Hassan et al. (1985), a characteristic such as independence would be condemned because it might threaten the harmony of the LA family and culture. As one subject stated, the LA believe that "it is not good to be independent, it shows a lack of respect to the family and social group who have supported the individual since birth." The contrasts come out clearly in what is not considered desirable in a leader. The LA attitude towards charisma, for example, is illustrated by the following interview response, "Charismatic leaders have something to hide, it is usually their ignorance to the task in hand." By contrast, AA subjects were just as strong in their views that a person's family and religion were not relevant to leadership ability. Among typical responses illustrating this view, one said, "Whether or not a leader has a family has nothing to do with their effectiveness", and another, "Religion has nothing to do with anything as far as successful leadership is concerned.

However, the lack of significant differences on 33 of the 48 items shows that the two cultural groups share many common perceptions of their leaders. Three items: taller, good at sport and attractive personal appearance, which are typically reported within descriptions of leaders (Robbins, 1994), were identified as not important by both the LA and the AA.

On the motivations for leadership, again differences appeared between LA and AA, and these differences were most notable on items where the LA evoked collectivist and religious values and the AA evoked individualistic values, such as personal promotion and advancement. Two motivating factors for leadership ranked high by both cultural groups were status and recognition.

However, the meanings attributed to each item were different. To illustrate, a LA said that status meant "One's place in the community, which helps to improve the image of the individual and the family." Compare this with the response by an AA to whom status meant "A position in society that has people looking up to you and helps you gain success, money and independence." The meaning of recognition also differed. For example, one LA subject stated, "Recognition is being appreciated and respected by others in your community for what you have done", whereas for the AAs recognition was expressed as "Being noticed by those around you which may aid later in personal promotion." Further research is required to measure and define the extent and generality of such differences in meaning.

Differences in the perception and motivation for leadership appeared between contexts for both the LA and the AA. Financial consideration was a strong motivator for the organizational context but low for the community context for both cultural groups. Fringe benefits was a stronger leadership motivator in the organizational than the community context, and more so for the AA than for the LA. Religion was a stronger motivator for the LA in the community context than in the organizational context, but was rejected in both contexts by the AA. The predominance of preferences for M-type leadership qualities in the LA subjects for both the organizational and the community contexts and in the AA for the community context suggests that contextual settings need to be taken into account for Misumi's (1985) PM theory of leadership.

The results have implications for community planning activities. For example, a planner may require information on activities which could be successfully conducted in the Parramatta or Bankstown areas in Sydney. Both of these areas house large numbers of LA people. On the basis of the current findings, the planner may save time and money and be assured of a degree of success by planning something associated with the family, religion or both. The findings also suggest cultural guidelines by which the community leader could guide the family therapist. For example, a leader may suggest the use of religion as a therapeutic avenue for a LA family, whereas such a suggestion for an AA family would not be made and time and effort would not be expended in attempting procedures that have little chance of success.

Practical implications are numerous when considering the differences found on leadership motivation between the community and organizational contexts for both the LA and AA. Although it is well known that in the organizational context leaders are recruited by offering financial rewards and fringe benefits, this research suggests that the LA candidate should also be offered the opportunity to work in teams, while the AA should be offered independence to implement their ideas. In the community context on the other hand, the LA will be attracted by the opportunity to be recognized for helping others, while the AA will be attracted by the opportunity for personal promotion.

The study has limitations in scope and sample. For example, the LA in this study were all drawn from the Christian community; no inferences can be made about the members of the Moslem LA who also comprise a significant number. However, the differences found were sufficient to suggest that additional research into the LA as a minority community in Australia would be valuable, especially if the LA relationships among other ethnic groups were also considered.

References

Brislin, R. W. (1970). Back-translation for cross-cultural research. *Journal of Cross-Cultural Psychology, 1,* 185-216.

El-Hayek, T. (1994). *Concepts of community leadership among Lebanese and Anglo-Australians.* Unpublished Third Year Independent Project, University of Newcastle, Australia.

Hassan, R., Healy, J., & McKenna (1985). Lebanese families. In D. Storer (Ed.), *Ethnic family values in Australia* (pp. 173-198). Sydney: Prentice Hall of Australia.

Hofstede, G. (1980). *Culture's consequences: International differences in work related values.* California: Sage.

Holt, J., & Keats, D. M. (1992). Work cognition in multicultural interaction. *Journal of Cross-Cultural Psychology, 23,* 151-159.

Humphrey, M. (1984). *Family, work, and unemployment: A study of Lebanese settlement in Sydney.* Canberra: AGPS.

McDonald, P. (1991). Migrant family structure. In K. Funder (Ed.), *Images of Australian families* (pp. 102-121). Melbourne: Longman Cheshire.

Misumi, J. (1985). *The behavioral science of leadership: An interdisciplinary Japanese research program.* Ann Arbor, MI: University of Michigan Press.

Misumi, J. (1992). PM Theory of leadership from a cross-cultural perspective. In S. Iwawaki, Y. Kashima, & K. Leung (Eds.), *Innovations in cross-cultural psychology* (pp. 18-27). Amsterdam: Swets & Zeitlinger.

Misumi, J., & Peterson, M. F. (1985). The Performance-Maintenance (PM) theory of leadership: Review of a Japanese research program. *Administrative Science Quarterly, 30,* 198-223.

Mullins, L. J. (1994). *Management and organisational behaviour.* London: Pitman.

Petzall, S. B., Selvarajah, C. T., & Willis, Q. F. (1993). *Management: A behavioural approach.* Melbourne: Longman Cheshire.

Ribeaux, P., & Poppleton, S. E. (1992). *Psychology and work: An introduction.* London: Macmillan.

Robbins, S. P. (1994). *Management.* New Jersey: Prentice-Hall.

Silin, R. (1976). *Leadership and values: The organisation of large-scale Taiwan enterprises.* Massachusetts: Harvard University Press.

Sinha, J. B. P. (1990). Further testing of a model of leadership effectiveness. In A. H. Othman & A. R. Wan Rafaei (Eds.), *Psychology and socio-economic development* (pp. 229-254). Malaysia: Universiti Kebangsaan.

Stogdill, R. M. (1948). Personal factors associated with leadership: a Survey of the literature. *Journal of Psychology, 25,* 35-71.

Stogdill, R. M. (1974). *Handbook of leadership: A survey of theory of research.* New York: Free Press.

Taft, R., & Day, R. H. (1988). Psychology in Australia. *Annual Review of Psychology, 39,* 375-400.

Waines, N. O., & Jenness, D. (1987). Mutual understanding between Lebanese and English parents and children. *Genetic, Social, and General Psychology Monographs, 113,* 165-191.

Socio-Cultural Environment, Work Culture, and Managerial Practices: The Model of Culture Fit

Rabindra N. Kanungo
McGill University, Canada

Zeynep Aycan
Koc University, Turkey

&

Jai B. P. Sinha
ASSERT, India

ABSTRACT

The Model of Culture Fit was tested in three cross-cultural studies. The model predicts that the socio-cultural environment and enterprise characteristics have significant influence on managerial assumptions about employee nature and behaviour and human resource management (HRM) practices. In the first study, workers in the United States, Canada and India completed a 45-item self-report questionnaire that enabled their comparison on six socio-cultural dimensions, eight work culture dimensions, and ten HRM practices. As predicted by the Model, Indian workers differed from those in both the U.S. and Canada on more dimensions than the U.S. workers differed from those in Canada. In the second study, new samples of Indian and Canadian participants responding to the questionnaire differed on dimensions similar to those found in the first study. In this study, relationships among societal and organizational culture and HRM practices were explored. A third, and previously published, study of differences between public and private sector organizations in India, was summarized for the additional evidence it provided consistent with the Model of Culture Fit. Research and practical implications of the three studies were discussed.

Organizations are complex structures that evolve within a dynamically interacting internal and external environment. Managing human resources in such complex systems requires an understanding of the economic, technological, political, legal as well as socio-cultural characteristics of the society. Although management scholars have examined the ways in which human resource management (HRM) practices are influenced by such forces, various streams of research in this area have not been integrated in the existing literature. The Model of Culture Fit presented in this paper aims at addressing this void by examining the impact of enterprise and socio-cultural environment on work culture and HRM practices.

The impact of culture on work values and behaviour in the organizational context has been demonstrated (e.g., Hofstede, 1980; Triandis,

1982; Trompenaars, 1993). In this research, cultural dimensions at the societal level (e.g., individualism/collectivism, power distance, uncertainty avoidance, masculinity/femininity, and universalism/particularism) were identified, and respondents in various countries compared their work values using these dimensions. At the organizational level, on the other hand, Schein (1992) has conceptualized the organizational culture as a product of prevailing managerial assumptions and premises about employee nature and behaviour. These assumptions include the relationship of employees to nature, time, space, and others in the organization. These two seemingly independent bodies of research have been incorporated into the work of Kanungo and Jaeger (1990) who described the connection between socio-cultural characteristics and internal work culture in a conceptual model, called the Model of Culture Fit. The model is presented in Figure 1.

The basic rationale underlying the Model of Culture Fit is that HRM practices are designed and implemented in congruence with managerial assumptions and beliefs about employee nature and behaviour. Such assumptions and beliefs constitute the foundation of the internal work culture. Managerial assumptions are, in turn, influenced by the social, cultural, economic, and political environment within which the organizations operate. In contrast to past research (e.g., Hofstede, 1980; Triandis, 1982), this model characterizes societal- and organizational-level values, assumptions, and beliefs as interacting rather than overlapping.

In the model depicted in Figure 1, there are two environmental forces influencing the internal work culture. First, there are enterprise variables such as the degree of competitiveness in the market, the nature of the organizational goal and mission, the state of organizational ownership and control, and the availability of resources (both technological and human). Secondly, there are socio-cultural variables characterizing the environment from which the organization draws its human resources. It should be noted that both the enterprise and socio-cultural environment are shaped by the continuous interaction among ecological, legal, political, historical, and social contextual variables.

Empirical support for the Culture Fit Model has been provided by the three independent studies described in this paper. All three studies utilized the same set of variables and measures. The first study, conducted by Kanungo and Aycan (1996), compared respondents from Canada, the United States, and India with regard to socio-cultural characteristics, internal work culture, and HRM practices. This study had two distinct purposes: (a) To compare the responses obtained within a developing country (India) with those from two developed countries in North America, with the expectation that Indian workers would differ

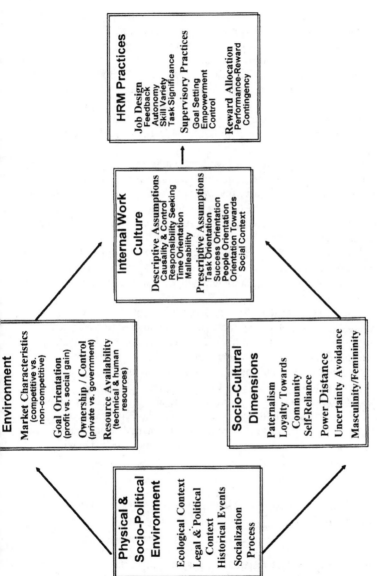

Figure 1. The Model of Culture Fit

Environment

Market Characteristics
(competitive vs.
non-competitive)

Goal Orientation
(profit vs. social gain)

Ownership / Control
(private vs. government)

Resource Availability
(technical & human
resources)

**Physical &
Socio-Political
Environment**

Ecological Context

Legal & Political
Context

Historical Events

Socialization
Process

**Internal Work
Culture**

Descriptive Assumptions
Causality & Control
Responsibility Seeking
Time Orientation
Malleability

Prescriptive Assumptions
Task Orientation
Success Orientation
People Orientation
Orientation Towards
Social Context

HRM Practices

Job Design
Feedback
Autonomy
Skill Variety
Task Significance

Supervisory Practices
Goal Setting
Empowerment
Control

Reward Allocation
Performance-Reward
Contingency

**Socio-Cultural
Dimensions**

Paternalism
Loyalty Towards
Community
Self-Reliance
Power Distance
Uncertainty Avoidance
Masculinity/Femininity

from those in Canada and the U.S. in perceived socio-cultural environment, work culture, and HRM practices, whereas such differences would
not be observed to the same extent between respondents from Canada and
the U.S.; and (b) to examine the relationship among dimensions of the
socio-cultural environment. The latter is particularly important because
various cultural dimensions are depicted as orthogonal in the extant
literature. However, it is our belief that such cultural dimensions are
interrelated, and a configuration among them that is common to all
cultures may provide a parsimonious framework to guide future cross-
cultural research.

In the second study by Kanungo and Sinha (1996), the relationship
between socio-cultural dimensions and characteristics of internal work
culture was tested. In addition, the way in which managerial assumptions
were related to HRM practices was examined. Finally, in the third study
Indian public and private sector organizations were compared to examine
the influence of the enterprise environment on the internal work culture
and HRM practices. Because this study has been published elsewhere
(Mathur, Aycan, & Kanungo, 1996), the results will be summarized in
this paper in order to present an integrated view of research related to the
Model of Culture Fit.

The three studies tested different propositions of the model. The first
two studies explored the link between socio-cultural environment and
internal work culture, whereas the third study examined the relationship
between the enterprise environment and the internal work culture. In the
first two studies, the emphasis was on the variance in socio-cultural
environment. However, in the third study, such variance was not
expected at the cultural level, because public and private sector organizations were compared within the same culture. This enabled us to explore
the influence of enterprise environment on internal work culture and
HRM practices by holding constant the socio-cultural environment.

STUDY 1
**Societal Culture, Managerial Assumptions and HRM Practices:
A Comparison Between Developed and Developing Countries**

Participants
A total of 838 individual respondents participated in this study: 200 from
Canada, 499 from India, and 139 from the United States. Canadian and
American respondents were lower- to middle-managers of various organi-
zations enrolled in two major business schools in North America. The
Indian data were collected from managers and employees of seven
different organizations.

The Questionnaire
The self-report "opinion" questionnaire consisted of three parts. In the first part, five socio-cultural dimensions (power distance, masculinity, uncertainty avoidance, paternalism, and individualism/collectivism) were assessed. Within individualism/collectivism two orthogonal dimensions were assessed (loyalty towards community and self-reliance) as suggested in the recent literature (e.g., Kim, Triandis, Kagitcibasi, Choi, & Yoon, 1994). The second part of the questionnaire assessed managerial beliefs and assumptions about employee nature on eight variables: Internal locus of control, obligation towards others, responsibility seeking, futuristic time orientation, malleability, proactive, reactive, and participative orientations. In the third part of the questionnaire, HRM practices were assessed in three areas: job design (four variables), supervision (four variables), and reward system design (two variables). Three of these ten variables (task significance, skill variety, and performance-extrinsic reward contingency) were measured using single items whereas the other eight variables were measured by two items each. The questionnaire con-sisted of forty-five statements with a six-point response format ranging from 1 (strongly disagree) to 6 (strongly agree). Questionnaires were self-administered, and took approximately twenty-five minutes to com-plete. The scales comprising the questionnaire have been found to be reliable and valid measures of the underlying constructs and its psycho-metric properties have been reported elsewhere (Mathur et al., 1996).

Results
The data from respondents in Canada, the U.S., and India were compared on 24 variables (six socio-cultural, eight internal work culture, and ten HRM practices) using a series of one-way analysis of variance tests. Differences between each country pair were then tested using a modified Bonferroni technique to enable us to control the type I error for planned comparisons (Keppel, 1991). Results are summarized in Table 1. Mean differences indicated that respondents from the countries differed on all but four variables: masculinity, futuristic orientation, responsibility seeking, and performance-extrinsic reward contingency. Pairwise compa-risons showed that respondents from Canada and the U.S. differed only on 9 out of 24 variables, whereas respondents from India differed from those from Canada on 18 and those from the U.S. on 16 dimensions.

With respect to the relationships among socio-cultural variables, in all three countries, paternalism was positively correlated with both power distance (Canada, $r = .23$, $p <. 001$; USA, $r = .26$, $p < .001$; India, $r = .18$, $p < .05$) and community loyalty (Canada, $r = .21$, $p < .01$; USA, $r = .30$, $p < .001$; India, $r = .25$, $p < .001$). Power distance had a positive relationship with uncertainty avoidance (Canada, $r = .33$,

Table 1. Comparison between Canada, U.S., and India on Dimensions

	Canada		U.S.		India	
	M	*SD*	*M*	*SD*	*M*	*SD*
Socio-Cultural Dimensions						
Paternalism	3.2	1.2	3.6	1.1	4.6	1.2
Power Dist.	3.1	1.1	3.9	0.9	3.9	1.1
Mas./Fem.	2.2	0.8	2.1	0.7	2.3	1.0
Uncert. avoidance	3.6	1.1	3.9	0.8	3.9	1.2
Community loyalty	3.3	1.1	3.6	0.8	4.0	1.1
Self-reliance	3.7	0.9	3.7	0.8	4.2	0.9
Organizational Culture						
Int. locus of control	5.1	0.9	5.1	0.9	4.1	1.3
Futuristic orientation	4.7	0.8	4.9	0.7	4.6	1.1
Malleability	4.6	1.0	4.5	0.8	4.1	1.3
Proact. orientation	3.9	1.0	3.6	0.9	3.2	1.2
React. orientation	4.0	0.9	4.2	0.7	5.0	0.8
Obl. tow. others	3.4	1.0	3.8	0.7	4.0	1.1
Respons. seeking	4.2	1.0	4.2	0.8	4.1	1.1
Part. orientation	4.8	0.9	4.4	0.7	4.9	0.9
Human Resource Management Practices						
Feedback	4.5	1.3	4.5	1.0	3.9	1.2
Autonomy	4.1	1.2	3.6	0.9	3.5	1.1
Skill variety	3.9	1.7	3.2	1.4	3.2	1.4
Task significance	3.9	1.6	3.9	1.3	3.5	1.3
Goal setting	3.4	1.3	3.5	1.1	3.9	1.1
Empowerment	4.4	1.2	4.6	1.0	3.9	1.2
Self-control	4.4	1.3	4.4	0.9	4.0	1.2
Laissez-a-faire	4.5	1.1	4.5	1.1	4.2	1.2
Perf. Ext. R-Cont.	3.3	1.7	3.3	1.5	3.5	1.4
Perf. Int. R-Cont.	3.4	1.2	4.2	1.1	3.7	1.1

Note. $*p < .01$; $**p < .001$; Mas./Fem. = Masculinity/Femininity; Uncert. avoidance = Uncertainty avoidance; Int. locus of control = Internal locus of control; Proact. orientation = Proactive orientation; React. orientation = Reactive orientation; Obl. tow. others = Obligation towards others; Respons. seeking = Responsibility seeking; Part. orientation = Participative orientation; Perf. Ext./Int. R-Cont. = Performance extrinsic/intrinsic reward contingency.

of Socio-Cultural Environment, Organizational Culture and HRM Practice

Difference between:	Can-US	Can-Ind	US-Ind	Overall
	$F(1,338)$	$F(1,698)$	$F(1,637)$	$F(2,836)$
Socio-Cultural Dimensions				
Paternalism	10.96*	187.69**	75.34**	107.22**
Power Dist.	45.96**	56.40**	0.36	34.13**
Mas./Fem.	0.03	4.20	4.88	2.96
Uncert. avoidance	11.42*	13.32*	0.04	7.50**
Community loyalty	7.34*	63.36**	24.20**	35.21**
Self-reliance	0.43	19.80**	26.32**	15.22**
Organizational Culture				
Int. locus of control	0.45	76.56**	58.52**	50.42**
Futuristic orientation	5.19	1.06	9.12*	4.36
Malleability	0.22	14.97*	12.18**	10.12**
Proact. orientation	8.52*	33.98**	9.36*	18.89**
React. orientation	5.33	102.01**	71.23**	61.15**
Obl. tow. others	14.82**	33.06**	3.42	16.80**
Respons. seeking	0.11	0.27	0.04	0.15
Part. orientation	20.07**	1.79	34.22**	15.20**
Human Resource Management Practices				
Feedback	0.18	21.06**	25.80**	16.77**
Autonomy	11.56*	30.91**	3.49	17.42**
Skill variety	18.15**	20.52**	0.16	14.15**
Task significance	0.06	8.41*	9.52*	6.50*
Goal setting	0.49	21.71**	14.59**	14.28**
Empowerment	0.81	19.19*	29.48**	16.97**
Self-control	0.03	8.41*	9.92*	6.64*
Laissez-a-faire	0.26	11.29**	6.81*	6.67*
Perf. Ext. R-Cont.	0.10	0.25	0.81	0.42
Perf. Int. R-Cont.	11.39*	0.19	13.69**	7.41*

$p < .001$; USA, $r = .19, p < .05$; India, $r = .38, p < .001$) and with community loyalty (Canada, $r = .25, p < .001$; USA, $r = .23, p < .01$; India, $r = .19, p < .01$). Finally, a negative correlation was found between community loyalty and self-reliance (Canada, $r = -.14, p < .05$; USA, $r = -.23, p < .01$; India, $r = -.20, p < .01$).

In addition to these relationships common to all countries, there were some relationships idiosyncratic to each country. For example, in the Indian sample, paternalism was negatively related to masculinity ($r = -.45, p < .001$), and power distance was negatively related to self-reliance ($r = -.18, p < .01$). For the two North American samples, uncertainty avoidance was positively associated with both paternalism (Canada, $r = .19, p < .01$; USA, $r = .23, p < .01$) and community loyalty (Canada, $r = .32, p < .001$; USA, $r = .29, p < .001$).

Discussion

This study compared respondents from the U.S., Canada, and India on various aspects of societal and organizational culture, and HRM practices. Results showed that, as expected, Canada and the U.S. did not differ as substantially as India did from both. These differences were especially apparent in managerial assumptions and HRM practices.

There are a number of intriguing findings. First, power distance and uncertainty avoidance were predictably higher in India than in Canada, but the United States sample unexpectedly scored high on these dimensions. Although this finding should be replicated with larger samples, it suggests that there is an invisible power distance in American organizations. High uncertainty avoidance, on the other hand, could be a function of recent downsizing in organizations.

Secondly, Indian respondents scored higher than North Americans on self-reliance. India, being a collectivist society, was expected to score low on self-reliance which is a manifestation of individualism. It appears that self-reliance may assume a different meaning in societies where there is poverty and scarcity of resources. Under such circumstances, it is important to be as self-reliant as possible in order not to burden other in-group members with one's demands. This suggests that individuals can be loyal to their communities, but this loyalty and concern for others may be at the root of self-reliance. The construct validity of self-reliance, therefore, should be examined more closely in the developing country context.

Finally, Indian and North American managers were, unexpectedly, similar in their assumptions regarding employee responsibility seeking and futuristic orientation. In addition, Indian managers valued participation and delegation at all levels as much as their North American counterparts did. These findings could be explained by India's rapid economic growth which has gained momentum in recent years. In order to maintain a competitive advantage, Indian managers seem to adopt 'Western' management techniques which emphasize planning and participation.

With respect to the relationship among dimensions of socio-cultural environment, the results indicated that paternalism, power distance, uncertainty avoidance, and loyalty towards community were orthogonal but related components of a larger construct such as 'vertical collectivism' (Chen, Meindl, & Hunt, 1997; Triandis, 1994). This overarching construct emphasizes the importance of fulfilling one's duties and obligations towards other in-group members, and sacrificing oneself for the good of the group. Future studies should further examine the relationship among cultural dimensions to formulate an encompassing scheme which could be validated in different cultural groups. In addition, idiosyncratic or culture-specific relationships among various dimensions should also be delineated.

STUDY 2
Cultural Values, Work Culture, and Managerial Practices:
A Test of the Culture Fit Model

Participants
Fifty-three Canadian and 73 Indian managers enrolled in MBA programs completed the same questionnaires as in the first study. Although enrolled as students, all respondents reported they were employed at the time of the study.

Results
Many of the results obtained in the first study with respect to differences and similarities between the respondents from Canada and India were replicated in this study (Table 2). The only difference between the results of the first and the present study was in the area of nature of supervision. In the present study, respondents from Canada and India did not differ with respect to task significance, empowerment, and supervisory control.

Although the data were collected in a single session, causal relations among socio-cultural environment, internal work culture, and management practices were explored through a series of multiple regression analyses. Canadian and Indian samples were pooled in the regression analyses. First, socio-cultural dimensions were regressed on each of the internal work culture variables (Table 3). Except for responsibility seeking and futuristic orientation, variance in all other dimensions of work culture was accounted for by socio-cultural characteristics. In turn,

Table 2. Comparison Between India and Canada on Dimensions of Socio-Cultural Environment, Organizational Culture and HRM Practices

	Canada		India		Diff. $F(1,124)$
	M	SD	M	SD	
Socio-Cultural Dimensions					
Paternalism	3.2	1.1	5.1	0.8	111.71**
Power Dist.	3.5	1.3	4.5	1.2	19.75**
Mas./Fem.	2.9	1.2	2.4	1.0	5.48
Uncert. avoidance	3.5	1.3	4.5	1.2	19.75**
Community loyalty	3.1	1.0	4.5	1.1	52.01**
Self-reliance	3.3	1.0	4.0	1.1	10.08**
Organizational Culture					
Int. locus of control	4.3	1.1	3.5	1.4	14.21**
Futuristic orientat.	4.3	1.0	4.7	1.0	3.63
Malleability	4.0	1.1	3.3	1.2	11.33**
Proact. orient.	3.9	1.2	2.7	0.9	43.25**
React. orient.	4.3	1.0	5.1	1.0	23.09**
Obl. tow. others	3.0	1.2	4.3	1.1	36.85**
Respons. seeking	4.1	1.2	4.0	1.3	0.13
Part. orientat.	5.0	0.8	4.8	1.1	0.78
Human Resource Management Practices					
Feedback	4.6	1.2	3.9	1.4	7.91*
Autonomy	4.3	1.3	3.0	1.2	33.04**
Skill variety	4.1	1.7	2.6	1.4	28.91**
Task significance	4.3	1.1	4.6	1.4	1.01
Goal setting	3.5	1.6	4.5	1.2	18.28**
Empowerment	4.8	1.0	4.6	1.1	0.97
Self-control	4.7	1.2	4.8	0.8	0.79
Laissez-a-faire	5.8	1.1	5.6	1.4	1.01
Perf. Ext.R-Cont.	3.4	1.6	2.5	1.4	10.49**
Perf. Int. R-Cont.	4.1	1.3	4.2	1.1	0.04

*$p < .01$; **$p < .001$. See Table 1 for an explanation of abbreviations.

most of the internal work culture dimensions predicted the nature of HRM practices. There were a few socio-cultural variables that directly influenced managerial practices, but their influence was weaker than that of work culture variables (Table 4).

Discussion
The pattern of differences between Canada and India was very similar to what was reported in the first study. The convergence of findings from two different data sets lend further support to the Culture Fit Model. Results pertaining to relationships among the three sets of variables were also encouraging. Paternalism, community loyalty, power distance, and uncertainty avoidance predicted low internal locus of control, low malleability and low proactivity, but high reactivity and high obligation towards others. An overview of the relationships seems to suggest that when both countries were taken together, meeting obligations to others at the cost of one's own interests is an important aspect of work culture which is influenced by a host of socio-cultural factors such as community loyalty, power distance, paternalism, and uncertainty avoidance. These socio-cultural dimensions individually or in different combinations also promote reactive orientation but depress internal locus of control, malleability, and proactive orientation.

Results revealed that HRM practices were mainly influenced by internal work culture variables. Those managers who believed that employees can improve their skills and take control of their future by being proactive provided enriched jobs (e.g., feedback, autonomy, skill variety, etc.). Goal setting, which requires a joint effort between supervisors and employees, is encouraged only when employees are assumed to seek responsibility on the job and fulfill obligations towards others.

The impact of the socio-cultural environment variables on managerial practices was less and weaker but in the expected direction. Loyalty towards community emerged as a strong predictor for lack of feedback, autonomy, and skill variety. It seemed that all these motivating behaviors were distracted by managers' loyalty towards the community and related status considerations. Uncertainty avoidance discouraged managers to get actively involved in goal setting. Paternalism had a negative impact on performance-extrinsic reward contingency probably because it may be directly associated with patronage rather than instant exchange of benefits. Taken as a whole, managerial practices were found to be influenced both by the internal work culture as well as the socio-cultural environment, the former having stronger impact than the latter.

Table 3. Socio-Cultural Values as Predictors of Work Culture

Predictor variables	β	t	R^2	F
Crit: Int. locus of control			.12	7.78**
Community loyalty	-.23	-2.33		
Power distance	-.20	-2.05		
Crit: Malleability			.07	8.18**
Community loyalty	-.26	-2.86		
Crit: Proact. orientation			.31	16.65**
Power distance	-.29	-3.44		
Paternalism	-.30	-3.57		
Uncertainty avoidance	-.17	-2.10		
Crit: React. orientation			.13	8.51**
Paternalism	.21	2.14		
Community loyalty	.20	2.05		
Crit: Obl. tow. others			.43	16.22**
Paternalism	.25	3.00		
Masculinity	-.25	-3.37		
Uncertainty avoidance	.22	2.97		
Self-reliance	.22	3.04		
Community loyalty	.22	2.63		
Crit: Part. orientation			.06	7.09**
Masculinity	-.24	-2.66		

Note. Only significant β weights are reported; **$p < .01$.
Crit = Criterion.

STUDY 3
Work Cultures in Indian Organizations:
A Comparison Between Public and Private Sector

In a study previously reported by Mathur et al. (1996), Indian public and private sector organizations were compared to test within a single socio-cultural environment the influence of enterprise environment on work culture and HRM practices. A total of 493 managers and employees from public and private sector organizations in India served as respondents to the same questionnaire used in the previous studies.

As members of the same social milieu, managers in both public and private sector organizations were in agreement with respect to their perceptions of the external socio-cultural environment, but this similarity was not observed in their beliefs and assumptions about their employees and their HRM practices. Private enterprises were characterized by an

Table 4. Social and Work Culture as Predictors of HRM Practices

Predictor variables	β	t	R^2	F
Crit: Feedback			.17	10.92**
Malleability	.32	3.54		
Community Loyalty	-.20	-2.23		
Crit: Autonomy			.31	11.38**
Proact. orientation	.44	4.64		
Community loyalty	-.30	-3.53		
Uncertainty avoidance	.24	2.68		
Masculinity	.18	2.13		
Crit: Skill variety			.14	8.64**
React. orientation	-.24	-2.57		
Community loyalty	-.22	-2.35		
Crit: Task signif.			.07	8.44**
Int. locus of control	.27	2.90		
Crit: Goal setting			.26	9.40**
Responsib. seeking	.33	3.99		
React. orientation	.26	2.99		
Obl. tow. others	.27	2.99		
Uncertainty avoidance	-.22	-2.44		
Crit: Empowerment			.11	6.43**
Int. locus of control	.22	2.45		
Futuristic orientation	.22	2.41		
Crit: Self-control			.05	5.37**
Futuristic orientation	.22	2.32		
Crit: Laisez-a-faire			.04	5.06*
Malleability	.21	2.45		
Crit: Perf. Ext. R-Cont.			.13	8.16**
Malleability	.25	2.74		
Paternalism	-.20	-2.19		

Note. Only sigificant β weights are reported; **p < .01. Crit = Criterion. See Table 1 for an explanation of the abbreviations.

emphasis on internal locus of control, futuristic orientation in planning, participation in decision making, and obligation toward others in the work context. These characteristics were observed to a much lesser extent in the public sector organizations. Similarly, in almost all areas of HRM practices including feedback, autonomy, task significance, empowerment, control, and performance-intrinsic reward contingency, differences were observed between public and private sector organizations in that the former was less effective in making employees more productive.

Observed differences in managerial assumptions and HRM practices between the public and private sectors, despite socio-cultural similarities, suggested that enterprise variables play an important role in determining what is expected from individuals in organizations. For example, in the private sector, companies are compelled to make long-term plans in order to survive in a competitive market environment. Similarly, the private sector work culture is less bureaucratic and less formal. It provides greater autonomy which, in turn, reinforces the belief that events are controllable by individuals and that people should be encouraged to participate in the decision-making process. Being less formal, such a culture also promotes meeting interpersonal obligations and provides mutual help at the workplace. In sum, this study demonstrated that within the same socio-cultural environment, work cultures and HRM practices may differ among organizations due to differing characteristics of the enterprise environment (Figure 1).

Conclusions and Implications

The three studies reported in this paper provided preliminary support for different aspects of the Model of Culture Fit. The first and the second study examined the connection between socio-cultural environment and managerial assumptions, while the third study explored the connection between the enterprise environment and organizational culture. Paternalism, power distance, uncertainty avoidance and community loyalty were the most salient cultural dimensions that differentiated respondents from India from those in North America. These cultural dimensions seem to form a cluster and predict a certain type of organizational culture. In a country high on these cultural dimensions, such as India, managers assume that employees, by nature, do not have control over the outcomes of their actions, their nature cannot be changed through training, they take a reactive rather than a proactive stance toward their job objectives, and their responsibilities towards others in the workplace are as important as their job performance. Such managerial assumptions result in less enriched jobs, and inappropriate supervision and rewards. A similar type of organizational culture and of HRM practices are observed in public sector organizations. Compared to the private sector, managers in the public sector discourage employee initiative-taking and participation. In public sector organizations, the job design and supervision practices make employees less productive compared to the private sector. Taken together, these results suggest that both socio-cultural and enterprise environments influence managerial assumptions that shape the organizational culture and resulting HRM practices.

There are a number of research and practical implications that can be drawn from these results. First, future cross-cultural research on work culture and HRM practices should be designed in such a way that various enterprise variables (e.g., organizational goal orientation, public versus private sector, type of industry, and market competitiveness) are controlled. Secondly, paternalism, which emerged as a salient cultural dimension for all three countries should be further examined. Paternalism is a unique construct that defines a specific relationship between the superior and the subordinate. The paternalistic authority figure provides care, guidance and protection for subordinates in exchange for their respect, loyalty and deference. As such, the 'respect to authority' component in paternalism is very different from that in authoritarianism. In the literature, paternalism has been portrayed as an aspect of authoritarianism. However, in our view, this is a misrepresentation. Paternalism, as a cultural dimension, has significant implications for organizations, and, this under-researched construct merits further attention in future studies.

Thirdly, findings reported in this paper suggest that self-reliance may have meaning other than its commonly assumed manifestation of individualism. Indian participants scored higher on self-reliance compared to North American respondents. This finding may imply that in collectivist countries where there is scarcity of resources individuals value self-reliance in order not to burden others with their demands. This potentially important finding requires replication in both collectivistic and individualistic cultures. Finally, various orthogonal cultural dimensions such as paternalism, power distance, loyalty towards community and uncertainty avoidance seemed to form a cluster in each of the three countries. Similar configurations of cultural dimensions as well as an overarching cultural construct could provide a parsimonious framework for future cross-cultural research.

Results reported in this paper have significant implications for global managers of multinational companies. Expatriate managers who are assigned for overseas posts often experience difficulties in adjusting to the new work environment in the host country. The difficulty mainly stems from a lack of understanding of the impact of culture on management assumptions and practices. Consequently, both the parent company and/or the expatriate try to impose 'Western' managerial assumptions and practices on the local workforce. The resultant mismatch poses a serious barrier to creating synergy, especially when the host unit is not receptive to such influence from the parent company (see Aycan, 1997, for a discussion on conflicting attitudes among the parent company, the local unit and the expatriate manager). For instance, in countries where there is high paternalism, employees expect clear guidance from their supervisors. Administering Western job enrichment techniques which emphasize individual autonomy and responsibility may yield unwanted results. Therefore, it is imperative for multinational companies to provide culture-specific training to their managers, so that employee expectations in the local unit could be better appreciated and met. Similarly, managing diverse workforces in US- or European-based companies requires an understanding of employees' cultural and ethnic backgrounds, so that successful HRM practices could be tailored and implemented according to employee needs.

References

Aycan, Z. (1997). Acculturation of expatriate managers: A process model of adjustment and performance. In Z. Aycan (Ed.), *Expatriate management: Theory and research, Vol. 4 of New Approaches to Employee Management Series* (pp. 1-41). Connecticut: JAI Press.

Chen, C. C., Meindl, J. R., & Hunt, R. B. (1997). Testing the effects of vertical and horizontal collectivism: A study of reward allocation preferences in China. *Journal of Cross-Cultural Psychology, 28,* 44-70.

Hofstede, G. (1980). *Culture's consequences: International differences in work-related values.* Beverly Hills, CA: Sage.

Kanungo, R. N., & Jaeger, A. M. (1990). Introduction: The need for indigenous management in developing countries. In A. M. Jaeger & R. N. Kanungo (Eds.), *Management in developing countries* (pp. 1-23). London: Routledge.

Kanungo, R. N., & Aycan, Z. (1996, August). *Role of socio-cultural environment in shaping work culture and HRM practices.* Paper presented at the 26th International Congress of Psychology, Montreal, Canada.

Kanungo, R. N., & Sinha, J. B. P. (1996, August). *Cultural values, work culture, and managerial practices: A test of Culture Fit Model.* Paper presented at the 12th Congress of International Association for Cross-Cultural Psychology, Montreal, Canada.

Keppel, G. (1991). *Design and analysis: A researcher's handbook.* Englewood Cliffs, New Jersey: Prentice Hall.

Kim, U., Triandis, H. C., Kagitcibasi, C., Choi, S., & Yoon, G. (Eds.) (1994). *Individualism and collectivism: Theory, method, and applications.* London: Sage Publications.

Mathur, P., Aycan, Z., & Kanungo, R. N. (1996). Indian organizational culture: A comparison between public and private sector. *Psychology and Developing Societies, 8,* 199-223.

Schein, E. H. (1992). *Organizational culture and leadership* (2nd ed.). San Francisco, CA: Jossey-Bass.

Triandis, H. C. (1982). Review of culture's consequences: International differences in work-related values. *Human Organization, 41,* 86-90.

Triandis, H. C. (1994). *Culture and social behaviour.* New York: McGraw-Hill.

Trompenaars, F. (1993). *Riding the waves of culture.* London: The Economist Books.

The Structure of Upward and Downward Tactics of Influence in Chinese Organizations

Haifa Sun and Michael Harris Bond
Chinese University of Hong Kong

ABSTRACT

This research established a structure for influence tactics used in Chinese organizations. A combined influence tactics inventory which included 25 items originating from the Chinese culture and 33 items originating from the American culture (Kipnis & Schmidt, 1982) was completed by 218 Chinese managers. Subjects were asked to indicate the frequency with which they used each tactic to deal with superiors or subordinates. After refining the inventory, researchers obtained an Influence Tactics Profile (ITP) of 34 items with 23 items from Kipnis and Schmidt and 11 from Chinese informants. The ITP was found to have two factors, labeled Contingent Control (CC) and Gentle Persuasion (GP), with high congruence across influence directions. Cluster analyses yielded 4-6 clusters within each factor, with most applicable across both upward and downward influence attempts. A few clusters were found to be distinctive depending on the influence direction. The rational basis and empirical evidence for the two-dimensional structure were discussed with respect to relevant findings from other research.

Fundamental in influence research is the empirical work of Kipnis, Schmidt and Wilkinson (1980). Kipnis et al. (1980) reduced 370 influence tactics, which were collected by interview from lower-level managers, into a 58-item questionnaire. They then asked respondents to describe on a 5-point scale how frequently during the past six months they had used each item to influence their bosses, co-workers, or subordinates at work. Factor analyses for the combined data yielded six interpretable factors: Assertiveness, Ingratiation, Rationality, Sanctions, Exchange of Benefits and Upward Appeal. When sub-samples were factor analyzed, four factors (Assertiveness, Ingratiation, Rationality and Sanctions) emerged as dimensions for all three influence directions. However, two factors (Exchange of Benefits and Upward Appeal) did not emerge in the factor analysis of influence tactics directed toward subordinates. Furthermore, Blocking and Coalition, did not emerge from the combined data, but the former appeared in upward influence and the latter in downward influence.

In accord with these analyses, Kipnis and Schmidt (1982) constructed the Profile of Organizational Influence Strategies (POIS), to be used across influence directions. The POIS consists of 33 influence tactics grouped into the following seven influence strategies: Assertiveness, Friendliness (Ingratiation), Reason (Rational Persuasion), Bargaining (Exchange of Benefits), Sanctions, High Authority (Upward Appeal) and Coalition.

The POIS has been the instrument of choice for studying the variables related to influence tactics. These studies have revealed that the frequency with which each influence dimension was used related to the status of the interactants (the influencer or the target), to the reasons for exercising influence, to the resistance offered by the target person, to some organizational context variables (Kipnis et al., 1980), and to the goals sought from superiors (Schmidt & Kipnis, 1984). Four broad styles of upward influence (Shotgun, Tactician, Ingratiation, and Bystander) were identified by using the POIS to evaluate managers (Kipnis & Schmidt, 1988). Employing another instrument based on the POIS, Yukl and his colleagues (Falbe & Yukl, 1992; Yukl & Tracey, 1992; Yukl, Falbe & Youn, 1993) studied the sequences and consequences of using various tactics. Schermerhorn and Bond (1991), using American and Hong Kong respondents, found differences across culture and direction of influence attempt on type of influence used. Although accepted as a valid measure, the POIS has some limitations in its measurement structure and its cross cultural generality is yet to be determined.

Some research has touched on both problems. Schmidt and Yeh (1992) used the POIS to examine the structure of leader influence among Australian, English, Japanese and Taiwanese managers. In spite of their claim that certain influence strategies were found across countries, they conceded that the specific tactics defining these influence strategies were not uniform across cultures. By checking factor loadings of the POIS items by nationality, the total number of items from the same dimensions in the POIS to the number of items from other dimensions is 15 to 10 for the Australian sample, 24 to 12 for the Taiwanese sample and 21 to 16 for the Japanese sample. Therefore, it is doubtful that the content of each dimension is equivalent across cultures. It is especially doubtful that the structure of the POIS has as many as seven independent dimensions. Schmidt and Yeh (1992) concluded both the Taiwanese and Japanese influence structures reflect the association of "hard" (assertiveness) and "soft" (reason) tactics, and suggested a fruitful avenue for future research would be to generate indigenous influence items.

Another study (Schriesheim & Hinkin, 1990), employed content and confirmatory factor analyses for the 27 items from the factors of Ingratiation, Exchange, Rationality, Assertiveness, Upward Appeal, and Coalition of the POIS. Content analyses identified six of the Kipnis et al. (1980) items that appeared weak and could perhaps be deleted, and the confirmatory factor analysis revealed that only the items of Rationality and Coalition loaded as predicted, whereas a considerable number of items from the four other sub-scales cross-loaded on two or more factors.

By contrast, some studies might seem to provide support to the factor structure established for the POIS (Yukl & Falbe, 1990). After reviewing this research (Schmidt & Yeh, 1992; Schriesheim & Hinkin, 1990; Yukl & Falbe, 1990), we concluded that the structural problems of the measure of influence tactics, namely, the incongruence across influence directions and their non-orthogonality, may be due to the use of liberal criteria in deciding the number of factors to extract from the POIS. We predicted that fewer factors would be extracted by using scree plots (Cattell, 1966) in deciding the number of factors. The factor structure could also be purified by deleting cross-loading items. We expect that these fewer and purer factors would have a better chance to be congruent across influence directions. Additionally, the problem of imposing the POIS as an etic can be solved by adding items derived from the Chinese culture to the POIS. The main objective of this research is to consider both the Western and Chinese cultures and to develop from these inputs an influence tactics inventory for use in Chinese organizations.

Method

Item Development
To identify the tactics used by Chinese managers to effect upward and downward influence at work, we interviewed a dozen Chinese scholars from the People's Republic of China who were studying in Hong Kong. Most of these scholars had managerial experience. Following an explanation of the POIS, we asked them to provide additional influence tactics from their own experience. From about 50 items, elicited in this way, 25 items were selected to be merged with the 33 items in the POIS, to construct an influence tactics questionnaire of 58 items.

Versions of the questionnaire were produced for upward and downward influence. Each version was prefaced by appropriate instructions. For upward influence, respondents were told that the items were to describe the tactics employed to influence a superior with whom they had difficulty dealing. For downward influence the questionnaire items and instructions replaced the word "subordinate" with the word "superior" in the instructions and items. Respondents were asked to use their experience at work to make a choice based on their real actions, not according to what others expect or what they felt they should do. There were seven response choices, ranging from always to never used.

We required the respondents to select a target with whom they had difficulty dealing in order to include as many tactics as possible in the final instrument. Yukl and Falbe (1990) had excluded the factor Sanction when they used the POIS as an instrument for research because they considered that the tactics involved in sanction had too low an endorsement rate. We expected that the endorsement rate of the tactics included in Sanction and possibility other types of tactics would be increased when the respondents dealt with "difficult" targets.

Respondents

The respondents were full-time employees who were attending a part-time management training workshop at two universities in Guangzhou. Respondents ($N = 219$) completed the questionnaire anonymously during class time. Fifty percent of the sample were between 20 to 29 years of age; 29% between 30 to 39, and another 14% between 40 to 49. The sample consisted of 135 supervisory staff, 49 middle class managers, and 9 upper class managers; 162 respondents had graduated from college, and 44 from senior high school. Males made up 60%, and females 32% with 8% failing to indicate their gender. Because a few respondents missed some answers, the percentages for some demographic categories were below 100.

Results

The Refinement of the Questionnaire

After collecting the data, interviews with some managers led to the deletion of eleven items that were considered to overlap in content or to not exactly reflect influence tactics in meaning. The remaining 47 items were factor analyzed using a principal components factor solution, followed by varimax rotation. Two-factor solutions were obtained for upward and downward influence according to their scree plots. Nine items with factor loadings under .30 on both factors were eliminated. The remaining 39 items were factor analyzed. Using the criterion that the secondary loading must be less than .35, five double loading items were deleted. This final version of the questionnaire of 34 items was named the Influence Tactics Profile (ITP).

Factor Structure

These 34 items were factor analyzed again, using a principal components factor solution with varimax rotation. According to the scree plots, two orthogonal factors were obtained. The two factors for upward influence accounted for 40.8% of the total item variance, while the two factors for downward influence accounted for 30%.

Table 1 lists the 34 items and their loadings on each of the two factors for both upward and downward influence. Nineteen items loaded on Factor 1 for both upward and downward influence. Seventeen of these items within Factor 1 came from Kipnis and Schmidt's POIS. These seventeen items were from factors such as Sanction, High Authority, Bargain, Coalition, and Assertive. Two items, "isolating the target" and "using organizational authority" originated from the Chinese culture. Most of the items in Factor 1 were characterized by the semantic format: "If you don't do X, I will punish you; if you comply, I will reward you." This factor was labeled Contingent Control (CC).

Fifteen items loaded on Factor 2. Six came from the factors Reason and Friendliness of the POIS. Nine items originated from the Chinese culture. The tactics in Factor 2 included items such as "acting humbly to make a request of the target", and "praising target behind target's back". All tactics involved making direct or indirect requests without associated promises or threats. Factor 2 was thus labeled Gentle Persuasion (GP).

Having obtained two-orthogonal-factor structures for upward and downward influence, a targeted or Procrustes rotation was carried out to check the congruence of factor structures between upward and downward influence (McCrae, Zonderman, Costa, Bond & Paunonen, 1996). The congruence coefficient was 0.97 (for CC) and 0.96 (for GP), thus supporting the congruence of factor structures between upward and downward influence.

Clusters

Hierarchical cluster analyses were performed within each factor separately. The complete linkage cluster method with Pearson correlations as the measure were adopted. The results for cluster analyses are presented in Tables 2 and 3.

Table 2 shows clusters within CC for upward and downward influence. For downward influence, five multi-item clusters (Contingent Punishment, Exchange of Benefits, Assertion, Organizational Authority, and Collegial Support) emerged and corresponded to the five factors (Sanction, Bargain, Assertive, High Authority, and Coalition) of the POIS. The items in each cluster came from the corresponding factor of the POIS, except for two items: "obtaining the support from superior" in the cluster Collegial Support came from the factor High Authority and "mentioning my help to target in the past" in Contingent Punishment came from the factor, Bargaining. The tactic "scolding the target" formed a single item cluster. From the items representing the Chinese culture, "isolating the target" went into the cluster Contingent Punish-

Table 1. Factor Loadings of the Influence Tactics in Contingent Control (CC) and Gentle Persuasion (GP) for Upward (up) and Downward (down) Influence

Influence tactics	Loading (up)			Loading (down)	
	CC	GP	CP	CC	CP
Giving target unsatisfactory appraisal	.81			.68	
Dismissing target	.79			.71	
@ Isolating target	.78			.63	
Not promoting target	.76			.71	
Setting work deadline	.75			.34	
Not raising target's salary	.66			.65	
Sending the case concerning target to superior	.67			.58	
Appealing to superior to deal with target	.63			.62	
Obtaining support from superior to request target	.68			.53	
Reporting the case concerning target to superior	.60			.72	
Providing job benefits to target	.61			.52	
Reminding target of my help to him in the past	.63			.68	
Scolding target	.60			.34	
Agreeing to target's request	.60			.47	
Obtaining support from peer	.55	.32		.46	
Specifying the thing for target's doing	.56			.35	
Using regulations of company	.56			.29	
@ Using organizational force	.49			.40	
Obtaining support from subordinate	.35			.32	

Table 1. (continued)

Influence tactics	Loading (up)		Loading (down)	
	CC	GP	CC	CP
Praising target to make him feel important		.58		.45
@ Knowing more information than target		.54		.54
@ Showing face-consideration		.51		.38
@ Working overtime		.60		.36
@ Demonstrating working skills		.66		.56
Requesting target with reason		.47		.51
Apologizing to target for requesting		.59		.48
Requesting with facts		.61		.49
@ Putting collective benefits first		.59		.38
@ Telling the target you value mutual relationship		.67		.56
Behaving friendly		.62		.60
Requesting target humbly		.67		.64
@ Behaving seriously before target		.56		.41
@ Praising target behind his back		.53		.51
@ Treating target fairly		.46		.47

Note. Only loadings > .30 are presented. Items with @ were indigenous Chinese tactics. Items without any marking were from the POIS.

Table 2. Clusters within Contingent Control for Upward and Downward Influence

Clusters	Upward Influence	Downward Influence
	Items within each cluster	
Contingent Punishment	*unsatisfactory appraisal *dismissing the target *not promoting the target *not raising target's salary scolding the target setting task deadline	*not promoting the target *dismissing the target remind him of my past help @isolating the target *not raising the target's salary *unsatisfactory appraisal
Exchange Benefits	*agree to his other request remind him of my past help support from superior @isolating the target *providing job benefits	*agree to his other request *providing job benefits
Organizational Authority	*appealing to superior *reporting to superior *sending target to superior *@using organizational force	*appealing to superior *sending target to superior *reporting to superior *@using organizational force
Assertion	*using company's regulation support from peer *specifying the request	*specifying the request setting task deadline *using company's regulation
Direct Superior's Support	direct superior's support	
Collegial Support		support from superior support from peer support from subordinate
Scolding		scolding the target

Note. * common items across influence directions; @ indigenous items.

Table 3. Clusters within Gentle Persuasion for Upward and Downward Influence

Clusters	Upward Influence	Downward Influence
	Items within each cluster	
Rational Persuasion	*requesting with facts *requesting target friendly *requesting with reason	*requesting target friendly *requesting with facts @knowing more information *requesting with reason apologizing for making request
Ideological Modeling	@valuing mutual relationship *@putting collective first @knowing more information *@behaving seriously	*@putting collective first *@behaving seriously
Feeling Management	*@showing face-consideration @praising target behind back *@treating target fairly	requesting target humbly @valuing mutual relationship *@treating target fairly *@showing face-consideration
Exemplification	*@working overtime *@demonstrating work skills *making target feel important requesting target humbly apologizing for making request	*@working overtime *@demonstrating work skills *making target feel important @praising target behind back

Note. * common items across influence directions; @ indigenous items.

ment and "using organizational force" into the cluster, Organizational Authority.

Within the factor CC for upward influence, four clusters emerged corresponding to the clusters Contingent Punishment, Exchange of Benefits, Organizational Authority, and Assertion for downward influence. The cluster Collegial Support in downward influence did not emerge in upward influence; two of the three items from Collegial Support in downward influence were distributed among the other clusters. The item "obtaining direct superior's support" formed a single-item cluster (Direct Superior's Support).

Table 3 presents the four clusters within GP for downward influence and the four clusters for upward influence. All three items in the Reason factor of the POIS went into cluster 1. The other two items in cluster 1, "apologizing to target" was from the Friendliness factor in the POIS, and "controlling more political, economic, and social information" was from the Chinese culture. Although this cluster could be said to correspond to the Reason factor from the POIS, it was gentler with the addition of the two extra tactics, and was named Rational Persuasion.

Cluster 2 named Ideological Modeling, involved the Chinese cultural tactics of "putting collective benefits first" and "dressing neatly and behaving seriously." Cluster 3, labeled Feeling Management, was characterized by feeling and impression manipulation. The tactic "requesting target in a humble and polite way" came from the Friendliness factor in the POIS and the other three items were from the Chinese culture. Tactics in Cluster 4, labeled Exemplification, focused on capability and the virtue of diligence. Among the three Chinese tactics, "working overtime", "showing diligence", and "grasping much working knowledge and skills" focused on capability, and "praising target behind target's back" also mainly related to capability. These three Chinese culture items merged with the item "informing target about his or her having capability and feeling important" which was from the factor Friendliness in the POIS.

The left hand side of Table 3 shows clusters within the factor GP for upward influence. These four clusters corresponded to the four clusters for downward influence. However, the cluster Exemplification included items "requesting target in a humble and polite way" and "requesting target with sympathy and apologies". These items made exemplifying towards the superior more indirect and milder than exemplifying towards the subordinate.

The tactics asterisked in both tables indicate tactics common between corresponding clusters across downward and upward influence directions. The extent of congruence can be seen from the ratio of tactics that are shared by corresponding clusters across influence directions. Although the clusters for upward and downward influence were basically congruent within factor CC, the single-item cluster Scolding and the cluster Collegial Support for downward influence, and the single-item cluster Direct Superior's Support for upward influence did not have corresponding clusters across different influence directions.

Discussion

The results of the factor analysis for the ITP provide a two-factor orthogonal structure. The first factor, Contingent Control, is mainly task-oriented. It reflects how managers get compliance from targets by using tactics such as contingent punishment, exchange of benefits, collegial support and assertiveness. The second factor, Gentle Persuasion, reflects tactics which give more consideration to the target's inner states and the relationship of the influencer with the target.

Similar two-dimensional structures can be found in other research on social behavior. Bond and Forgas (1984) established a two-factor structure for the behavior intentions of both Chinese and Australians. They labeled the first factor trust. The second factor in their study was named association. We believe that the factor, trust, in their research corresponds to GP, and the other factor, association, corresponds to CC.

Two similar structures of interpersonal behavior also relate to the present findings. Wiggins (1979) developed a two-dimension circumplex of interpersonal variables. The first component of the circumplex was Ambitious-Dominant against Lazy-Submissive and the second was Warm-Agreeable against Aloof-Introverted. Later, these two dimensions were referred to as Dominance and Nurturance (Wiggins & Pincus, 1989). In the management area, Smith, Misumi, Tayeb, Peterson and Bond (1989) found the generality of a two dimensional leadership style, P (Performance) and M (Maintenance) across four different cultures. We believe that Dominance and Performance correspond to CC, while Nurturance and Maintenance correspond to GP.

The two-factor structure is not only parsimonious in conceptualization but also shows congruence across upward and downward influence directions. Additionally, we have successfully identified clusters derived from the Chinese culture such as Ideological Modeling and Feeling Management. The Ideological Modeling cluster consisted of items such as "putting collective benefits first" and "dressing neatly and behaving seriously". The Feeling Management cluster consisted of items such as "showing face-consideration" and "treating target fairly". These four items were employed across downward and upward influence by Chinese informants. These items reflect relationship orientation and authority concern (Yang, 1994) and involve behavioral strategies important in the Chinese collective culture.

The clusters in the current study corresponded somewhat to the factors of the POIS. However, the clusters within each factor were more likely to correlate with each other than with the factors CC and GP. Such correspondence provides indirect evidence that the factors in the POIS are not independent. The generality of the clusters is lower than the factors in the current study, the items of some clusters are not correspondent across influence directions. Items "obtaining support from subordinate", "obtaining support from peer" and "obtaining support from superior" form a cluster in downward influence. But, these items distribute themselves into other clusters in upward influence. A few items were not shared by the clusters with the same label and their belonging to clusters depends on the influence direction. For example, "praising the target behind target's back" was found in the cluster Exemplification in downward influence, but found in the cluster Feeling Management in upward influence. In the Chinese culture, praising a subordinate is the role of the superior, whereas for a subordinate to praise a superior is a tactic of feeling or impression management.

The theories, concepts and measures of Western psychology could be enlarged by incorporating various cultural heritages (Bond & Pang, 1991). By including indigenous measures, we may determine empirically the degree of overlap and uniqueness among the various cultural inputs, and thereby reach a less culturally-bound psychology. In this sense the present research has taken a first step toward creating the theories and instruments of influence reflecting the Chinese as well as the Western culture. The two-orthogonal-factor structure of the ITP is only preliminary and needs to be confirmed by further empirical studies. Furthermore, it is necessary to test the stability and comprehensiveness of clusters involving items from the Chinese culture.

References

Bond, M. H., & Pang, M. K. (1991). Trusting to the *Tao*: Chinese values and the re-centering of psychology. *Bulletin of the Hong Kong Psychological Society, 26/27*, 5-27.

Bond, M. H., & Forgas, J. P. (1984). Linking person perception to behavior intention across cultures: The role of cultural collectivism. *Journal of Cross-Cultural Psychology, 15*, 337-352.

Cattell, R. B. (1966). The meaning and strategic use of factor analysis. In R. B. Cattell (Ed.), *Handbook of Multivariate Experimental Psychology* (pp. 174-243). Chicago: Rand McNally.

Cattell, R. B., & Jaspers, J. A. (1967). A general plasmode for factor analytic exercises and research. *Multivariate Behavioral Research Monographs*.

Falbe, C. M., & Yukl, G. (1992). Consequences for managers of using single influence tactics and combinations of tactics. *Academy of Management Journal, 35*, 638-652.

Kipnis, D., & Schmidt, S. M. (1980). Intraorganizational influence tactics: Explorations in getting one's way. *Journal of Applied Psychology, 65*, 440-452.

Kipnis, D., & Schmidt, S. M. (1988). *Profiles of organizational influence strategies*. San Diego, CA: University Associates.

Kipnis, D., & Schmidt, S. M. (1988). Upward-influence styles: Relationship with performance evaluations, salary, and stress. *Administrative Science Quarterly, 33*, 528-542.

McCrae, R. R., Zonderman, A. B., Costa, P. T. Jr., Bond, M. H., & Paunonen, S. V. (1996). Evaluating replicability of factors in the revised NEO Personality Inventory: Confirmatory factor analysis versus procrustes rotation. *Journal of Personality and Social Psychology, 70*, 552-566.

Schermerhorn, J. R., & Bond, M. H. (1991). Upward and downward influence tactics in managerial networks: A comparative study of Hong Kong Chinese and Americans. *Asia Pacific Journal of Management, 8*, 147-158.

Schmidt, S. M., & Kipnis, D. (1984). Managers' pursuit of individual and organizational goals. *Human Relations, 37*, 781-794.

Schmidt, S. M., & Yeh, R. S. (1992). The structure of leader influence: a cross-national comparison. *Journal of Cross-Cultural Psychology, 23*, 251-264.

Smith, P. B., Misumi, J., Tayeb, M., Peterson, M., & Bond, M. H. (1989). On the generality of leadership style measures across cultures. *Journal of Occupational Psychology, 62*, 97-109.

Schriesheim, C. A., & Hinkin, T. R. (1990). Influence tactics used by subordinates: A theoretical and empirical analysis and refinement of the Kipnis, Schmidt, and Wilkinson sub-scales. *Journal of Applied Psychology, 75*, 246-257.

Wiggins, S. (1979). A psychological taxonomy of trait-description terms: The interpersonal domain. *Journal of Personality and Social Psychology, 37*, 395-412.

Wiggins, J. S., & Pincus, A. L. (1989). Conceptions of personality disorders and dimensions of personality. *Psychological Assessment: A Journal of Consulting and Clinical Psychology, 1*, 305-316.

Yukl, G., & Falbe, C. M. (1990). Influence tactics objective in upward, downward, and lateral influence attempts. *Journal of Applied Psychology, 75*, 132-140.

Yukl, G., Falbe, C. M., & Youn, Y. Y. (1993). Patterns of influence behavior for managers. *Group & Organization Management, 18*, 5-28.

Yukl, G., & Tracey, J. B. (1992). Consequences of influence tactics used with subordinates, peers, and the boss. *Journal of Applied Psychology, 77*, 525-535.

Yang, K. S. (1996). The psychological transformation of the Chinese people as a result of societal modernization. In M. H. Bond (Ed.), *The handbook of Chinese psychology* (pp. 479-498). Hong Kong: Oxford University Press.

Educational / Developmental Psychology

Cross-cultural Challenges to the Development of a Culture-Sensitive Pedagogy within an Emerging 'Global Culture'

Elwyn Thomas
University of London, UK

ABSTRACT

A culture sensitive pedagogy actively reflects the culture specific knowledge, behavior, attitudes, and skills to complement the basic learning requirements common to all schooling. To develop a pedagogy that is richer and more relevant in content and style to both teachers and learners requires a thorough analysis of the cultural context and a selection of those ideas and practices unique to the culture to enrich curriculum planning At the same time there is a strong emerging 'global' culture that cannot be ignored. Fueled by the Internet, computers in the classroom, English as the dominant language, and universal standards for teacher training, it is creating demands for a form of teaching that accommodates both global ideas and contextual needs. It is concluded that an emic-etic balance is the challenge for the culture sensitive pedagogy that meets the demands of an emerging global culture.

Cross-cultural studies of behaviour are becoming more salient as potential contributors to the policy and practice of education. This higher profile of cross-cultural research, is also occurring at the same time educators and other professionals face challenges posed by increasing globalization. This paper focuses on developing a culture sensitive pedagogy that attempts to balance the demands for educational change felt by learners and teachers. A culture sensitive pedagogy should be of interest to all those who are concerned with improving communication between teachers and learners throughout the world. In view of the fact that cross-cultural pedagogy is relatively new, the approach in this paper will be exploratory rather than prescriptive. Considerable research is needed before a substantive and workable paradigm can be accepted for a culture sensitive pedagogy. This paper is just the start of this process.

Cross-Cultural Pedagogy: A Neglected Area

It is well documented that whatever their origins, students are potentially capable of achieving most learning objectives. However, what is not so well documented is the learners' approach to the learning task. For instance, information about the styles, methods, and idiosyncrasies learners employ to solve problems can tell us more about the context of learning and teaching than just knowing the learner has been successful in getting the correct answer. Even less well documented, is the content and specific approaches to learning content that need to be considered as essential components of a pedagogy that addresses cultural needs, and how teachers should be trained to implement such a pedagogy effectively. Cross-cultural and educational research carried out mostly in developing countries has shown how meaningful and effective a culturally-rooted pedagogy can be (Aikman, 1994; Nunes, 1994; Teesdale & Teesdale, 1994).

Research that identifies different cultural pedagogies, and describes the impact they may have on improving educational quality, will be a welcome antidote to a possible global standardisation. By building on this research, it should be possible to provide a meaningful and interesting pedagogy, that bridges the new with existing knowledge and skills.

A Pedagogical Model and Influencing Factors

The origins of the concept of pedagogy can be traced to the time of the Greeks. Many recent pedagogical ideas have come from psychologists such as Piaget (1971), Brunei (1966), Shulman (1986), and Gagne (1975). More recently the work of Schon (1983) and Zeichner (1983) have added insights into developments in pedagogy with particular reference to teacher education. Little has emerged in the way of workable theories of teaching. However, indicators from educational research point to the fact that pedagogy is no longer considered just an instructional process with broadly accepted methods of delivery and predictable learner-teacher interactions. Pedagogy is far more complex: The author's view of pedagogy is that there are four main components that interact with one another (see Figure 1).

The *epistemological component* refers to the knowledge base that all teachers need, and includes a philosophical framework as a guide to what and how subjects are taught (e.g., a child-centred or subject-centred approach). The second is the *process component* and includes activities such as planning, instructing, managing, evaluating, reflecting and prioritising linked with decision making in the classroom. The third component is *contextual* and includes the socio-cultural matrix of which language, religion, and cultural traditions provide a unique profile to the practice and development of pedagogy. The *personalistic component* refers to the part played by a teacher's self growth, motivation and commitment to improve teaching and learning.

There are six principal factors that affect in varying ways, and determine the form, style and success of each of the components of the pedagogical model. The *political* and the *economic factors* have the most

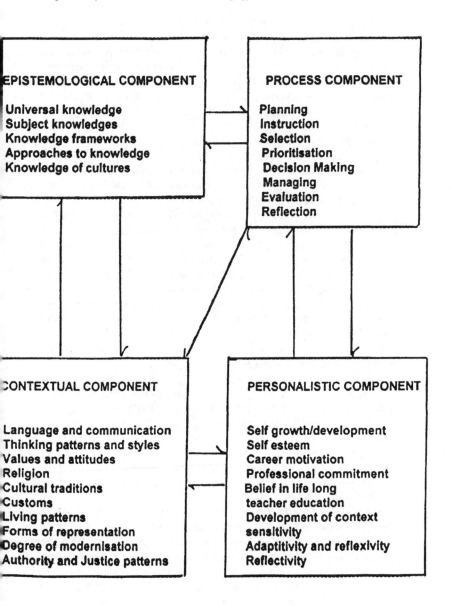

Figure 1. The Pedagogical Model and Its Influencing Factors

powerful effect on the development and even the existence of a particular pedagogy. Political factors are particularly important when it comes to selecting an educational philosophy or providing the appropriate climate for a teacher's personal development. Economic determinants become paramount when a pedagogy is perceived to be over teacher-resourced (which it rarely is), and whether the increased use of educational technology would make teaching more efficient and effective.

Societal factors can also be powerful in influencing pedagogy, often through the school curriculum. For instance, the world of work has a crucial stake in what is taught in school and increasingly how it is delivered. *Professionalism* and the need for *research and innovation* affect the epistemological and personalistic components of the pedagogical model. Professionalism activates both the process and personalistic component of teaching, while continuous updating from research into knowledge and skills about pedagogy contributes to the quality of education. Finally, *cultural factors* have an important role in the development of a meaningful and effective pedagogy. The drive by developing countries to modernise their educational systems and to look elsewhere (mainly to the West) has impoverished their own cultural base. However, it is increasingly evident that traditional ways of communication, existing values, and beliefs have a pivotal role for the future of society as well.

Pedagogy as a Set of Cultures
The act of teaching is increasingly being perceived as a culture or set of subcultures. It is interesting to note that in the third edition of the American Educational Research Association Handbook on Research on Teaching (Wittrock, 1986), attention was given to the culture of teaching. Since then, interest in the subject has intensified and there has been considerable research generated (Feiman-Nemser & Floden, 1986; Little, 1982; Metz, 1978; Zeichner & Tabachnik, 1983). The work of Schon (1983) on the concept of the reflective teacher has provided added interest to the subject.

Hargreaves' (1992) perspective is that teaching cultures might be better explained if we distinguished between the *content* of a culture of teaching and its *form*. According to Hargreaves (1992), the content includes knowledge, substantive attitudes and values, habits and ways of doing things. Form includes pervasive features: (a) *individualism*, which emphasizes the isolation of teachers in the classroom; (b) *balkanization*, in which teachers work in separate groups often in competition with one another; (c) *collaborative cultures*, which emphasise professionality between teachers, such as compatible initiatives to improve practice; and (d) *contrived collegiality*, binding teachers in time and space to meet certain demands by their superiors. Therefore, teaching is increasingly seen to be a set of universal features but sustaining a variety of sub-cultures that interrelate with each other. Teaching is also a contextual activity, which has the potential of being flexible and adaptable.

A Culture Sensitive Pedagogy

A culture sensitive pedagogy is one in which each of the four pedago-gical components discussed above are so structured and integrated with one another that they actively reflect culture specific knowledge, behaviours, attitudes, and skills. These culture-specific attributes should complement the basic learning requirements common to all schooling. An examination of the influencing factors, shows that all six factors would play their part in the development of a culture sensitive pedagogy. There is need for a thorough analysis of a particular culture, coupled with an enlightened approach to selecting those parts of the culture that would provide stability, alongside those elements of a curriculum that are necessary for meaningful schooling in the next millennium. What is advocated is pragmatism in the form of prerequisites that would enable educators to embark upon the development of teaching and learning strategies. There are two prerequisites that need to be considered when developing a culture sensitive pedagogy: a thorough *cultural analysis* and what may be called the process of *cultural selectivity*.

Cultural Analysis

A cultural analysis is an extensive examination of the cultural context of a community, small group, or individual. It is a process that requires rigorous research and study of the background influences and cultural history. A cultural analysis that involves school children would probe in depth what each pupil would bring to the classroom in terms of culture. It would also seek to find out as much as possible about cultural interactions between pupils during the school day (e.g., friendship patterns, rule-following in games and play). Cultural analysis should also seek to enrich curriculum planning, through the adaptation of ideas and practices specific to a particular cultural group, which would hopefully benefit both learner and teacher (Thomas, 1994). A cultural analysis aims to explore current and changing attitudes toward what is taught in school and where possible, attitudes of the home and community. The outcome of the analysis would hopefully result in the development of a pedagogy that is richer and more relevant in content and decisive in style. The pedagogy might also provide greater opportunities for schooling to be intimately involved in community development.

The outcome of a series of cultural analyses should provide much of the knowledge and experience for making each component of the model more culturally enriching and sensitive to the cultural needs of learners and teachers. The effect of employing such an analysis would be to reinforce the influence of the culture factor on the various pedagogical components.

Cultural Selectivity

The task of selecting appropriate data to be used in developing the knowledge and instructional base for a culture sensitive pedagogy will be formidable, especially in cultures that are rich, substantive and complex. Criteria for cultural selection would assist matters. The greatest challenges in the application of cross-cultural principles will be encountered at the stage of cultural selectivity. For instance, let us examine the case of developing a school curriculum. Certain essentials such as learning mathematics, and how to read and write are considered universal needs for all children. However, the way children engage in different learning styles and strategies to achieve success in reading, writing and mathematics are likely to be culture-specific. There is in effect an etic (cross-cultural), and an emic (intra-cultural) dimension to both the learning and teaching processes. The work of Nunes (1994) with Brazilian street children concerning mathematics shows these dimensions vividly. Nunes's sample of children were able to achieve considerable success in addition and subtraction using methods they themselves used on the streets in their business transactions. What is more remarkable is that these street children out-performed school pupils of the same age who used formal and traditional methods of solving mathematical operations taught in school.

Developing an Epistemological Base for a Culture-Sensitive Pedagogy

Every teacher is expected to have knowledge of the teaching subject or subjects (e.g., language, mathematics). An increasing emphasis on teacher professionalisation has resulted in the teacher's knowledge base being widened and deepened considerably. This is particularly evident when consulting the contents of teacher preparation programmes in different countries (e.g., Singapore and Malaysia). More teachers are now required to have studied educational courses such as educational psychology and philosophy, curriculum theory and practice as well as more subject content and general knowledge. This has meant for teachers in developing countries that indigenous knowledge about the society's cultural traditions and ways of thinking and processing of knowledge have been sacrificed to more universalistic prerogatives.

It has been shown that both the form and content of knowledge characteristic of certain cultures have an important place in the teaching of language, history, social studies, and mathematics. There are, however, three major problems with making epistemological components more culture relevant. The first problem is the need to know more about the nature and realms of knowledge that reflect a particular culture. The second relates to the inclusion of the appropriate knowledge in school and college curricula. The third problem and probably the most difficult, is to convince teachers, learners and parents that their culture really has special knowledge that is important to be learned.

For example, Thomas (1980) found that Nigerian Hausa primary school children explaining social and physical causality provided interesting responses. Their responses reflected how causes of family quarrels, marriage problems, and petty theft are resolved within the family. It took an effort for some of these findings to be included into the science and social studies curricula. Similarly, in much of Chinese culture the deep knowledge and experience gained over the centuries about respect for family and community through the enduring concept of filial piety, was absent from most school curricula in social studies in Malaysia and Singapore. It was only in the mid 1980s that Confucianism became part of values education in secondary schools for ethnic Chinese in Singapore. Family discussions about business ventures, profit making and profit sharing, the hierarchical nature of family decision making (mainly male dominated), and prioritising financial or religious targets contribute to the rich and fascinating epistemology of both Afro-cultures and Sino-cultures. In most cultures, there can be substantial indigenous knowledge relating to traditional science, health, and medicine, as well as a literature, and language. These 'indigenous' knowledges are often side-stepped by the growing need for knowledge and skill subsumed under the so called 'global culture'.

Exploring Culture-Specific Pedagogical Processes

The process component of pedagogy includes managing, decision making, instructing, teaching and learning styles, evaluation, planning, selection, and prioritisation. All these activities are characterised by features that are common across most cultures, but there are also culture-specific elements that need to be identified in the search for a culture sensitive pedagogy. For example, *teaching styles* can often be culture-specific. In teaching Chinese alphabetical characters, most teachers favour a strongly didactic approach. In fact, it is almost impossible to teach Chinese in any other way. It is also clear that the teacher's awareness of childrens' individual learning styles, usually neglected by teachers and curriculum planners, can play a valuable part in making instruction more sensitive and effective (Little, 1994; Nunes, 1994; Teesdale & Teesdale, 1994).

Recent research has shown the need to develop good *planning strategies* that are sensitive to everyday cognition. The work of Tanon (1994) in the Ivory Coast showed how informal planning of weaving tasks can transfer successfully to other school related tasks that require planning skills. Research focussing on the skill of carefully selecting those culture specific behaviours that are perceived to improve teaching and learning effectiveness, and those behaviours that do the opposite, would also be included. An example of positive sensitivity would be the work of Nunes (1994) using the methods of Brazilian street mathematics. Being sensitive to the more negative side of certain cultural influences is discussed in the work of Kean-Terry (1994). She has shown in Singapore how culture-specific teaching styles associated with rote learning of Mandarin, can transfer across to other subjects of the curriculum, probably having a negative effect on developing creative, original and analytical thinking generally.

Exploring Cultural Context as a Basis for a Culture-Sensitive Pedagogy

Knowing and being able to select the appropriate context is the key to the development of a culture sensitive pedagogy. The contextual component is likely to include knowledge about customs and traditions, use of local languages, modes of thinking, communication through drawing, different forms of social discourse, specific kinship agendas, and ways of judging group members. The role of spiritual and religious beliefs as part of a community's value system, and a school values education programme would be another crucial focus of this component. These are the contextual inputs into the pedagogical components model that would be part of a prototype for a culture-sensitive pedagogy.

There are several questions that need to be addressed when assessing the role a contextual component can play in developing a culture sensitive pedagogy. The first relates to the extent of knowledge about a particular context, and whether an adequate cultural analysis has been carried out. The second is what form of cultural selectivity has been applied? A third is who selects, is it the teacher or are those decisions made by policy makers and planners? The fourth issue relates to the question of acceptability. Parents and teachers, particularly in the emerging economies of the Pacific rim, might see it as unnecessary to include any culture-specific knowledge and skills into the school curriculum. In this case, parents may be concerned that extra content included in the school curriculum could detract from the pupils' academic achievements. In most instances, parents would hold the view that homes already provide a sufficient cultural and religious base for their children.

Let us consider some examples of how a particular use of context can be implemented in developing a more meaningful and sensitive pedagogy. In several parts of Central Africa, such as Zimbabwe and Malawi, it is quite common to see children construct the most intricate wire toys (Gilbert & Lovegrove, 1968). In the author's experience, most representations were of cars and trucks. Some of these wire toy cars were so true to the original that one could even recognise the make of car (e.g., the British Mini or the Japanese Toyota). Also, the steering and gear constructions were all in place and usually worked well. Here is a case of a context extremely rich in the deployment of motor skills, precise modelling techniques, and a clear understanding of the mechanics of the car. Unfortunately, teachers use a pedagogy which ignores this rich experience, using instead explanations exclusively from textbooks emphasising mainly Western examples.

Among the ethnically diverse school population of Malaysia, the author noted that little was selected by curriculum planners from a rich aesthetic and artistic cultural context which typifies the Chinese, Indian, and Malay ethnic groups. There is an extremely rich endowment among these ethnic groups in art, story telling, dance and music. This endowment is given every opportunity to flourish outside the school in evening clubs and during the many public festivals held throughout the year. However, curriculum planners for the most part, tend to downplay the important contribution that could be made to the study of art, drama, and aesthetics from this rich multicultural heritage.

The Teacher's Role as a 'Cultural Bridge'

A major problem which the author has encountered in training teachers in developing countries, is that they do not appreciate the enriching effect their own culture may have. The reason for this lies partly in the way teachers are trained and partly in the way society values its cultural traditions. However, both teachers and the society at large should be prepared to be open and critical about some of the constraints produced by its culture/s, and be prepared to adapt to change when it is necessary. It is unlikely that the view of Kean-Terry (1994) in Singapore on language learning would be welcomed by the die hard Chinese Mandarin scholars. On the other hand, the government of Singapore does recognise the fact that over-zealous didactic teaching, can be a barrier to more analytical, open and creative learning.

The quality of an educational system is only as good as the quality of its teaching force. For teachers to be active, credible, and effective, they need to feel that their context matters and that developing more sensitivity to the needs of their learners is an integral part of their role as a "cultural bridge" (Thomas, 1994). This analogy of a "bridge" is intimately linked to the recognition that the personalistic component of the model plays a vital part in raising expectations of pupils, and initiating and maintaining high levels of motivation during their years of schooling. Through constant encouragement by teachers, children will achieve a sense of self-esteem and a sense of competence which prepares them for living in a fast and ever changing world. Teachers who are "in tune" with the old and the new cultures will be able to help children adapt and adjust to such changes. This is also an essential ingredient of a culture sensitive pedagogy.

It must be emphasised that a culture sensitive pedagogy can complement existing pedagogies. It is not envisaged that there would be total replacement of modern methods of teaching and learning by indigenous forms. The essence of a culture sensitive pedagogy would incorporate the best ideas and practices from all types of teaching, but it would ensure that the cultural context of teaching and learning would be pivotal.

Cross-Cultural Challenges of a Culture-Sensitive Pedagogy
In developing a culture sensitive pedagogy, there are two concerns. The first concern is, the emergence of a so called 'global culture' and its impact on schooling. A second concern is, the need for educators to achieve a balance between selecting knowledge and skills for teaching and learning that will meet the demands of the 'global culture' (and its strong overtones for standardisation), and to ensure that culture-specific features are retained as part of the curriculum. Two key cross-cultural issues have direct relevance to a discussion about these concerns. The first concern is the nature of psychological universals, and the second, is the relationship between emic and etic influences in researching cross-cultural problems.

Psychological Universals, 'Global Culture,' and a Culture-Sensitive Pedagogy
The relationship between the existence of universals and the effects of globalization will be an issue of immense importance for educationalists. This is especially so, when it comes to planning educational programmes that have to take into account the cultural context of different cultural groups as they operate in an increasingly global culture. The inevitability of the globalization process and it's effect on attitudes and behaviour will need checks and balances built into future educational strategies. One way of meeting this need is to develop effective and culturally sensitive approaches to learning and teaching (Thomas, 1997).

The task of seeking out psychological universals or common principles will not only be problematical but controversial as well (Thomas, 1992, 1994). However, that is not to say we should abandon the search, because it is clear that the transnational nature of the school and the schooling process has become a natural locus for the identification of common and essential goals in learning and teaching. As Triandis (1978, 1979) and Longer (1980) have pointed out, one of the functions of universals would be to enhance international understanding. Another function would be to provide a guide and benchmark for international comparisons in education and particularly in student and teacher performance (Thomas, 1989). If these two functions were realised, much common ground would emerge in the establishment of universals or common principles in the globalization process.

The advent of the Internet has meant that globalization has become intensified. The speed of access is also making information readily available and in some cases cheaper than using facsimile, postal, and telegraphic forms of communication. Developments in CD Rom could also mean a complete rethinking of the production and use of teaching materials. These developments are certain to influence the way we learn and the way teachers will instruct in the future. In fact, changes are already taking place as more children have access to personal computers.

Promoting a different form of teaching which accommodates both global ideas and contextual needs (i.e., cultural needs) of both learners and teachers will not be easy. However, it is not possible to ignore the effects of globalization. The intensity of globalization, as far as cultural interaction is concerned, is likely to increase rather than diminish. 'Global culture' is essentially about a myriad of social interactive encounters, some of which will be transient, and others more enduring. These encounters will be characterised by communication systems that are not only varied in themselves, but are speedy in delivering information over a wide area of the world. The global culture can also involve many persons interacting simultaneously, yet scattered about in different places on the globe. Another factor is the 'universalising' effect of computerisation, as evident in the adoption of keyboard conventions and the dominance of certain international languages, especially English. These and other influences are key agents in the spread of the 'global culture.'

Teachers will find that coping with the massive amounts of information will be a formidable task. However, the main battleground will be the way teachers can develop positive yet critical attitudes toward the effects of the 'global culture' on teaching practices in the classroom. Teachers who are trained to have positive attitudes towards the benefits of the 'global culture' for their pupils would have considerable advantages over those who are not willing to accept change and who avoid innovating and experimenting. A teacher training regimen with strategies that allow teachers to adapt in the face of change, will also be developing mental sets in which cautious attitude change towards new ideas becomes a feature of sound praxis. Teachers are going to be melding the positive effects of this new 'global culture' with the existing cultures of knowledge and teaching. It is hoped that the meld will result in a culture sensitive pedagogy that will improve not only the quality of teaching, but will lead to learning outcomes that can ultimately benefit all.

Developing an Emic-Etic Balance as a Challenge for a Culture-Sensitive Pedagogy and the Demands of a Global Culture

The important contributions that emic and etic approaches to the study of cross-cultural behaviour could make to the quality of schooling and curriculum planning, has been discussed elsewhere (Thomas, 1989, 1992). For example, it has been shown that emic approaches to the study of values at primary and secondary school levels in Singapore and Malaysia relating to Chinese values such as *Hsiao* (filial piety), *Ren* (righteousness), and *Yi* (human heartedness), are better understood by using the tools of cultural analysis to study these concepts from within the culture (Thomas 1990, 1997a, 1997b). Such studies should hopefully prepare the ground for the development of strategies that will have more meaning for those who teach, and for those who learn about values in their own culture. What the emic dimension does for a culture sensitive pedagogy is to provide the necessary culture specific context for teaching and learning.

On the other hand, the etic dimension could also play a part in the consolidation of a values education. In Asian countries there has been a concerted attempt to develop teaching and learning strategies that not only address culture- or country-specific issues in the teaching of values, but a move to have a more regional approach to the subject. A start has been made by countries of the Asian region to achieve this by creating what is called Affective Development Education (UNESCO, 1992). Affective Development Education aims at embracing a set of commonly shared values which provides an etic dimension to values education. This could be perceived as a type of *regional eticism*. It would not be difficult to envisage the emergence of a *global eticism* where the impact of a global culture could result in values education having a world wide appeal.

The task for those who would develop a culture sensitive pedagogy, would be to employ a series of rigorous cultural analyses of, and selections from, indigenous, 'regional', and 'global' cultural contexts. The most challenging task facing educationalists who have a sound knowledge of cross-cultural techniques, field methodologies and relevant research findings is how to apply these in the quest to build a pedagogy that is balanced in terms of culture specific elements, while addressing the pressing needs for all teachers and learners to survive in the global village of the future.

References

Aikman, S. (1994). School curriculum as a forum for articulating intercultural relations with particular reference to the Peruvian Amazon. In E. Thomas (Ed.), *International perspectives on schooling and culture: A symposium proceedings* (pp. 197-218). London: Institute of Education, University of London.

Brunei, J. S. (1966). *Toward a theory of instruction.* Cambridge, MA: Harvard University Press.

Feiman-Nemser, S., & Floden, R. E., (1986). The cultures of teaching. In M. C. Wittrock (Ed.), *Handbook of research on teaching* (3rd ed., pp. 505-526). New York: Macmillan.

Gagne, R. M. (1975). *Essentials of learning for instruction.* Hinsdale, IL: Dryden Press.

Gilbert, W., & Lovegrove, N. (1968). *Science education in Africa.* London: Longmans.

Hargreaves, A. (1992). Cultures of teaching: A focus for change. In A. Hargreaves & M. G. Fullan (Eds.), *Understanding teacher development* (pp. 216-240). London: Cassell.

Kean-Terry, A. (1994). Culture and learning: A Singapore case study. In E. Thomas (Ed.), *International perspectives on culture and schooling: A symposium proceedings* (pp. 261-277). London: Institute of Education, University of London.

Little, A. (1994). Learning for all: Bridging cultures. In E. Thomas (Ed.), *International perspectives on culture and schooling: A symposium proceedings* (pp. 65-75). London: Institute of Education, University of London.

Little, P. W. (1982). Norms of collegiality and experimentation: Workshop conditions of school success. *American Education Research Journal, 19,* 325-340.

Lonner, W. J. (1980). The search for psychological universals. In W. H. Triandis & W. E. Lambert (Eds.), *Handbook of cross-cultural psychology* (Vol. 1, pp. 143-204). Rockleigh, NJ: Allyn & Bacon.

Metz, M. H. (1978). *Classrooms and corridors: The crisis of authority in desegregated secondary school classrooms.* Berkeley: University of California.

Nunes, T. (1994). Cultural diversity in learning mathematics: A perspective from Brazil. In E. Thomas (Ed.), *International perspectives on schooling and culture: A symposium proceedings* (pp. 357-370). London: Institute of Education, University of London.

Piaget, J. (1971). *Science of education and the psychology of the child.* London: Longmans.

Schon, D. (1983). *The reflective practitioner.* New York: Basic Books.

Shulman, L. (1986). Paradigms and research programmes in the study of teaching. In M. Wittrock (Ed.), *Handbook of research on teaching* (3rd ed., pp. 3-36). New York: Macmillian.

Tanon, F. (1994). A cultural view on planning: The case of weaving in Ivory Coast. *Cross-Cultural Psychology Monographs, 4.* Tilburg: Tilburg University Press

Teesdale, R., & Teesdale J.(1994). Culture and schooling in Aboriginal Australia. In E. Thomas (Ed.), *International perspectives on culture and schooling: A symposium proceedings* (pp. 174-196). London: Institute of Education, University of London.

Thomas, E. (1980). *Causal thinking in Hausa primary school children.* (Research Report). London: Institute of Education, University of London.

Thomas, E. (1989). Curriculum planning, cultural context and theories of human development: An identity challenge. In D. M. Keats, D. Munro, & L. Mann (Eds.), *Heterogeneity in cross-cultural psychology* (pp. 314-331). Amsterdam: Swets & Zeitlinger.

Thomas, E. (1990). Filial piety, social change and Singapore youth. *Journal of Moral Education, 19,* 192-205.

Thomas, E. (1992). Schooling and the school as a cross-cultural context for study. In S. Iwawaki, K. Yoshisa, & K. Leung (Eds.), *Innovations in cross-cultural psychology* (pp. 425-441). Amsterdam/Lisse: Swets & Zeitlinger.

Thomas, E. (1994). Overview. *International perspectives on schooling and culture: A symposium proceedings* (pp. 4-30). London: Institute of Education, University of London Publication.

Thomas, E. (1997). Developing a culture sensitive pedagogy: Tackling a problem of melding "Global Culture" within existing cultural contexts. *International Journal of Educational Development, 17,* 13-26.

Thomas, E. (1997a). Teacher education and values transmission: Cultural dilemmas with difficult choices. In K. Watson (Ed.), *Educational dilemmas series* (pp. 246-259). London: Cassell.

Thomas, E. (1997b). Values old and new: Curriculum challenges. In J. Lynch, C. Modgil, & S. Modgil (Eds.), *Education and development: Vol. 3. Tradition and innovation* (pp. 154-169). London: Cassell.

Triandis, H. C. (1978). Some universals of social behaviour. *Personality and Social Psychology Bulletin, 4,* 1-16.

Triandis, H. C. (1979). The future of cross-cultural psychology. In A. J. Marsella, R. G. Tharp, & T. J. Ciborowski (Eds.), *Perspectives on cross-cultural psychology* (pp. 389-410). New York: Academic Press.

UNESCO (1992). *Education for affective development: A guidebook on programmes and practices.* Bangkok: UNESCO.

Wittrock, M. C. (1986). *Handbook of research on teaching* (3rd ed.). New York: Macmillian.

Zeichner, K. M., & Tabachnik, B. R. (1983). *Teacher perspectives in the face of institutional press.* Paper presented at the American Educational Research Association, Montreal.

Zeichner, K. M. (1983). Alternative paradigms of teacher education. *Journal of Teacher Education, 34,* 3-9.

Primary Schoolchildren's Social Competence in Three Countries

Paul Vedder
Leiden University, The Netherlands

ABSTRACT

Children's social competence was measured in three countries: The Netherlands, the Netherlands Antilles, and Sweden. The data, collected with the *Revised Class Play* scale, were analyzed to discern whether or not this scale measures the same aspects of social behavior in different cultures and whether children give a comparable definition of socially competent behavior. Two hundred and three children from the Netherlands Antilles, 221 Dutch and 291 Swedish children in grades 4-6 participated. The results show that the *RCP*-scale measures comparable aspects of social behavior in all three countries. The definition of socially competent behavior, however, varies slightly.

Children influence each other's social behavior in accordance with the meaning they attach to particular types of social behavior (Kurtines & Gewirtz, 1987; Rubin, 1990), and in accordance with their own motivation for specific social behavior (Ogbu, 1993; Kromhout & Vedder, 1996). Using the categories of social behavior explored with the *Revised Class Play* scale (*RCP*; Masten, Morison & Pellegrini, 1985) we investigated whether or not children from different countries or cultural backgrounds attach the same meaning to descriptions of social behavior. The three categories of social behavior investigated were sociability/leadership, aggressive/disruptive, and sensitive/isolated.

Earlier studies showed minor differences between cultures. Chen, Rubin, and Sun (1992) reported that the factor structure in a sample of Canadian children and in a sample of Chinese children was generally comparable to the original factor structure. Krispin, Sternberg, and Lamb (1992) studied the *RCP*'s cross-cultural validity in Israel. The three factors found in North-American studies were also found in Israel, but 'sensitivity/isolation' was the second most important factor in the subsample of boys. Moreover, the researchers found that the item "Too bossy" was placed on the sociability/leadership factor, suggesting that for Israeli children leadership consists of assertive behavior. The authors suggested that these two findings may reflect the acceptability of aggressive behavior for men and the unacceptability of "feminine" sensitivity.

Like these earlier studies, the present study attempted to show that attaching meaning to a description is a process in which listeners or readers "tie the utterance to features of the context in which it is embedded, and to various unstated background propositions" (Shweder & Much, 1987, p. 207). The context and background propositions to a large extent will be filled in on the basis of children's socialization experiences.

Children from three cultures
The Netherlands and Sweden are both wealthy, liberal European countries well-known for their social welfare systems. Curaçao is the main island of a group of small islands in the Caribbean that together form the Netherlands Antilles. It is a former Dutch colony with its own government, although it is still quite dependent upon the Netherlands. Below I will discuss a few aspects of child-rearing in the three countries.

The Netherlands
Super et al. (1994) showed that social competence and independence are two important educational goals of Dutch parents with respect to young children. Children should be capable of playing, or more generally being on their own, without direct adult attention and support. Children should learn to get along well with peers, without adult interference (Eldering & Vedder, 1992; Vedder & Bouwer, 1996). A recent national survey on the home education of 0 - 18 year olds (Rispens, Hermanns, & Meeus, 1996) shows that social competence and independence are seen as the most important goals for older children as well. Respect or obedience and academic achievements are seen as far less important than getting along with each other in a harmonious way. Generally, parents in the Netherlands do not have different educational goals for boys and girls, and at home, gender-specific socialization is not obvious, apart from the fact that most mothers are the primary educators.

The Netherlands Antilles (Curaçao)
The first rule of Curaçaoan education is that children are expected to respect adults, especially their mothers. Respectful behavior is defined as being polite, not arguing, and doing as adults say (Vedder & Kook, 1993). Independence as a goal also is important, but clearly has a different meaning for girls and boys. About half of the children live in families in which the mother is the only parent. Girls are brought up with the idea that later in life they should be able to manage without a male companion. They learn to feel responsible for themselves and for their offspring. They are fostered to earn their own living as adults. Boys, on

the other hand, are left more on their own. Once they begin school, they get considerably more freedom to move around than do girls.

Beginning early in life, education in Curaçao is gender-specific. Girls are seen and treated more as children who can be dressed up nicely and who can be shown off, while parents wish their boys to be active. These child-rearing practices foster a certain amount of macho and extravert behavior in boys, even when they are less than four years old. There is a widespread fear in this society of boys becoming "softies", a trait that is almost synonymous with homosexual. Child-rearing practices encourage boys to develop behavior that cannot be interpreted as "softie" behavior (Vedder, 1995).

Sweden

In 1985, Ekstrand and Ekstrand reported that Swedish parents wish their children to be independent, active and to take initiative. They also have to be tolerant and obedient (Pétursson & Jonsson, 1994). Swedish parental goals resemble the goals that Dutch parents stress. In Sweden, however, the impact of non-home education seems to be larger, since Sweden has a much higher percentage of women in the labor force (United Nations, Eurostat & Statistics Sweden, 1995). While parents work, the children are taken care of by professional educators. Ekstrand (1994) states "It is, of course, important for adults in a society where almost everybody works outside the home that their children enjoy being in a group and are able to keep themselves occupied. Swedish children are consciously trained to be loyal to their peer group" (p. 10). In general, parents and educators seem to be rather successful in this respect. In her study, Ekstrand (1994) showed that "getting along well with peers" is seen by Swedish children as an important aspect of "good behavior". Sweden has done much in the last half century to bridge the gender gap in almost all social settings. Swedish children, in contrast to Dutch children, have both mothers and fathers who follow courses and are trained to pursue a professional career (O'Dowd, 1996).

In summary, this short description of child-rearing practices, ideologies, and settings in the Netherlands, Curaçao, and Sweden shows that education in the three countries differs on important points, especially regarding the values that influence the education of children in these countries. With this in mind, the *RCP*-study reported here should clarify whether or not children's socialization affects the meaning or value they attach to particular role descriptions used in the *RCP*.

Method

Subjects

In Curaçao, 203 children participated as voters (the choosing children in a class): 92 boys and 111 girls. They voted 231 candidates (the sum of all classmates who could be chosen). The children attended grades 4 - 6 of an elementary school in Otrobanda, a part of the capital of Curaçao, Willemstad. Their ages ranged from nine to fifteen years. The children came from a lower socio-economic background.

In the Netherlands, the voters were 221 Dutch children (110 boys and 111 girls), and the candidates were 505 classmates in the grades 6 - 8 of elementary school, which is equivalent to grades 4 - 6 in the Antillean and the Swedish system. Their ages ranged from nine to thirteen years. The children attended nine elementary schools in five cities in the densely populated Western part of the Netherlands. Some 75% of the pupils had a lower socio-economic background.

In Sweden, the study was conducted in grades four, five, and six in six elementary schools in the Stockholm region and in three schools in Gotland, an island southeast of Stockholm in the Baltic sea. The voters were 149 Swedish girls and 142 Swedish boys and the candidates were 421 classmates. The children's ages varied between ten and thirteen years. The children came largely from a lower socio-economic background.

In all countries the difference between the number of voters and candidates is due to the fact that we focus on the voters, who are either Curaçaoan, Dutch or Swedish children, whereas the candidates are all children in the participating classes, including many immigrant children. In the Swedish study we established that Swedish children attached the same meaning to descriptions of social behavior irrespective of whether the candidates were Swedish children or immigrant children (Vedder & O'Dowd, 1996). We suppose that the same holds for Curaçaoan and Dutch children.

Instrument

The *RCP* consists of thirty one-sentence descriptions of behavior. Fifteen of these describe behavior that is socially competent according to Western norms, labeled "sociability/leadership". Fifteen other items describe behavior that is socially incompetent according to Western norms, labeled either "aggressive/disruptive" or "sensitive/isolated". Examples of items in the three categories are "Makes new friends easily", "Picks on other kids" and "Rather plays alone than with others" respectively.

On Curaçao a Dutch version of the *RCP* was used. It was a version translated and adapted from the Masten version by Aleva (1993). Twenty-four items were directly translated, and six were adapted. The version that was used in the Netherlands contained 32 items. One item from the original American version and one of Aleva's adapted items were added to the version used in Curaçao. For the Swedish version the 32 Dutch role descriptions were translated and back-translated to ensure comparability with the Dutch version.

Procedure
The *RCP* was administered in school classes. Each of the children received a paper on which the items were listed and a list of the names of their classmates. This list served as a reminder, so that children did not forget to include classmates who were not present when the *RCP*-scale was administered. The children were asked to pretend to be directors of a play. Each item represented a role, such as "teases other children too much". For every role the children were to write down the numbers corresponding to one boy and one girl who most closely resembled the description. Children were not allowed to choose themselves or anyone who did not belong to the class.

In Curaçao and in the Netherlands children were instructed and supervised by a researcher. In Sweden teachers administered the *RCP*, because the main researcher was not proficient in Swedish. The teachers received extensive written instructions giving them background information on the scale and supplying them with the text that they should read to the children. During the administration the teachers were assisted by a member of the research team.

Scoring/Analyses
Scoring was undertaken in two steps. How often children were voted for a particular role description and who voted for them was determined first. The resulting scores were standardized by class and sex through a z-score transformation procedure, to control for variations in the number of voters (the choosing children in a class) and the number of candidates (children of the same sex who could be chosen). Z-scores greater than 2.5 were truncated (compare Masten et al., 1985; Krispin et al., 1992). These z-scores were further analyzed in factor analyses (Principal Component Analysis, rotation Varimax).

Results

In the Netherlands, the PCA resulted in five factors with eigen-values higher than one. The first three factors were the same as the three distinguished in the Masten et al. (1985) study. Their order was the same. The explained variance was 20.1%, 15.2% and 7.7% respectively. Factor 4 had two items which originally were part of the factor aggressive/disruptive (explained variance 4.2%), and factor 5 was a one-item factor. The total explained variance was 50.8%.

On Curaçao, the data also yielded five factors, of which the first three were the same as in the Dutch studies and in the North-American studies. Factor 4 was a selection of three items from the sociability/leadership factor, and one item with a negative loading from the factor aggressive/disruptive. Factor 5 was a combination of two items which originally referred to sensitivity/isolation, one item from the aggressive/disruptive factor and one from sociability/leadership. We termed this factor "touchy". The explained variance was 21%, 15.8%, 10.6%, 5.4, and 5.1% respectively (total 58%).

In Sweden, the PCA resulted in six factors, of which the first three were again the same as in the other studies, although the order of the factors was different. In Sweden the most important factor was aggressive/disruptive, the second was sociability/leadership and the third was sensitivity/isolation. The fact that the first factor is aggressive/disruptive behavior may be the outcome of a socialization process in which there is a strong emphasis on being kind. Deviation from this norm was conspicuous. The additional three factors mainly concerned specifications of the first three factors. The explained variance was 22.6%, 19.5%, 7.7%, 4.2%, 3.9%, and 3.3% respectively (total 59.2%).

Table 1 shows at item level the differences between the samples. The values in columns 2, 3, and 4 are the loadings on the factor as specified in columns 5, 6, and 7. They are the highest loadings of that item from the rotated factor matrix. Values lower than .40 are not included. To make comparison easier, the order of the first and second factor in the Swedish sample has been reversed, so that factor 1 refers in all samples to sociability/leadership, and factor 2 to aggressive/disruptive behavior.

For 16 items their distribution among factors was similar across the three countries. The Curaçaoan sample created most differences. Most of these were not really indicative of differences of meaning attached to the items. One clear exception concerned item 19. In Sweden and the Netherlands, this item refers to aggressive/disruptive behavior, while the Curaçaoan children see it as socially competent behavior.

Tabel 1. Distribution of RCP-Items and Factors in Samples of Dutch (Nl), Curaçaoan (Cu), and Swedish (Sw) Children (a Selection from the Three Rotated Factor Matrices)

	Loadings			Factor		
	Nl	Cu	Sw	Nl	Cu	Sw
1. Gets into a lot of fights	.71	.56	.73	2	2	2
2. Rather plays alone than with others	.75	.67	.75	3	3	3
3. Has good ideas for things to do	.65	.61	.60	1	4	1
4. Loses temper easily	.62	.69	.61	2	5	2
5. Shows off a lot	.47	.46	.63	2	1	2
6. Someone you can trust	.55	.47	.56	1	4	1
7. Interrupts when other children are speaking	.59	.73	.67	4	2	2
8. Does not obey the teacher	.53	.74	.68	2	2	2
9. Has trouble making friends	-.58	.61	.61	5	3	3
10. Has many friends	.74	.73	.85	1	1	1
11. Feelings get hurt easily	.64	.62	.87	3	5	4
12. Everyone listens to	.62	.79	.69	1	1	1
13. Plays fair	*	.48	.61		3	6

	Loadings			Factor		
	Nl	Cu	Sw	Nl	Cu	Sw
14. Helps other people when they need it	.49	**	.63	1		6
15. Always tries to get attention	.52	.78	.72	2	2	2
16. Can't get others to listen	.46	.73	.61	3	3	3
17. Good leader	.70	.77	.67	1	1	1
18. Makes new friends easily	.63	.66	.79	1	1	1
19. Too bossy	.70	.58	.75	2	1	2
20. Often left out	.69	.54	.61	3	3	3
21. Talks a lot	.67	.76	.68	4	2	2
22. Usually sad	.67	.56	.81	3	5	4
23. Everyone likes to be with	.67	.71	.83	1	1	1
24. Good sense of humor	.52	**	.59	1		5
25. Sticks nose in things that are not his/her concern	.68	.67	.73	2	2	2
26. Very shy	.76	.74	.75	3	3	3
27. Can get things going	.75	.76	.61	1	1	1
28. Teases other children too much	.67	.63	.76	2	2	2
29. Doesn't react to teasing	.66	.67	.64	3	3	3
30. Usually happy	.55	.72	.54	1	4	5
31. Picks on other kids	.73	-.48	.78	2	4	2
32. Likes to play with other kids than alone	.44	.41	.56	1	5	1

Note. * value lower than .40; ** item not included in scale used on Curaçao.

Gender Differences

We did comparable analyses for subsamples: boys voting for boys, boys voting for girls, girls voting for girls, and girls voting for boys. The PCA's in the Dutch and the Swedish subsamples yielded outcomes comparable to those in the complete samples. Some interesting differences, however, were found between the Curaçaoan total sample and subsamples. The PCA-outcomes in the subsamples in which the candidates were girls were similar to those in the complete Curaçaoan sample and in the Dutch and Swedish samples. The PCA on the data of the Curaçaoan subsample boys voting boys yielded nine factors. The first five are: 1. sensitivity/isolation (16% explained variance), 2. aggressive behavior/leadership (11.4% explained variance), 3. disruptive behavior I (9.9% explained variance), 4. sociability/leadership (6.6% explained variance), and 5. sociability/happiness (5.1% explained variance). The fact that sensitivity/isolation is such an important factor for boys can easily be interpreted as reflecting the fear of being considered a "softy." This fear is a strong force in manifesting macho-behavior. The second factor (aggressive behavior/leadership) indicated that leadership for Curaçaoan boys might be strongly related to aggressive behavior.

The PCA on the data of the subsample of girls voting boys resulted in eight factors with an eigen-value higher than one (total explained variance of 64.8%), of which only the first four could be labeled and interpreted easily. The first factor, labeled boys' sociability/leadership (explained variance of 19.6%), suggested that Curaçaoan girls see a combination of socially competent and aggressive behavior frequently in Curaçaoan boys. Factor 2 (11.1%) referred to sensitivity/isolation, factor 3 (10.7%) was about disruptive behavior, and factor 4 (7.1%) could be interpreted as the complement to factor 1. It combined "Someone you can trust," "Plays fair," and "Can't get others to listen." The sensitivity/ isolation factor in second place suggests that this kind of behavior of boys is more conspicuous than plain disruptive behavior.

The findings lead to the conclusion that the meaning attached to *RCP*-items by Dutch and Swedish children and by Curaçaoan children voting girls is largely comparable. Differences exist between these samples and the subsamples of Curaçaoan children with Curaçaoan boys as candidates. When voting boys Curaçaoan children easily combine socially competent and aggressive behavior.

The Three-Factor Solution

In addition to the PCA's with more than three factors, we also tried a three-factor solution in each (sub)sample. As was reported elsewhere, we found that the three-factor structure as originally identified by Masten et al. (1985) and reported in earlier studies (Chen et al., 1992; Aleva,

1993), that is, the factors sociability/leadership, aggressive/disruptive and sensitive/isolated, can be adequately used in the Swedish sample (Vedder & O'Dowd, 1996). In the present study, the three-factor structure also appeared to be rather strong in all Dutch and Curaçaoan (sub)samples. Apart from a few exceptions the items loaded on the factors as expected. The amount of variance in *RCP*-scores which can be explained by the three factors ranged between 36% and 47.4%. The reliability of the sub-scales (Cronbach's alpha coefficient), were generally as good in Curaçao (.67 to .89) as in the Netherlands (.76 to .85).

Discussion

In three countries, the Netherlands Antilles (more precisely Curaçao), the Netherlands, and Sweden the Revised Class Play scale was used to measure social competence in elementary school children. The main question of this study was: Do children from countries with different socialization traditions with respect to children's social behavior attach a different or a comparable meaning to the role descriptions used in the *RCP*?

The children came from cultures with different socialization traditions. A strong emphasis on gender differences and macho-behavior were described as typical of Curaçaoan socialization. Dutch socialization was described as geared toward children's capability to enjoy themselves without adult guidance or support. Gender differences do not play an important role in Dutch socialization. Swedish education is characterized by a strong appeal to children to be kind and by explicit attention to gender equality.

The findings of the present study at least partly correspond to these differences in socialization. In Sweden the most important factor is aggressive/disruptive. This behavior may be more obvious, or more conspicuous in a country with a strong emphasis on getting along well, and where kindness is seen as an important characteristic of children. Gender specific socialization traditions on Curaçao and stressing macho behavior in boys were easily recognized in the findings. On Curaçao, boys, and even to a larger extent girls tended to evaluate boys in terms of macho-behavior. The findings from Curaçao were partly comparable to the findings from the Israeli sample reported by Krispin et al. (1992). In subsamples with boys as candidates sensitivity/isolation is more important than in North-American samples, and sociability/leadership may include aggressive or assertive behavior. The same subscales, measuring sociability/leadership, aggressive/disruptive behavior, and sensitive/isolation, with largely the same role descriptions can be reliably used in Curaçao, Sweden, and in the Netherlands. The outcomes of the studies presented in this paper illustrate the notion that descriptions of social behavior derive meaning within a particular cultural context. The present study suggests topics for future research. To a large extent, interest in measuring children's social competence stems from a justified fear that maladjusted behavior in childhood raises the risk of emotional and social problems in later life (Parker & Asher, 1987; Morison & Masten, 1991). The present study as well as other studies on the *RCP*'s cross-cultural validity suggest the appropriateness of exploring the *RCP*'s predictive validity in a variety of cultures, as well as the processes that underlie the predictive validity or its lack.

There is evidence that Afro-Caribbean and Afro-American children and youngsters have much in common in terms of their socialization experiences (Suarez-Orozco, 1991; Dickerson, 1995). Given this comparability and given the outcomes of this study, it seems important to take a closer look at the validity of the *RCP*-scale in relation to Afro-American children as well as other minority and immigrant children.

References

Aleva, L. (1993). Beoordeling van sociale interacties op de basisschool: Betrouwbaarheid en validiteit van de Revised Class Play [Assessing social interactions in elementary school: Reliability and validity of the Revised Class Play]. *Tijdschrift voor Ontwikkelingspsychologie, 20,* 175-194.

Chen, X., Rubin, K., & Sun, Y. (1992). Social reputation and peer relationships in Chinese and Canadian children: A cross-cultural study. *Child Development, 63,* 1336-1343.

Dickerson, B. J. (Ed.) (1995). *African-American single mothers: Understanding their lives and families.* London: Sage.

Ekstrand, G. (1994). *Children, norms and values in three countries on three continents.* Miniprints no. 823. Malmö: School of Education.

Ekstrand, G., & Ekstrand, L. (1985). *Patterns of socialization in different cultures: The cases of India and Sweden.* Miniprints no. 513. Malmö: School of Education.

Eldering, L., & Vedder, P. (1992). *OPSTAP, een opstap naar school-succes?* [Hippy, good for better school achievement?] Amsterdam: Swets & Zeitlinger.

Krispin, O., Sternberg, K., & Lamb, M. (1992) The dimensions of peer evaluation in Israel: A cross-cultural perspective. *International Journal of Behavioral Development, 15,* 299-314.

Kromhout, M., & Vedder, P. (1996). Cultural inversion in children from the Antilles and Aruba in the Netherlands. *Anthropology and Education Quarterly, 27 (4),* 1-19.

Kurtines, W., & Gewirtz, J. (Eds) (1987). *Moral development through social interaction.* New York: John Wiley.

Masten, R., Morison, P., & Pellegrini, D. (1985). A revised class play method of peer assessment. *Developmental Psychology, 21,* 523-533.

Morison, P., & Masten, A. (1991). Peer reputation in middle childhood as a predictor of adaptation in adolescence: A seven-year follow-up. *Child Development, 62,* 991-1007.

O'Dowd, M. (1996). *Expectations, education, and human lives. A longitudinal study of a welfare state generation in a gender perspective (1938-1994).* Stockholm: Stockholm University, Institute of International Education.

Ogbu, J. U. (1993). Differences in cultural frame of reference. *International Journal of Behavioral Development, 16,* 483-506.

Parker, J., & Asher, S. (1987). Peer relations and later personal adjustment. *Psychological Bulletin, 102,* 357-389.

Pétursson, P., & Jonsson, F. (1994). Religion and family values. In T. Pettersson & O. Riis (Eds.), *Scandinavian values.* Uppsala: Uppsala University Press, 151-165.

Rispens, J. , Hermanns, J., & Meeus, W. (Eds) (1996). *Opvoeden in Nederland* [Child-rearing in the Netherlands]. Assen: Van Gorcum.

Rubin, K. H. (1990). Introduction: Peer relationships and social skills in childhood - an international perspective. *Human Development, 33,* 221-224.

Shweder, R., & Much, N. (1987). Determinations of meaning: Discourse and moral socialization. In W. Kurtines & J. Gewirtz (Eds.), *Moral development through social interaction* (pp. 197-244). New York: John Wiley.

Suarez-Orozco, M. (1991). Migration, minority status, and education: European dilemmas and responses in the 1990s. *Anthropology and Education Quarterly, 22,* 99-120.

Super, C., Harkness, S. Van Tijen, N., Van der Vlugt, E., Fintelman, M., & Dijkstra, J. (1994). The three Rs of Dutch childrearing and the socialization of infant arousal. In S. Harkness & C. Super (Eds.), *Parents' cultural belief systems: Their origins, expressions, and consequences.* New York: Guilford Press.

United Nations, Eurostat & Statistics Sweden (1995). *Women and men in Europe and North America.* Geneva: United Nations Publications.

Vedder, P., & Kook, H. (1993). Early childhood care and education in Curaçao. *International Journal of Early Years Education, 1,* 29-34.

Vedder, P. (1995). *Antilliaanse kinderen.* (Antillean children) Utrecht: Jan van Arkel.

Vedder, P., & Bouwer, E. (1996). Consensus as a prerequisite for quality in early child care; the Dutch case. *Child & Youth Care Forum, 25,* 165-182.

Vedder, P., & O'Dowd, M. (1996). *Social competence in Swedish elementary schools: The validity of the RCP.* Stockholm: Stockholm University, Institute of International Education.

Author Note

The study in Sweden was made possible by the Nils-Eric Svensson stipend granted in 1995 to the author. This stipend is given every year by the Bank of Sweden Tercentenary Foundation to a non-Swedish, European scientist to enhance European scientific cooperation. The author gratefully acknowledges the collaboration of Hetty Kook, Mariska Kromhout, and Mina O'Dowd in the studies described in this paper. Address for correspondence: Paul Vedder, Center for Intercultural Pedagogics, P.B. 9555, 2300 RB Leiden, Netherlands.
E-mail: vedder@rulfsw.leidenuniv.nl

Conceptual / Methodological Issues

Psychological Anthropology and the "Levels of Analysis" Problem: We Married the Wrong Cousin

William K. Gabrenya, Jr.
Florida Institute of Technology, USA

ABSTRACT

The "Levels of Analysis" problem in Cross-Cultural Psychology reflects our discipline's difficulty in conceptualizing the place of the individual in culture and society. Early in our history, we borrowed an ecological orientation from certain of our cousins in Psychological Anthropology that interpreted cultural differences in personality in terms of human adaptation to the natural environment. In recent decades, we have begun, implicitly and sometimes naively, to follow the theorizing and methodologies of the early, highly personological models of Culture and Personality and of the modern, cognitive idealist approaches of cognitive anthropology. I argue for a materialist, situational approach that places causal primacy on ecological and infrastructural factors rather than on symbolic, idealist, and mentalistic phenomena.

The Levels of Analysis problem in cross-cultural psychology (CCP), as well as in other social science disciplines, is a series of difficult questions: Should we study culture and psychology by focusing on individual or on collective phenomena? What accounts for the recurring finding that we obtain different results when we look empirically at seemingly similar phenomena at these two levels? Can we understand the interaction of culture and psychology through methods that begin with the thought and behavior of the individual, or must we begin with culture-level analysis using methods developed in the "institutional social sciences"? Can we understand the intrapsychic processes of the individual if we start from a macroscopic, cultural level?

Cross-cultural psychologists have taken distinctly different approaches to grappling with these issues. Some focus on sophisticated statistical methods that could be used to perform multi-level research with individual level data (e.g., Schwartz, 1996), while others see the problem as a conceptual or interpretational issue. I argue in this article that the Levels problem is essentially metatheoretical and has its roots in the manner in which we have inherited our basic conceptual orientations from our cousins in psychological anthropology (PA). These orientations form the (often unexamined) implicit assumptions underlying our work and guide us to a particular level of analysis.

My starting point is the assertion that the Levels problem is essentially theoretical, and cannot be solved through statistical slights-of-hand. The theoretical problem is the old one we have long failed to solve: What is culture? Where is it? Not only have we failed to specify our defining construct, we have produced few theories that illustrate its relationship to psychology. In 1984, the *Journal of Cross-Cultural Psychology* (JCCP) published a special issue on defining culture (Lonner, 1984). I believe that that issue was the most important issue ever published. Perhaps it is time to revisit this fundamental question.

Psychology and Anthropology
I have always been confused about the relationship between CCP and cultural anthropology, particularly PA. We have failed to confront what I believe is a problem of disciplinary identity: IS CCP indeed an errant branch of anthropology, rediscovering and rehashing the theoretical problems addressed by PA since the era of Boas and Freud? Will theoretical advances in our field take place only if we complement the methodological sophistication we have inherited from our siblings in experimental psychology with the cultural sophistication of our cousins on the other side? Gustav Jahoda explored this relationship in his book *Psychology and Anthropology* (1982); I hope to do something similar in this paper, albeit less ambitious and from a different perspective.

The two are close kin: I propose that CCP can be viewed as an extension of the classical culture and personality schools of PA (Piker, 1994). These schools, in diverse ways, ask questions such as: What is the relationship between psychological processes and cultural processes? Does personality differ across cultures? How much of human behavior is shaped by culture and how much by biology? If one accepts a slightly broad view of personality, encompassing individual values, behavioral styles, world views, and the like, one can browse through *JCCP* and see that most articles are indeed studies of culture and personality, reporting two- and multi-culture comparisons of personality-like dependent variables: "DV in C_1 and C_2: A cross-cultural perspective." If we are performing culture and personality studies, how is our work linked to that of our kin in anthropology?

Tracing the Family Tree
Historically, various traditions in CCP have developed under the influence of one or more schools of culture and personality—even though many of us currently active in CCP are unaware of these schools and their problems. My contention, as expressed in the title of this chapter, is that CCP originally was "married" to what I characterize as "good

cousins" in PA, but has recently fallen in with the bad side of the family, influencing our choice of level of analysis and our implicit metatheory.

Who are these cousins, good and bad? Robert LeVine (1973) and Philip Bock (1988) have attempted to organize conceptually the schools of culture and personality and the distinctions I will make are based on a synthesis of their ideas. By "schools" I am following the terminology used by LeVine, Bock and others to indicate general theoretical approaches to the culture-and-person relationship, each of which is represented by one or more specific theories, models, or research programs. My intention in reviewing these schools is not to duplicate the excellent works of those referenced herein, but to show how the anthropologists and psychologists who formulated the schools were elucidating metatheoretical orientations that directly or indirectly have come to be represented in modern CCP. Rather than a microanalysis of the philosophical epistemology or assumptions underlying various approaches to CCP (such as Eckensberger (1979) has done for psychology), I pursue a more molar analysis at the level of schools in CCP. My analysis places an emphasis on relationships and commonality of functioning across schools that can be useful for understanding the broad ancestral heritage of various approaches to CCP.

Figure 1 illustrates the culture and personality schools in a highly simplified manner. At the outset, the reader should note the contrasting positions of "P" in the schools. "P" can be of fundamental importance (Psychological Reductionist), contributory importance (Mediational), or simply a dependent variable (Materialist). The goals of PA are first to understand culture better by employing psychological constructs and secondarily to help us understand psychology better by examining its place in culture. The latter goal is often attributed to CCP and to cultural psychology. The schools of culture and personality provide a broad map of the various ways the place of psychology in culture can be conceptualized and, as I argue below, have passed to CCP legacies of thought that have contributed to its theoretical development. Several of the schools are described in more detail in the following sections. For a more thorough treatment, please refer to the sources cited below.

Leslie White's 3-level pyramidal conceptualization of culture (White, 1959) provides a useful heuristic for understanding these schools. White and his students, notably Marvin Harris (1968, 1979), thought of culture as organized in three parts or levels: material culture or *infrastructure*, a society's subsistence technology; *social structure*, including both political and domestic economy; and ideology or *superstructure*, cultural elements including ideology, values, religion, myth, games, art, and so on (see *Figure 2*). Materialist, ecological and some Marxist theories of culture emphasize causality running *up* the pyramid, placing primacy on material

Psychological Anthropology: A Map

$P \to C$
Psychological Reductionist
Freud, Róheim, Spain, Spiro,
Fromm, McCelland

Culture developed through
Psychological Processes of
Individuals

$C1 \to P \to C2$

Mediational
Kardiner, DuBois,
Whiting, Child

Childhood Determinism
Personality Processes determine
Expressive Parts of Culture
(Ideology, Myth, etc.)

$S \to P$
$C \to S \to P$
Situationist
Personality
G.H. Mead: Role theorists

$C2 \to C1$
$C2 \to P \to C1$
Cognitive
Goodenough

Emic methods
Mentalistic, Idealist

$C = P$
Configurationist
Mead, Benedict

Extreme relativism
Culture and Personality not
Distinguishable

$C \to P$
$C \to S \to P$
Materialist
Harris, White

Personality Adapts to
Requirements of Ecology,
Technology, Social Structure,
and Ideology

$C \to S \to P$
Social Structure and

Sociology: Role theorists
House, Kohn, Inkeles

$P \leftrightarrow C$
Cultural
Schweder

People as Active Agents
Culture and Personality
Mutally Determinative

Figure 1. Psychological Anthropology: A Map of Schools of Culture and Personality (P = Personality or Psychological Processes; C = Culture, and S = Context or Situation)

Note. The schematic by the author is based on the writings of Bock (1983), D'Andrade (1995), and LeVine (1973).

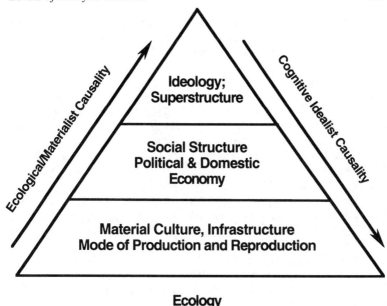

Figure 2. Leslie White's Pyramidal Conception of Culture. Culture is defined as comprising Three Components, Material Culture (technology), Social Structure, and Ideology

subsistence technologies. On the other hand, idealist, psychological reductionist, and cognitive approaches see causality running *down* the pyramid, holding ideas, symbolic aspects of culture, or psychological processes as determining factors in cultural evolution. This contrast is fundamental in social science and is reflected in important societal activities such as the formation of domestic political beliefs (e.g., is poverty caused by infrastructural inequities or by deficient belief systems among the poor?).

Although there has been a two-way dialog between PA and CCP from their respective beginnings, some of which involved the interdisciplinary work of the founding members of IACCP, it appears that most of the influence has been from anthropology to psychology. Thus, many of our research traditions, metatheoretical orientations, and in some cases specific theories, can be traced back to schools of culture and personality. I refer to these influences as our "legacies" because some are historically remote, some have contributed to the zeitgeist of CCP without being actually known to a majority of its practitioners, and still others are riding a wave of metatheoretical change in social science alongside CCP. "Legacy" is also meant to communicate the idea that CCP has adapted each of the schools' positions to fit its needs in a process analogous to cultural diffusion.

The Good Cousin

The earliest legacy in CCP seems to be ecological, sharing roots with at least two schools of culture and personality. The ecological legacy is most clearly represented in Berry's (1976) Ecocultural Framework. "Ecology" is generally used to mean "any combination of natural conditions that affects food-production techniques, which are clearly fundamental to the functioning of society" (Segall, Dasen, Berry, & Poortinga, 1990, p. 19). Anthropologists have always been concerned with the ecological setting of the cultures they studied, but the formal inclusion of this concern in theories focusing on psychological processes may have begun with the Mediational School. The mediational approach in PA seeks to explain the ideological and symbolic realms of culture—essentially White's superstructure, represented by C_1 in Figure 1—by calling on psychological processes that are said to mediate the effects of infrastructure and structure on superstructure. The psychoanalyst Kardiner's neo-Freudian Basic Personality theory initiated this line of theorizing in its attempt to explain and predict the "basic" or "modal" personalities (P in Figure 1) and superstructural elements (C_2) of individual societies from their economies, social structures, and child-rearing practices (C_1) (Kardiner & Linton, 1939). Subsequently, Whiting's neo-Kardinarian model (Whiting & Whiting, 1974) approached the relationship of ecology, economy, social structure with child-rearing, personality and superstructure (termed "projective expressive systems") in a cross-cultural manner employing the technology of holocultural research facilitated by the Human Relations Area Files.

Holocultural/Area Files research uses quantitative data coded from ethnographies to calculate cross-cultural correlations among societal-level variables such as subsistence economy and modal child-rearing practices. In the classic Whiting and Child (1953) study, for example, an attempt was made to show that personality mediates the relationship between child-rearing practices and ethnotheories about illness. Holocultural research has produced some impressive cross-cultural findings concerning the relationships among ecological, cultural and personality variables (e.g., see Segall, 1983). The Mediational School guided the famous Six Cultures Study, in which links among ecology, subsistence methods, domestic economy, and behavioral measures of personality were identified. The Mediational School is closely linked by theory, methods and adherents to the classical ecologically-inspired work of John Berry (1976), William Lambert (1971), Ruth and Lee Munroe (e.g., Munroe &

Munroe, 1975), and Marshall Segall (e.g., Segall, Campbell, & Herskovits, 1966) among others.

The most explicit ecological statement among the schools is found in the Materialist approach (Harris, 1979). LeVine (1973) includes this approach in the so-called Anti-Culture and Personality School, and technically it is outside PA because of its minor interest in psychological processes. Harris is a student of White, and both of their theorizing reflects the materialism of Marxism without its Hegelian components. Harris' "principle of ecological determinism" paraphrases much of Whiting's and Berry's models: "The etic behavioral modes of production and reproduction probabilistically determine the etic behavioral domestic and political economy, which in turn probabilistically determine the behavioral and mental emic superstructures" (Harris, 1979, pp. 55-56). The ecological legacy is an *up*-the-pyramid conceptualization, that is, ideology and social structure are viewed as causally dependent on infrastructure.

Although in CCP we are more interested in understanding the characteristic behavior of people in societies rather than the ontogeny of superstructure, some of our work appears to adopt the logic of the Mediational School in the way it places personality in a central position. Conditions of life, including child-rearing experiences, are said to contribute to the development of generally similar personalities or values among members of a society. These common personalities are in turn evidenced in the behavior of individuals and then at the collective level in institutions and culturally-widespread practices. For example, Inkeles' (1983) model of modernization maintains that industrialization produces modern values and modern behaviors that contribute to the development of modern institutions. Triandis' (1995) collectivism theorizing posits a collectivist society that produces people with collectivist personalities which are in turn expressed as collectivist behaviors and in the development of collectivist institutions (although the latter institutions may be seen as an aspect of the collectivist society at the beginning of the loop). Stretching White's pyramid a bit, the causal direction is *up* then *down*. CCP investigators who are interested primarily in understanding the projective-expressive system are not likely to conceptualize the causal process in this way, as discussed below.

I argue that these are our good cousins. To anticipate my defense of this statement, presented in a later section, the ecological approach provides a superior strategy for understanding the behavior of individuals and the evolution of cultural forms because it adopts an etic, scientific approach with a solid starting point in invariant laws of nature and the relationship among nature, human subsistence techniques, and the adaptation of societal and psychological characteristics to these exigencies.

The Relativist Cousin

The Configurational or "Culture-is-Personality" School, most closely associated with Ruth Benedict and Margaret Mead (Benedict, 1934; Mead, 1935), viewed the cultural elements of each society and its members' personalities as a gestalt-like whole that is irreducible and indeterminate. Cultures are irreducible to component parts such as economic, social structural, personality, or ideological subsystems. They are indeterminate because universal biological, ecological, or culturological causal processes that could account for the observed worldwide variability in culture and personality in a nomothetic manner are rejected; we are asked to appreciate each culture's unique configuration rather than understand it (LeVine, 1973).

Despite the prominence of some of the members of the Configurational School, such as Margaret Mead, it does not seem to have had a direct impact on CCP outside of the relativism it shares with some other schools. However, a configurational legacy seems to appear in two ways in modern CCP. It is evidenced in some of our too-frequent imprecise or shallow theorizing, published research in which causal links are not spelled out and differences are described but not really explained. It also can be found in the use of psychometric measures which are taken as indices of both culture and personality simultaneously. Complicating the Levels problem, self-report measures are used to infer something about the "culture" at the same time that they indicate something about the individuals in the culture. Much of the published research involving collectivism seems to suffer from this theoretical lapse. The Configurational School's gestaltist approach defies the White pyramid heuristic, but its relativist orientation is evident in the third cousin.

The Wrong Cousin

The implicit conceptualization of culture and personality held in CCP appears to have drifted from the ecological approach to a cognitive idealist style, paralleling similar shifts in anthropology. The cognitive idealist legacy in CCP has roots in the Reductionist School of culture and personality and in the cognitive anthropology field within modern PA. "Idealist" is used to indicate the ideational and symbolic aspects of culture and their representation at the individual level in cognitive content and process. This concept is elaborated in the following sections.

Psychological Reductionism

The Reductionist School of culture and personality, attributed to Freud and carried to the present by anthropologists such as Spain (1982), seeks to explain cultural phenomena by recourse to psychological processes, that is, culture is "reduced" to psychology. McClelland's extensive research on need for achievement and economic development (McClelland, 1971) is reductionist in that a societal-level phenomenon—economic prosperity—is explained by changes in the achievement values of individual members of society. Causality runs *down* the pyramid in this school. Although little psychodynamic theorizing can be discerned in CCP, an implicit Reductionist legacy may be identified in our excessive psychologizing (in my opinion) and our inattention, except in a descriptive and superficial manner, to the cultural origins of the psychological dependent variables on which we focus.

Cognitive Anthropology

Cognitive anthropology developed in the mid-1950s as anthropology's definition of culture shifted from behavior and events in the physical world to a cognitive system to which observable behavior is only probabilistically related (Casson, 1994). The "great paradigm shift" (D'Andrade, 1995) toward a cognitive idealist perspective was accompanied by the decline of behaviorism in psychology and the early development of psychology as a cognitive science, seen in the work of Jerome Bruner, Noam Chomsky and George Miller. The focus of cognitive anthropology is on understanding the characteristics of this cognitive system through an emic research strategy that seeks to understand the world from respondents' points of view. A relativist orientation predominates. Culture is viewed generally as an idea system, either resident collectively in the cognitive mechanisms of individuals, or in the collective representations of the society, or both; individuals are presented with maps or schemas of the surrounding world and with rules to live by. Research focuses on people's self-reported conceptions or on the collective ideology of the society. Examples of this approach include analyses of myth and explorations of folk taxonomies (D'Andrade, 1995). Causal priority is *down* the pyramid.

The idealist legacy can be seen in CCP's emphasis on values, attitudes, beliefs, attributions, and personality traits of individuals, to the widespread exclusion of behavioral measures (Gabrenya, 1994; see below). Cognitive anthropology employs intensive, highly structured interview methods to identify mental structures characteristic of a culture (indeed, the mental structure *is* the culture), while in an analogous fashion, CCP uses self-report instruments and multivariate data analysis to reveal the structure of values, personality traits, conceptions of intelligence, and so on among individuals. This structure is subsequently attributed to a "society" or "culture" at a higher level of analysis. American social psychology, perhaps primed by its fascination with social cognition, appears ready to embrace a cognitive idealist form of cultural psychology and to reject much of the extant CCP (Markus, Kitayama & Heiman, 1996). The ecological approach to social perception promoted by Leslie Ziebrowitz (McArthur & Baron, 1983) has had seemingly little impact on this movement.

J'Accuse

Why is the cognitive idealist legacy the wrong cousin, and why is this marriage a bad idea? A long and difficult debate between the ecological and cognitive idealist approaches might fail to settle the issue of which is a superior metatheory, but I will present the ecological case in this article. Many of my arguments in this section are derived from Harris (1968, 1979). A more in-depth discussion would require exploring epistemological issues, making value judgments about the ultimate goals of social science, and addressing the Levels problem of distinguishing between situationist approaches to individual personality and materialist approaches to cultural evolution.

The argument for an ecological or materialist metatheory begins with the thesis that culture is ultimately grounded in nature, not in ideas. Human cultures evolved in a barefisted struggle for survival in which the harsh realities of subsistence production and the inherent problems of excessive reproduction presented powerful contingencies. For example,

Nature is indifferent to whether God is a loving father or a blood-thirsty cannibal. But nature is not indifferent to whether the fallow period in a swidden field is one year or ten (Harris, 1979, p. 57).

The biochemical nature of agricultural production, taking place until recently in the absence of chemical fertilizers and farm price supports, has dictated people's activities independently of their cosmological conceptualization of nature and the universe. The idealist approach, in contrast, denies this link to nature:

... the nonrational suppositions, ideas about worth, and classifications of a people (... a pig is not an animal to eat ...) are not derivable from reason or direct experience with nature—one must be "let in" on the secret, one must, somehow, receive the "frame" of understanding from others (Shweder, 1984, p. 49; in Miller, 1996).

In the "Information Age," comprising just the most recent .1% of the history of our species, perhaps 25% of humans are fairly distant from this "culture/ nature interface" (all Western psychologists are in this set).

However, even for humans living in this new and unusual situation, the material bases of technological innovation and the transformation of energy in all its forms shape social institutions and propel ideological change. Infrastructural conditions influence not only political and economic structures but also components of these structures proximally related to the productive activities of many individuals —notably the industrial corporation. Ongoing transformations of these cultural elements are the dynamic behind worldwide changes in other areas such as individual modernity and social values. Radical changes in infrastructural and structural conditions can lead to abrupt shifts in ideology in only one generation, particularly when these ideas are functionally related to such changes (Inkeles, 1983, Yang, 1986), suggesting that the ideological basis for culture is not *a priori* constant and stable. Whereas some idealist theories hold that people create culture through activity, from an ecological perspective cultures are seen as presenting individuals with limited sets of options from which they are "free" to choose. It is this freedom that may give individuals the illusion that they are creating culture by their choices.

Idealist approaches seek to describe the values and beliefs of cultures but often leave the person lost in thought, failing to link values and beliefs to antecedent social conditions or consequent observable behavior. Gaines and Reed (1995), for example, demonstrate how Gordon Allport's conceptualization of racial prejudice, coming out of the individualist, cognitive tradition of American social psychology, fails to place White attitudes in a social context. They contrast Allport's theory with the African-American sociologist W. E. B. DuBois' attempt to trace racism to its economic and societal origins. At its extreme, a highly relativist idealist approach abandons a scientific, nomothetic approach to social science by rejecting the possibility of a universal process that can generate and explain the nature of ideology in all its cultural forms.

The central goal of cognitive anthropology is discovering the rules that govern behavior. In CCP, the emphasis is often on implicit goals, such as values and social beliefs. The link between rules or values and behavior is highly distal because such idealist elements are often inconsistent with each other, vaguely understood by actors, and clouded by a host of situational exceptions. However, as social psychologists have long known, behavior is multiply determined by situational contingencies, costs, and values and attitudes, and attitudes and beliefs themselves are often determined by behavior, which is in turn strongly guided by costs and benefits.

Idealist approaches seem to implicitly commit the ecological fallacy, that is, identifying idealist elements such as beliefs or values and implying that there is considerable uniformity in these elements among individuals in the society. CCP shares with the American psychology it loves to criticize an inattention to societal conflict, deviance, and social structure, each of which contribute to value dissensus in all but the simplest societies. In this regard, it evidences the legacies of all the culture and personality schools that posited common underlying psychological characteristics to members of a cultural group.

The ecological approach differs from the idealist approach in the way it treats mentalistic phenomena such as ideology and its psychological correlates of values and personality. The ecological approach seeks to understand these phenomena from the perspective of the ecological foundation of the natural environment, linked to cultural-level phenomena such as technologies, institutions, history, and social structure. Such a research style is *multi*-leveled, and a serious attempt is made to understand how these levels are mutually causative.

Deconstructing Cognitive Idealism

Intellectual currents in CCP have not received much attention by social scientists (Eckensberger, 1994), so the following analysis of the multiple determinants of the idealist legacy is a rather speculative starting point (see Figure 3). On the one hand, there are powerful forces in psychology that lead us to idealist thinking, such as the ever-emerging "self" movement (Markus & Kitayama, 1991) and the dominant social cognition orientation in American social psychology. Self-theorists focus on the subjective, self-focused experiences of individuals while social cognition emphasizes the cognitive processing of individuals. Coming from anthropology are research strategies emphasizing emic methods aimed at capturing the respondent's point of view and even retreating from field work itself. Also coming from anthropology is the current trend towards cultural relativism.

I believe there are also powerful non-intellectual roots to the idealist legacy in CCP. The oft-cited individualist bias (Gabrenya, 1989) and liberal, middle-class values (Hogan & Emler, 1978) of American psychology may have promoted this idealist CCP, as "postindustrial" middle class people have moved from producing things to producing information. From an ecological perspective, this phenomenon could be analyzed by looking at the nature of the "cognitive ecology" (Gabrenya, 1989) of the cross-cultural researcher. I suggest we live in a niche in which the types of research that are possible and valued lead to an idealist orientation.

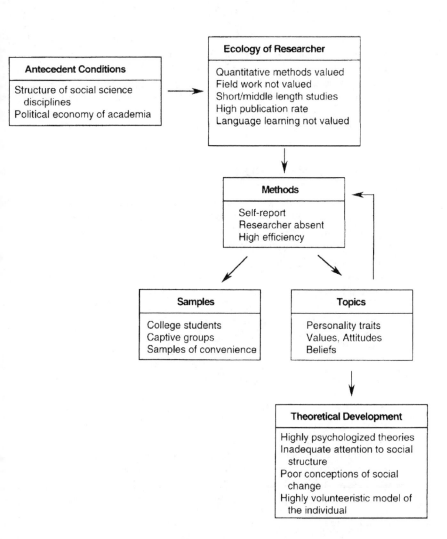

Figure 3. The "cognitive ecology" of the Cross-Cultural Psychologist

Figure 3 illustrates one model of the relationships among theory, methods, and niche characteristics. The researcher is conceptualized as occupying an ecological niche that presents powerful contingencies to which he/she must accommodate in order to survive in the discipline. One set of responses to these contingencies is the methods chosen for research, which in turn shape the manner of respondent sampling and the research topics that can be studied most efficiently. Research topics feed back to shape methods. The ecology of the researcher reflects the manner in which the social sciences have organized themselves over the last century, and the political economy of academia in the nation in which the researcher works.

Research in an Idealist Metatheory

What are some results of this idealist orientation? Since behavior is less important than intrapsychic concepts, much research in CCP compares a personological dependent variable across two or more cultures, typically assessing values or beliefs. We look at what people say they value or think, or say they do, or say they would do, rather than what they actually do. In my own area, Chinese Studies, this idealist orientation can be found in the prevalent research styles, including my own.

This style is clearly evident in our journal. I conducted a content analysis of 17 years of the *Journal of Cross-Cultural Psychology* (1979 to 1995) and identified 127 articles that reported studies which included Chinese, Japanese, or Korean participants (the focus of the content analysis was on East Asians). Self-report methods (e.g., value surveys) and experiments in which both the independent variable manipulation and dependent variable measures were performed on paper (e.g., scenario studies) comprised 78% of the articles. A disproportionate number of our studies used intellectually sophisticated, middle class college student respondents to tap idealist cultural phenomena. In a separate content analysis of 25 years of JCCP through 1994 (Öngel & Smith, 1994), more than half of the articles with Chinese samples were found to include at least one sample of college students (Üsten Öngel & Peter Smith, personal communication, March 29, 1994). The ultimate result of our idealist orientation is a level of analysis focused on the ideologies of individual college students.

Solutions

By making these charges against my own academic field, I place myself in the uncomfortable position of being obligated to offer some solutions to the problem. I will offer six practices that I feel might improve the quality of our work.

1. Stop pretending that your independent variable is culture

As Beatrice Whiting and others said many years ago, "culture" is too big to be treated as a unitary construct in empirical research (Whiting, 1976). Let us use the term at lunch and in bars and bistros, but in serious research specify the component parts of interest: family structure; industrialization; economic system; wealth; even "collective representations." This practice may force us to specify processes and causal effects rather than make vague "cultural" comparisons, and to work with independent variables at the societal level of analysis.

2. Pay more attention to sociology

We should learn more about the structure and dynamics of modern societies. Here the sociologists are more useful than the anthropologists because most of our research is conducted in comparatively modern, complex societies. It would be useful to take a look at the small area known as "psychological sociology" or "social structure and personality" (House, 1977) or the smaller area termed "societal psychology" (Himmelweit, 1990). The work of Melvin Kohn and his associates (Kohn & Schooler, 1983) on social class and personality is a classic example of sophisticated work linking social structure and psychological variables.

3. Take another look at role theory

The most promising but least active area within the social structure and personality school of sociology is role theory. My dissertation advisor wrote the definitive work in the area while I was a student (Biddle, 1979), but it took me a long time to realize that this level of analysis may be the path we missed. Social positions are the central organizing facts of people's lives in both modern and traditional societies, forming the link between the situational conditions of interest to ecologists and psychological phenomena and behavior.

4. Read more psychological anthropology

Back in the 1980s, I tried to estimate the amount of reading one would have to do to remain current as a well-informed cross-culturalist (Gabrenya, 1988). It was quite discouraging, essentially impossible. One would have to read in dozens of journals and over several disciplines.

However, in some way we need to maintain contact with our cousins in anthropology, good and bad, if the cultural sophistication of CCP is to show any improvement.

5. Do field work

I wonder if we can ever be good cross-cultural or cultural psychologists by following the training and disciplinary model of mainstream psychology. Appreciation of a culture cannot be obtained without prolonged "on the ground" experience. Such experiences are not easy to come by for most psychologists and, even when they do obtain them, there is a danger that the manner in which they do so (e.g., sabbaticals or personal ties to particular societies) may promote a single- or within-culture style and expertise seemingly at cross-purposes with CCP. However, idealist thinking would be well-tempered by an understanding of the ecological context of respondents' daily lives.

6. Take a walk in the woods

I suggest that humans are not fundamentally different in some key respects from the trees in your local park. Cultures, people, and trees are adapted to a real world with real implications for life and death, success and failure, pleasure and pain. Our research, lost in thought as it has become, has severed its connection to real things, the natural world and the situations in which most people live. What is it that allows or encourages us to assume the arrogant attitude that we humans have transcended the lot of all other living organisms on the planet? Perhaps it is intrinsic to the middle class ecological niche in which we psychologists dwell. As others have charged in deconstructing G. H. Mead and symbolic interactionism (e.g., see Meltzer, Petras & Reynolds, 1975), our middle class professional lives are focused on ideas and resplendent with opportunities, detached from the experience of nature and from the lives of people who do not live in our world of abstraction and reflection.

Now there's an idea.

References

Benedict, R. (1934). *Patterns of culture*. Boston: Houghton Mifflin.
Berry, J. W. (1976). *Human ecology and cognitive style: Comparative studies in cultural and psychological adaptation*. New York: Sage/Halsted/Wiley.
Biddle, B. J. (1979). *Role theory: Expectations, identities, and behaviors*. New York: Academic.

Bock, P. K. (1988). *Rethinking psychological anthropology: Continuity and change in the study of human action.* New York: W. H. Freeman.

Casson, R. W. (1994). Cognitive anthropology. In P. K. Bock (Ed.), *Psychological anthropology* (pp. 61-96). Westport, CT: Praeger.

Cross-Cultural Psychology Bulletin (1995, March). Melbourne, FL: International Association for Cross-Cultural Psychology.

D'Andrade, R. (1995). *The development of cognitive anthropology.* New York: Cambridge University Press.

Eckensberger, L. H. (1979). A metamethodological evaluation of psychological theories from a cross-cultural perspective. In L. H. Eckensberger, W. J. Lonner, & Y. H. Poortinga (Eds.), *Cross-cultural contributions to psychology* (pp. 255-275). Amsterdam: Swets and Zeitlinger.

Eckensberger, L. H. (1994). On the social psychology of cross-cultural research. In A. M. Bouvy, F. J. R. van de Vijver, P. Boski, & P. Schmitz (Eds.), *Journeys in cross-cultural psychology* (pp. 31-40). Amsterdam: Swets and Zeitlinger.

Gabrenya, W. K., Jr. (1988, February). *Cross-cultural psychology as culture broker: A journal citation analysis.* Society for Cross-Cultural Research, El Paso, TX.

Gabrenya, W. K., Jr. (1989). Social science and social psychology: The cross-cultural link. In M. H. Bond (Ed.), *The Cross-cultural challenge to social psychology* (pp. 48-66). Beverly Hills, CA: Sage.

Gabrenya, W. K., Jr. (1994, June). *Issues in studying the Psychology of the Chinese.* International Conference on Chinese Psychology, Chinese University of Hong Kong.

Gaines, S. O. Jr., & Reed, E. S. (1995). Prejudice: From Allport to DuBois. *American Psychologist, 50,* 96-103.

Harris, M. (1968). *The rise of anthropological theory: A history of theories of culture.* New York: Thomas Y. Crowell.

Harris, M. (1979). *Cultural materialism: The struggle for a science of culture.* New York: Vintage Books.

Himmelweit, H. T. (1990). Societal psychology: Implications and scope. In H. T. Himmelweit & G. Gaskell (Eds.), *Societal psychology* (pp. 17-45). Thousand Oaks, CA: Sage.

Hogan, R. T., & Emler, N. P. (1978). The biases in contemporary social psychology. *Social Research, 45,* 478-534.

House, J. S. (1977). The three faces of social psychology. *Social Psychology Quarterly, 40,* 161-177.

Inkeles, A. (1983). *Exploring individual modernity.* New York: Columbia University Press.

Jahoda, G. (1982). *Psychology and anthropology: A psychological perspective.* New York: Academic.

Kardiner, A., & Linton, R. (1939). *The individual and his society*. New York: Columbia University Press.

Kohn, M. L., & Schooler, C. (1983). *Work and personality: An inquiry into the impact of social stratification*. Norwood, NJ: Ablex.

Lambert, W. W. (1971). Cross-cultural backgrounds to personality development and the socialization of aggression: Findings from the Six Cultures study. In W. W. Lambert & R. Weisbrod (Eds.), *Comparative perspectives on social psychology* (pp. 49-61). Boston: Little, Brown.

LeVine, R. A. (1973). *Culture, behavior, and personality*. Chicago: Aldine.

Lonner, W. J. (1984). Special section: Differing views on culture. *Journal of Cross-Cultural Psychology, 15*, 107-162.

Markus, H. R., & Kitayama, S. (1991). Culture and the self: Implications for cognition, emotion, and motivation. *Psychological Review, 98*, 224-253.

Markus, H. R., Kitayama, S., & Heiman, R. J. (1996). Culture and "basic" psychological principles. In E. T. Higgins, & A. W. Kruglanski (Eds.), *Social psychology: Handbook of basic principles* (pp. 857-913). New York: Guilford.

McArthur, L. Z., & Baron, R. M. (1983). Toward an ecological theory of social perception. *Psychological Review, 90*, 215-238.

McClelland, D. C. (1971). *Motivational trends in society*. New York: General Learning Press.

Mead, M. (1935). *Sex and temperament in three primitive societies*. New York: Morrow.

Meltzer, B. N., Petras, J. W., & Reynolds, L. T. (1975). *Symbolic interactionism: Genesis, varieties and criticism*. London: Routledge & Kegan Paul.

Miller, J. G. (1996). Theoretical issues in cultural psychology and social constructionism. In J. W. Berry, Y. Poortinga, & J. Pandey (Eds.), *Handbook of cross-cultural psychology: Theoretical and methodological perspectives* (Vol. 1, pp. 85-128). Boston: Allyn and Bacon.

Munroe, R. L., & Munroe, R. H. (1975). *Cross-cultural human development*. Monterey, CA: Brooks/Cole.

Öngel, Ü., & Smith, P. B. (1994). Who are we and where are we going? JCCP approaches its 100th issue. *Journal of Cross-Cultural Psychology, 25*, 25-53.

Piker, S. (1994). Classical culture and personality. In P. K. Bock (Ed.), *Psychological anthropology* (pp. 1-17). Westport, CT: Praeger.

Schwartz, S. (1996, August). Individual and cultural value dimensions: Statistical improvements yes, but conceptually as confused as ever! In F. van de Vijver & K. Leung (Chairs), *Individual and Cultural Traits* in *Multilevel Inferences*. Symposium conducted at the XIII Congress of Psychology, Montreal, Canada.

Segall, M. H. (1983). Aggression in global perspective: A research strategy. In A. P. Goldstein & M. H. Segall (Eds.), *Aggression in global perspective* (pp. 1-43). New York: Pergamon.

Segall, M. H., Campbell, D. T., & Herskovits, M. J. (1966). *The influence of culture on visual perception*. Indianapolis: Bobbs-Merrill.

Segall, M. H., Dasen, P. R., Berry, J. W., & Poortinga, Y. H. (1990). *Human behavior in global perspective*. Boston: Allyn and Bacon.

Shweder, R. A. (1984). Anthropology's romantic rebellion against the enlightenment, or there's more to thinking than reason and evidence. In R. A. Shweder & R. A. LeVine (Eds.), *Culture theory: Essays on mind, self, and emotion* (pp. 27-66). New York: Cambridge University Press.

Spain, M. E. (1982). *Oedipus in the Trobriands*. Chicago: University of Chicago Press.

Triandis, H. C. (1995). *Individualism and collectivism*. Boulder: Westview Press.

White, L. A. (1959). *The evolution of culture: The development of a civilization to the fall of Rome*. New York: McGraw-Hill.

Whiting, B. B. (1976). The problem of the packaged variable. In K. F. Riegel & J. A. Meacham (Eds.), *The developing individual in a changing world* (Vol. 1). Chicago: Aldine.

Whiting, B., & Whiting, J. B. (1974). *Children of six cultures*. Cambridge, MA: Harvard.

Whiting, J. W. M., & Child, I. L. (1953). *Child training and personality: A cross-cultural study*. New Haven: Yale.

Yang, K. S. (1986). Chinese personality and its change. In M. Bond (Ed.), *The psychology of the Chinese people* (pp. 106-170). Hong Kong: Oxford University Press.

Cross-Cultural Research Ethics:
Personal-Historical Observations

Harry C. Triandis
University of Illinois, USA

ABSTRACT

This brief report provides a personal account of the events surrounding cross-cultural psychology's early interest in research ethics. The subsequent formation of a committee and the publication of guidelines which became the focus of discussions within IACCP are related. Although the guidelines posed a number of questions and raised the consciousness of researchers, they were never adopted by the Association as an ethical code.

Because the International Association of Cross-Cultural Psychology revisits the topic of ethics every 20 or so years, and I will probably not be around next time that happens, I will give you my personal account of the history of the topic in cross-cultural psychology.

The first discussions on cross-cultural ethics took place in December 1966 to January 1967. I attended a conference in Ibadan, Nigeria that was organized by Herb Kelman and Henri Tajfel, in which this topic was discussed. My awareness of the topic was stimulated by the presentations of some of the Tunisian social scientists who complained about "intellectual colonialism." They argued that collecting data in another culture without consulting local social scientists was wrong, both from the point of view of science and ethics. I found their argument convincing, and introduced a segment on the ethics of cross-cultural research into my book, The Analysis of Subjective Culture (Triandis, 1972, pp. 36-37; 48-53).

In 1971 Roger Russell, then President of IUPsyS and Chair of the Committee on International Relations in Psychology of the American Psychological Association, asked June Tapp to chair a committee that would develop guidelines on the way to do ethical cross-cultural research. Kelman hosted our meeting at Harvard, and we developed a draft. We then presented the draft at various international meetings, for example in Japan in 1972 and in South America in 1973, and were told by members of the audience that our guidelines were much too strict, and in fact unrealistic. I remember one Japanese professor, whose name I did not catch, saying "I do so much for my students, that the least they can do is to participate in my research and do what I tell them to do."

In spite of the objections we heard at international conferences we published the guidelines (Tapp, Kelman, Triandis, Wrightsman, & Coelho, 1974). The Tapp report was supposed to be advisory. Its main concerns were to avoid ethnocentrism, to do methodologically sound research, to be fair to the individuals and communities studied, to the collaborators, and to the discipline.

In 1974, the IACCP Executive Committee asked Ron Taft to chair an ethics committee to see if the Tapp report could be adopted by the IACCP. Taft had difficulties forming a committee and getting answers from the committee members through the mail. In 1976, he presented a preliminary report at the Tilburg IACCP meeting, with contributions from Russell McArthur (Canada), James Ritchie (New Zealand), Ernest Boesch (Germany), and Durganand Sinha (India). Noting that some regions of the world were not represented in the committee, the IACCP Executive asked Michael Durojaiye to obtain further contributions on the subject, especially from the less economically developed parts of the world. Michael did not have much more luck than Ron in getting input on the subject. The October 1977 issue of the IACCP Cross-Cultural Newsletter included an article by Taft (1977) which evaluated the Tapp report, argued that it was too strict, and presented a number of critical incidents showing the difficulties of arriving at satisfactory standards of ethics.

Finally, Ron Taft prepared a report in 1978, which was adopted by IACCP on July 29th 1978. The report raises questions, but did not provide many answers. Here are some of the questions that were raised:

1. Are the principles in the Tapp report ethnocentric?
2. Are the guidelines of the Tapp report realistic (i.e., can one actually do research or are they too restrictive for the conduct of the research)?
3. Can cross-cultural researchers do all the things that are suggested by the report? For example, can they always give something of value to the community that provided the data?
4. How can we deal with situations where the values of the researcher and the culture under study are drastically different? Are such situations always to be considered as "intellectual imperialism?"
5. How can we study people who do not understand the meaning of "research" and cannot give "informed consent?"
6. When the values of the researcher clash with the values of the local community, can the research be done?
7. How can the value of publication be reconciled with the value of privacy, or secrecy?

These latter two points raise a host of problems that require special attention. For example, the researcher wants to report a practice that the local community finds embarrassing because the community says "outsiders see it out of context"; or the researcher wants to publish AIDS statistics and the local government wants to avoid panic. Or the researcher wants to report the high frequency of female infanticide and the local government does not want such information to become available. Note that this is a general problem: When a researcher finds something uncomplimentary about a culture, scientific ethics say that the information must be published, but good relations with the community require that it not be published, For example, the researcher wants to publish that the Hopi rain dance does not result in more rain, and the Hopi community wants to keep all information about the rain dance secret.

Taft concluded his report by arguing that the Tapp report raises our consciousness, but that it cannot be used to guide the actions of cross-cultural researchers. Yet the report raised very serious questions, and our association has the responsibility to develop guidelines for researchers. For example, when I find something uncomplimentary, I bury it around complimentary information, and try to publish it in places that are not widely read by the public. A newspaper or magazine is definitely not the place to publish such information. Is that way of dealing with the dilemma ethical, realistic, recommended? The association should deal with such issues and take a stand.

References

Taft, R. (1977). Comments on the 1974 "Tapp" report on the ethics of cross-cultural research. *IACCP Cross-Cultural Newsletter, 11,* 2-8.

Tapp, J. L., Kelman, H. C., Triandis, H. C., Wrightsman, L. W., & Coelho, G. V. (1974). Continuing concerns in cross-cultural ethics: A report. *International Journal of Psychology, 9,* 231-249.

Triandis, H. C. (1972). *The analysis of subjective culture.* New York: Wiley.

Short-Comings in Cross-Cultural Research Ethics: The Tapp et al. (1974) Report Revisited

Graham Davidson
Central Queensland University, Australia

ABSTRACT

This paper provides an overview of Tapp et al. (1974) and subsequent IUPS symposia and resolutions on cross-cultural research ethics. Various ethical guidelines, including recommendations that researchers "engage only in activities abroad that are ethically acceptable at home" *and* that they recognize meanings attributed to those research activities by the host community, are considered. It is argued that these guidelines do not provide researchers with ways of resolving ethical dilemmas that arise from (a) research in their own culture and (b) conflicting Western and non-Western systems of ethics. Examples of dilemmic cross-cultural research, including studies of community attitudes and responses to HIV, suicide ideation, substance misuse, and child sexuality, and contrasting ethical approaches to these dilemmas are discussed.

The most extensive, extant statement on the ethical responsibilities of cross-cultural research psychologists arose out of the work of a sub-committee of eminent cross-cultural researchers established in 1971 by the International Union of Psychological Sciences (then called IUPS; currently the Union is known by its modern acronym IUPsyS) and the American Psychological Association's (APA) Committee on International Relations in Psychology. The work of the committee was discussed and revised at a number of international symposia held between 1971 and 1973, resulting in the publication of a set of *Advisory Principles for Ethical Considerations in the Conduct of Cross-Cultural Research* (Tapp, Kelman, Triandis, Wrightsman, & Coelho, 1974). While acknowledging that the establishment of the subcommittee and ensuing symposia were mainly North American initiatives, Tapp et al. argued strongly that there was a need to recognize "the 'universal' value of mutually acknowledging social and scientific responsibility and [for] raising psychological consciousness about the impact of research on individuals and groups." (p. 235)

Ethical Principles in Cross-Cultural Research
The 13 major clauses that constitute the Tapp et al. (1974) guidelines are an elaboration of the following four general principles. First, researchers

should not conduct any investigation that is ethically unacceptable in their own research community *or* that violates the values of the culture(s) in which the research will be conducted. Cross-cultural researchers from Australia, for example, should only conduct research that conforms with the commonly accepted code of research conduct adopted by institutional ethics committees (National Health and Medical Research Council, 1988), *and* with Section E on Research of the Australian Psychological Society's (APS) Code of Professional Conduct (1994), *and* that is ethically acceptable to the host community. The latter may be judged in terms of the cultural meaning of the research topic, the research procedures, the personal conduct and behavior of the researcher, the methods of reporting, and ways in which findings may be used. Thus, the first principle requires researchers to behave in an ethically responsible manner according to the standards of their own research culture, and to be sensitive to the value systems of cultures in which they conduct their research. The corollary is that researchers must seek to know the values of the host culture as well as they know the values of their own research culture.

This need for cross-cultural understanding leads to the second general principle that researchers should seek consultation and collaboration with knowledgeable members of host communities. Local researchers and advisors can offer advice about whether research topics and practices are consistent with the value orientations in their own communities, about whether research measures and techniques give a fair and culturally unbiased appraisal of the behavior under investigation, and about whether findings are collated and presented in a manner that makes them accessible to host communities. The ideal collaborative arrangements in any cross-cultural endeavor are (a) an equal partnership between researchers from all the host cultures or communities, including the culture from which the research originates and (b) inclusion of a training component for new researchers.

Cross-cultural research partnerships also assist with the identification of local research needs and potential local benefits from research participation. With respect to this third principle, there is an expectation that research will have potential benefits for participant cultures and communities. This has obvious ramifications for reporting results, but less obvious, though just as important consequences for the formulation of cross-cultural research questions and initial contacts between researchers and host communities.

Field work approaches that are designed to produce research questions mutually agreed upon by visiting researchers and host communities have been investigated by Davidson (1980) and André (1981). Where research benefits are concerned, I have so far focused mainly on the direct benefits of the research for the host culture(s). It goes without saying that participant communities should not be worse off, or disadvantaged *in any way*, by their participation in cross-cultural research. Researchers therefore need to consider the broader political consequences of the research they plan to conduct and, wherever possible, identify potential political advantages and disadvantages that might accrue to the researcher's and participants' cultural groupings.

A fourth broad ethical principle underlying the Tapp et al. (1974) guidelines is respect for the rights and protection of the welfare and dignity of individual participants. This principle is embodied in the researcher's responsibilities to (a) negotiate free and informed consent, (b) respect confidences, (c) anticipate any harmful consequences that might be associated with participants' involvement in the research project, and (d) effectively debrief participants.

There was evidence of interest within the IUPS at about the same time, to provide guidelines for psychologists working cross-culturally. The report by Holtzman (1976) on the IUPS Executive Committee meeting in Paris included a number of resolutions concerning the need for professional psychologists to protect the "inviolable rights of human beings" set down in United Nations Charters, and the International Union's commitment to support affiliated groups and their members who are required to act in defense of others' human rights. The resolutions are equally applicable to research that has the potential to infringe on the rights of individuals and groups who differ from the researcher in terms of their "race, religion, or ideology" (p. 310). There was further elaboration on ethical standards for practicing researchers and professionals in a series of articles introduced by Holtzman (1979) in the *International Journal of Psychology*. Issues that pertained specifically to cross-cultural research closely reflected the guidelines developed by Tapp et al. (cf. Durojaiye, 1979).

Early Critiques
The Tapp et al. (1974) guidelines preceded, and to some degree generated, further discussion about ethical principles and approaches underpinning cross-cultural psychological research. In 1976, the IACCP held a symposium to further consider the content and application of the guidelines (Taft, n.d., 1977). Taft's summary (a) accentuated the difficulty of achieving culturally representative decision making about a code of conduct for cross-cultural researchers, (b) pointed to problems that can arise when making judgments about the beneficial effects of research, (c) considered problems associated with the negotiation of informed consent, and (d) strongly recommended that the guidelines, and other similar codes, be afforded the status of aspirational guidelines, that should be

applied flexibly to specific research studies. Therefore, the guidelines would "serve as consciousness-raising exercises to shake up the researcher from time to time so that he (sic) does not too easily settle down to accepting his compromise stance as being ethically satisfying" (Taft, 1977, p. 6).

Problems Inherent in Principle Ethics

Although the heuristic value of the Tapp et al. (1974) guidelines should not be underestimated when the ethical conduct of cross-cultural research studies is being considered, there has been little progress during the intervening two decades in the debate about (a) whether such a code that is based on principle ethics provides adequate protection of the interest and well-being of individuals and communities who become participants in cross-cultural projects, and (b) how researchers set about to resolve the problems that have arisen - and will continue to arise - from inevitable conflicts between different sets of cultural values and the competing best interests of all stakeholders in their research studies. In their current form, the guidelines do not provide researchers with ways of resolving conflicts that arise from (a) the juxtaposition of Western, scientific and non-Western systems of ethics, and (b) the complexity of, and overlap between, stakeholders' cluster rights and duties. These limitations of the Tapp et al. (1974) guidelines which are inherent in all guidelines that are based on principle ethics are explored further using examples of ethical dilemmas that have been drawn from the cross-cultural research literature.

The focus first of all is on the likelihood of conflict between Western, scientific and non-Western ethics and value systems. This type of conflict stems from Tapp et al.'s (1974) first principle that researchers should not conduct research that is ethically unacceptable in their own research community *or* that violates the values of the culture(s) in which the research will be conducted. Two examples of cross-cultural research serve to illustrate this conflict. Barry (1988) described a number of problems arising from attempts to conduct epidemiological studies of HIV infection in Tanzania. The problems arose as a result of the Tanzanian government's insistence that blood samples be obtained without the informed consent of the women who were to be tested and that donors not be informed of the results of blood tests. These research practices were deemed by the researchers to be in violation of the rights of donors, and of regulations for research with human participants within the researchers' culture, and thus the study did not proceed.

This was not the case for the study by Herdt (1990) of nose bleeding rituals and secret practices of pedaphilic fellatio amongst the Sambia of New Guinea's Eastern Highlands region, where initiation of boys into male cults begins between the ages of 7 and 10 years. Herdt's account of fieldwork undertaken in the 1970s appeared to be a benign acceptance of child physical abuse and sexual practices which, despite being a custom in the host culture, would otherwise result in mandatory reporting and criminal charges being laid, and certain rejection by institutional ethics committees in present-day North American or Australian society. Here is an example of two systems of legal and moral responsibility in conflict. In the American or Australian system the researcher has a responsibility to protect young boys from sexual exploitation and, depending on State law, may be mandatorily required to report sexual abuse of minors. In the Sambian system pedaphilic fellatio in the men's houses was the social norm. The conflict is not resolved by consultation with knowledgeable Sambian males, or by having their consent to study these initiation rites, protecting the identity of the participants, using noninvasive research procedures, and debriefing participants. In summary, the research was conducted in a way that was consistent with the ethical principles of the scientific community and the social standards of the host community, but side-stepped the legal and moral responsibilities on North American and Australian scientists who conducted research in their communities.

Christakis (1992) argues that any set of guidelines that is premised on cross-cultural research meeting the ethical standards of different, host cultures is unworkable. He suggests that the two-systems approach fails in its bid to address the following questions: (a) which standards must the research meet, given that, if judged by a third standard, it might be deemed ethically unacceptable, (b) who should decide whether *all* guidelines are met, and (c) who should act as arbiter if standards collide?

Principle codes, on which the Tapp et al. (1974) guidelines are premised, contain inherent conflicts and necessary compromises between stakeholders' cluster rights and duties. There are numerous examples of these ethical dilemmas in the literature. What is known as the Barrow Alcohol Study (Klausner & Foulks, 1982; Foulks, 1989) led to extensive socio-political and scientific debate about which stakeholders' interests are served by applied social research into dysfunctional behavior in cultural minorities. The controversy about the study's research findings was sparked initially by host community leaders' disagreements with the researchers' interpretation of reasons for excessively high levels of alcohol use by members of the host community. This led to a number of public statements and exchanges involving community leaders, community organizations and independent researchers and academics condemning the research methods and findings and questioning the motives of the researchers and funding bodies (Foulks, 1989). The debate demonstrates that cross-cultural research can be shown to have both beneficial and harmful consequences for host communities, and challenges the assumptions that proper, informed consent can be obtained under circumstances where the wider political and social consequences of social research are unknown prior to the commencement of the research. It raises doubts about the principle of consultation and collaboration under circumstances where there is an unequal power relationship between the researcher's culture and the host culture. Finally, the Barrow Alcohol Study was illustrative of the disagreements that can arise as a result of the different ways that cultural groups socially construct dysfunctional behavior (see Manson, 1989).

In cross-cultural health and mental health research, studies of suicide and suicidal thinking (e.g., Reser's, 1990, large-scale study of suicidal ideation and self-harm among Aboriginal people in Australia's Far North-East) present researchers with very difficult decisions. On the one hand, researchers have a duty of care for persons who otherwise may not seek, or even know about, help available from mental health professionals that may conceivably lead to the disclosure of information about suicidal research participants. On the other hand, it is frequently argued that the quality of research data is improved if data are collected anonymously or if confidentiality is maintained; and research ethics policies such as that of the National Health and Medical Research Council (1988) serve to protect the confidentiality of participants' identity. Cross-cultural studies of safe sex practices and epidemiological studies of sexually transmitted diseases (STDs) in communities thought to have high instances of STDs pose similar dilemmas (Last, 1991). These ethical dilemmas are no different in nature from those confronting applied and professional psychology generally (Davidson, 1995). However, if the interests of science and scientific ethics are put ahead of the immediate health and well-being of research participants the consequences for individuals and families in host communities may be serious, and even fatal.

Finally, dual relationships between visiting researchers and host communities and colleagues are ethically problematic. This applies particularly to cases where researchers volunteer their services or are contracted to provide expert evidence or to advocate for communities, while research agreements are being negotiated or research is being carried out. It also applies in cases where promises of cross-cultural collaboration and provision of research support appear to offer unusually generous privileges and advantages to local researchers (compare Sartorius, 1988). The principles in question are the quality of the consent obtained from individuals, communities, and gatekeeper researchers who are in a dependent relationship with the researcher, the possibility of unduly large and inappropriate incentives being offered to those parties for their participation, and the "objectivity" of the researcher under circumstances where conflicts of interest may arise between the research role and personal or other professional roles. The Tapp et al. (1974) guidelines that are based on set principles do not address these ethical dilemmas. Where might cross-cultural researchers turn, therefore, in search of workable ethical approach? Two possible alternatives will be considered.

Alternative Ethical Approaches

Christakis (1992) has written about the application of contextual approaches to ethical thinking that have their origins in social constructionism. According to Christakis, meta-ethical and ethical precepts, including the precept of conflict, are contextually and culturally constructed. Decisions about ethical issues that arise when different cultural constructions of these precepts exist must be negotiated between parties, with equal privilege being afforded to each party's ethical system. Discourse ethics (also see Benhabib & Dallmayr, 1990) differs from ethical relativism, in that (a) dialogue between the parties is ongoing, (b) negotiation is context-specific, (c) all parties engage in both self-examination and mutual comparison, and (d) disagreement and unresolved conflict are accompanied by tolerance of other parties' positions.

Ethical contextualism as Christakis (1992) has described it does not seek to eliminate ethical dilemmas. When ethical principles conflict or where the best interests of the researcher and the host community are incompatible with one another, instead of seeking to remove the conflict the researcher, along with others in the research community who have responsibility for ethical surveillance, and host community leaders should seek to negotiate a course of action that is held by all parties to be an agreeable settlement of the differences. Agreement on a course of action is limited to that piece of research in that particular research setting. Beneficial and harmful consequences of adopting the negotiated course of action are recognized and tolerated as such. If the research proceeds, as these consequences emerge subsequent research activities are renegotiated. When the agreed course of action is completed, and the final results are to hand, the actions themselves and the findings have the imprimatur of the parties, because all have acted in accordance with the agreed settlement. The particular situational issues that underpinned the negotiated course of action and reasons for tolerating the ethical conflicts that remain are acknowledged when each party gives its imprimatur to the research. Placement of emphasis on negotiation of conflicting values and interests of researchers and host communities, and on the acceptance of their continuing existence in specific circumstances are implicit in Foulks's retrospective acknowledgment that "difficulties [in the Barrow Alcohol Study] might have been avoided had we obtained better insight into the community's beliefs regarding the nature of the problem, and had we been able to ensure more total community participation in deciding how the results of the study were to be used" (Foulks, 1989, p. 7).

A negotiated course of action is an unlikely outcome if ethical imperatives are pursued. The ethical problems that emerged during the study of HIV infection in Tanzania (Barry, 1988) were not eliminated by the researchers' decision that the study should not proceed. On the contrary, the researchers' insistence that the host culture apply "ethical standards as stringent as those applied to research carried out within the developed country" and "defend the principle of autonomy" (Barry, 1988, p. 1085) had the same public health outcomes that were associated with anonymous serum sampling and nondisclosure. Specifically, there was no health promotion or medical treatment of persons testing HIV positive. Further negotiation of a long term research and education plan might only improve this outcome.

Notwithstanding the appeal of Christakis's ethical contextualism, or pluralism, there is little likelihood that the psychological sciences on mass will relinquish ethical universalism. There is a need, therefore, to explore ethical frameworks in the Western tradition that view rights and duties as coextensive and conditional. I am currently exploring the applicability of *prima facie* duty theory (Ross, 1930) for resolving the types of ethical dilemmas confronting professional and research psychologists that arise as a result of national codes of conduct that are premised on a principle ethic. Put simply, *prima facie* means conditional, and the foundation of any *prima facie* duty, and also right, is the relationship that exists between the parties who are involved. In the words of Ross (1930), "When I am in a situation ..... in which more than one of these *prima facie* duties is incumbent on me, what I have to do is study the situation as fully as I can until I form the considered opinion (it is never more) that in the circumstances one of them is more incumbent than any other; then I am bound to think that to do this *prima facie* duty is my duty *sans phrase* in the situation." (p. 19) Ross's intuition theory also states that our *prima facie* duties in a loosely prioritized order are fidelity, reparation, gratitude, justice, beneficence, self-improvement and non-maleficence. Acts that result in us fulfilling our duties are right acts, but in the end the right act is the one that is, as Ross (1939, p. 53) described it, "the most suitable of those possible in the circumstances." Within such a theory, *prima facie* professional duties to all parties, including oneself, can be weighed and a course of action that discharges one's professional duties, according to various criteria that Ross (1930) also discussed, can be adopted.

Ethical decision making in research may proceed along the following steps:

1. How should the researcher act toward research participants in order never to lie to or mislead participants?
2. How ought the researcher act toward research participants in virtue of the researcher's other duties toward them?
3. How ought the research act in virtue of the researcher's duties to other stakeholders in the research, whether they be members of the researcher's or the host culture?
4. If fulfilment of a duty to participants contravenes the fulfilment of other duties to those participants or to other stakeholders, how may the researcher discharge those other duties ethically by making reparation to participants or other stakeholders where necessary?
5. What other relevant circumstances might influence the researcher's decision about the action to be taken?
6. How then *will* the researcher act?
7. As the research progresses what other action is required so that the researcher's duties to all parties are discharged ethically?

If a promise of confidentiality given to research participants can not be kept because to do so would jeopardize the health and safety of a research participant or third party, or if negotiation of fully informed consent can not be achieved prior to the commencement of the research, then those duties to participants must be discharged by the researcher in other ways if the researcher is to act ethically. Speculation about how researchers might have acted in those cross-cultural studies highlighted by this paper is made difficult by Ross's insistence that prima facie duties have a relational foundation. One would need to know more about the relationships between the researchers and their host communities and about the implicit and explicit promises inherent in those relationships before such speculation is possible.

Conclusion

Universalistic solutions offered by the Tapp et al. (1974) guidelines to the ethical conflicts that arise from attempts to combine different systems of values, and to negotiate cluster rights and duties of stakeholders in cross-cultural research, just don't work. Discourse ethics and *prima facie* approaches, although philosophically incompatible with one another, at least offer distinctive solutions to these ethical disputes.

References

André, R. (1981). Multi-cultural research: Developing a participative methodology for cross-cultural psychology. *International Journal of Psychology, 16,* 249-256.

Australian Psychological Society. (1994). *Code of professional conduct.* Melbourne, VIC: Author.

Barry, M. (1988). Ethical considerations of human investigation in developing countries. *The New England Journal of Medicine, 319,* 1083-1086.

Benhabib, S., & Dallmayr, F. (Eds.). (1990). *The communicative ethics controversy.* Cambridge, MA: Massachusetts Institute of Technology Press.

Christakis, N. A. (1992). Ethics are local: Engaging cross-cultural variation in the ethics of clinical research. *Social Science and Medicine, 35,* 1079-1091.

Davidson, G. R. (1980). Psychology and Aborigines: The place of research. *Australian Psychologist, 15,* 111-121.

Davidson, G. R. (1995). The ethics of confidentiality. *Australian Psychologist, 30,* 153-157.

Durojaiye, M. O. A. (1979). Ethics of cross-cultural research viewed from third world perspective. *International Journal of Psychology, 14,* 137-141.

Foulks, E. F. (1989). Misalliances in the Barrow alcohol study. *American Indian and Alaska Native Mental Health Research, 2*(3), 7-17.

Herdt, G. (1990) Sambia nosebleeding rights and male proximity to women. In J. W. Stigler, R. A. Shweder, & G. Herdt (Eds.), *Cultural psychology: Essays on comparative human development.* (pp. 401-423). New York: Cambridge University Press.

Holtzman, W. H. (1976). Report of the meetings of the General Assembly and Executive Committee of the I. U. P. S. *International Journal of Psychology, 11,* 305-312.

Holtzman, W. H. (1979). The IUPS project on professional ethics and conduct. *International Journal of Psychology, 14,* 107-109.

Klausner, S., & Foulks, E. F. (1982). *Eskimo capitalists: Oil, alcohol and social change.* Montclair, NJ: Allenheld and Osmun.

Last, J. M. (1991). Epidemiology and ethics. *Law, Medicine and Health Care, 19*(3-4), 166-174.

Manson, S. M. (Ed.) (1989). The Barrow Alcohol Study [Special issue]. *American Indian and Native Alaska Mental Health Research, 2*(3).

National Health and Medical Research Council. (1988). *Statement on human experimentation and supplementary notes*. Canberra, ACT: Author.

Reser, J. P. (1990). *A perspective on the causes and cultural context of violence in Aboriginal communities in North Queensland: Commissioned report to the Royal Commission into Aboriginal Deaths in Custody*. Townsville, QLD: James Cook University of North Queensland.

Ross, W. D. (1930). *The right and the good*. Oxford: The Clarendon Press.

Ross, W. D. (1939). *Foundations of ethics*. Oxford: The Clarendon Press.

Sartorius, N. (1988). Experience from the mental health programme of the World Health Organization. *Acta Psychiatrica Scandinavia, 344,* 71-74.

Taft, R. (1977). Comments on the 1974 "Tapp" report on the ethics of cross-cultural research. *IACCP Cross-Cultural Psychology Newsletter, 11*(4), 2-8.

Taft, R. (n.d.). *A symposium on the "Tapp report": Report of the I. A. C. C. P. Ethics Committee*. Melbourne, VIC: Monash University.

Tapp, J. L., Kelman, H. C., Triandis, H. C., Wrightsman, L. S., & Coelho, G. V. (1974). Continuing concerns in cross-cultural research: A report. *International Journal of Psychology, 9,* 231-249.

Previous book in the series:
Selected papers from the International Conference of the International Association for Cross-Cultural Psychology (IACCP)

Diversity and Unity in Cross-Cultural Psychology
5th International Conference, Bhubaneswar India, 1981
Editors: R. Rath, H.S. Asthana, J.B.H. Sinha and D. Sinha
1982, 380 pages, ISBN 90 265 0431 4

Expiscations in Cross-Cultural Psychology
6th International Conference, Aberdeen Scotland, 1982
Editors: J.B. Deregowski, S. Dziurawiec and R. C. Annis
1983, 460 pages, ISBN 90265 0450 0

From a Different Perspective
7th International Conference, Acapulco Mexico, 1984
Editors: I. Reyes Lagunes and Y. Poortinga
1985, 396 pages, ISBN 90 265 0672 4

Growth and Progress in Cross-Cultural Psychology
8th International Conference, Istanbul Turkey, 1986
Editor: Ç. Kagitçibasi
1987, 418 pages, ISBN 90 265 0852 2

Heterogeneity in Cross-Cultural Psychology
9th International Conference, Newcastle Australia, 1988
Editors: D.M. Keats, D. Munro and L. Mann
1989, 592 pages, ISBN 90 265 1018 7

Innovations in Cross-Cultural Psychology: Selected Papers
10th International Conference, Nara Japan, 1990
Editors: S. Iwawaki, Y. Kashima and K. Leung
1992, 492 pages, ISBN 90 265 1232 5

Journeys into Cross-Cultural Psychology
11th International Conference, Liège Belgium, 1992
Editors: A.M. Bouvy, F.J.R. van de Vijver, P. Boski and P. Schmitz
1994, 410 pages, ISBN 90 265 1403 4

Key Issues in Cross-Cultural Psychology
12th International Conference, Pamplona-Iruña, Navarra, Spain, 1994
Editors: H. Grad, A. Blanco and J. Georgas
1996, 386 pages, ISBN 90 265 1441 7